COUNSELING CLIENTS WITH HIV DISEASE

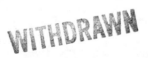

Counseling Clients with HIV Disease

Assessment, Intervention, and Prevention

MARY ANN HOFFMAN

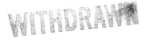

THE GUILFORD PRESS
New York London

©1996 The Guilford Press
A Division of Guilford Publications, Inc.
72 Spring Street, New York, NY 10012

Author's Note
The names and identities of the people written about in this book have been carefully disguised in keeping with their rights to priviledged communication with the author and in accordance with professional standards of confidentiality.

Printed in the United States of America

This book is printed on acid-free paper.

Last digit is print number: 9 8 7 6 5 4 3 2 1

Library of Congress Cataloging-in-Publication Data

Hoffman, Mary Ann.
    Counseling clients with HIV disease : assessment,
intervention, and prevention / Mary Ann Hoffman.
        p. cm.
    Includes bibliographical references and index.
    ISBN 1-57230-063-9
    1. HIV infections—Patients—Counseling of. I. Title.
RC607.A26H6 1996
362.1'969792—dc20   95-37282
                                                CIP

To Damon and Jennifer
and in loving memory of my niece,
Lauren Elizabeth Hoffman, earth's sweetest dancer

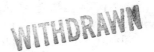

Acknowledgments

There have been rare moments in my life when I have known, with absolute certainty and with great clarity, that something very important and significant was happening, or about to happen. One of those moments came in 1983. I was seeing a client and something was very wrong. Anthony, a vibrant, lively, and engaging 19-year-old, was getting sick. We had heard about a new, devastating disease that seemed to be primarily affecting gay men. It hit both of us that afternoon, with a sense of absolute certainty, that this was what was making Anthony sick. At this moment of realization, we were intensely and mutually engaged in our therapeutic work so we knew that this would be a journey we would both be taking, although not always together and not for the same reasons.

Anthony's journey soon led to a confirmation of his fears when the HIV antibody test became available for the first time and his disease, initially called human T-lymphotropic virus type III (HTLV-III), was officially identified and named. Eventually, after an emotionally, physically, and spiritually challenging and exhausting bout with his disease, Anthony died. I believe that he went directly to the heaven he so strongly believed in and that had sustained him through his pain and through the fear, stigma, and disinterest he experienced from others.

My own journey and interest in learning more about HIV disease began with Anthony. There was something about this young man, and the way he viewed his life and having HIV disease, that touched me on a deep level and that I found compelling. I was drawn to understand more about this new disease. As trite as this sounds, Anthony put a face on HIV disease and personalized it for me. Because of Anthony I would never be able to dismiss HIV disease as irrelevant to my work and to my life, or as something that affected others but not me or my own world. I could not walk away from this disease.

Although Anthony was truly the catalyst that compelled me to pay attention and to know, in a profound way, that HIV was important, I have ultimately learned, and continue to learn, from a number of other people. First and foremost, I want to thank my clients and research participants who have willingly and poignantly shared with me their experiences of living with HIV disease. Without their words and stories, there would not have been a book.

I am fortunate to have in my husband, Damon Silvers, Ph.D., the benefits of a live-in, gifted therapist. Damon read drafts of many of the chapters, offered numerous clinical insights and perspectives, and willingly let me interrupt him time after time to listen to my ideas, to provide input when I felt stuck, or to offer moral support. I am also indebted to Damon and to our daughter Jennifer for the love, support, and patience they gave me during the writing process. Writing is typically a solitary activity that absences the writer from the center of the family. I am sure that it was difficult for them to see so much of my back as I sat at my computer during this process.

I cannot think of a more difficult task than reading early drafts of a book. I will always be indebted to my student and colleague, Jeanine Driscoll, who read the entire first draft. Jeanine is a talented and experienced clinician and teacher who has long worked with persons with HIV disease. She has a gift of skillfully pairing knowledge with compassion and humor. She shared this gift with me many times as she offered her own experiences and perspectives in a way that deepened my understanding of issues, provided her insights about themes in the clinical material, and gently suggested that I must have been "really tired" when I wrote garbled passages.

I am also indebted to many other friends, colleagues, students, and family members who offered invaluable assistance and support during the process of writing this book. James Croteau, Ph.D., read an earlier draft and provided a number of astute observations and suggestions that significantly strengthened the manuscript. Charles Gelso, Ph.D., Janet O'Keeffe, Ph.D., and my students, Cynthia Breaux, M.A., Shirley Hess, M.Ed., and Shari Willis, M.S., read drafts of various chapters or provided research support. I want to thank Jim Donnelly for his skill in helping me prepare the tables and figures for this book. I am also deeply appreciative of the vision and guidance of my editor, Kitty Moore. Again and again I was reminded of the value of multiple perspectives in helping me articulate my views and in polishing this manuscript.

I am grateful for the support and insights provided by my friends and colleagues, Clara Hill, Ph.D., Hedy Teglasi, Ph.D., and Barbara

Wood, Ph.D., who shared their experiences with managing the process of writing a book while working full-time and being a parent. I am also grateful to Sharon Spiegel, Ph.D., who I can always count on for support and inspiration. My niece, Rachel Stein, and my daughter, Jennifer, helpfully provided me with several important insights about adolescents and HIV disease.

Finally, I want to thank my parents who taught me to believe that being human means to view what happens to others as having implications and meaning for all of us. From them I learned that interest, caring, and compassion are important and necessary qualities.

Contents

CHAPTER 1

Introduction: Counseling Clients with HIV Disease

My soul is fighting my body's instinct to live.
My body requires life; my soul, flight. There
is no reconciling these two.
— MENDELSON (1995, p. F1)

What the human immunodeficiency virus (HIV) has clearly shown is that health epidemics are rarely, if ever, just about disease. Epidemics thrust the specter of death, with all of its meanings and implications, into the midst of the living. In this way, diseases such as HIV profoundly affect the psychosocial, cultural, and political aspects of communities and countries. Moreover, the meaning attached to a particular disease, such as HIV, affects how those who are afflicted perceive themselves and are perceived by others. Given the enormity of the impact of HIV, it has become the most intensively studied virus in history (Greene, 1993). This worldwide pandemic has enormous implications for the health and psychosocial well-being of individuals, their family structures, and their community structures, for the delivery of psychosocial and medical services, and responses by governmental agencies. What we learn about the HIV pandemic has the potential to serve as a "blueprint" to guide responses to future health epidemics.

Although many issues that persons living with HIV disease face are similar to those faced by persons with diseases such as cancer, the complex sociocultural aspects of HIV disease and its transmission set it apart. First, HIV is transmitted through behaviors that are usually private and are often associated with norms and values of a subculture. Disclosing one's HIV status can reveal intimate aspects about one's life and can result in stigma and discrimination from others. Second, this disease is the leading cause of death in young adults and appears to be terminal. Many young people are facing a progressive, debilitating disease at the same time that their contemporaries are looking forward to a long future. Third, given the progressive nature of HIV, nearly all aspects of the individual's life are affected, including physical and emotional well-being, social supports, and life roles. Finally, many subcultures and communities have also been profoundly altered as a result of HIV disease.

HIV disease's impact on subcultures and communities in the United States can best be illustrated by examining the demographics of this epidemic. HIV disease was first observed in the United States in 1981, when a small number of gay men became ill with diseases that did not usually occur in young people (e.g., Kaposi's sarcoma) and that did not respond as expected to treatment. Initially, this epidemic primarily affected gay men. Over time, large numbers of injecting drug users also became infected. Presently, the majority of the cumulative cases of AIDS are comprised of injecting drug users and men who have sex with men (Centers for Disease Control and Prevention, 1995).

These statistics tell one story about the impact of HIV disease. Other statistics reflect different aspects of this epidemic. For example, African Americans and Latinos are disproportionately affected in AIDS cases for both men and women. The vast majority of people with AIDS are young (in their 20s to 40s), which has multiple implications about the impact of this epidemic on family structures and on lost years of productivity. Finally, AIDS cases represent just one end of the disease continuum. An additional 1.5 to 2 million Americans are estimated to have HIV disease. Moreover, recent cases of HIV infection show an increasing number of cases of heterosexual transmission (especially among women), which suggests that HIV disease now has a strong foothold in multiple populations. What these statistics show are that HIV disease affects many groups or subcultures of people in the United States, that multicultural factors, such as race and sexual orientation, are important defining variables in this epidemic, and that HIV disease, in terms of who is affected, continues to shift. These factors contribute to the psychosocial impact of HIV disease.

One of the most powerful ways to address the psychosocial aspects of this disease is through counseling interventions. In one review on positive behavior change in persons with HIV, Selwyn (1986) concluded that one predictive theme emerged: the importance of a comprehensive and ongoing counseling component. This is valuable because as HIV disease progression occurs, individuals are also undergoing major changes in numerous aspects of their lives, other than their health. Therefore, it is helpful to view HIV as a disease that has important psychosocial consequences as well as medical consequences. Counseling interventions help clients learn to live with these psychosocial consequences.

What do counseling interventions offer that other forms of support may not? Ferrara (1984), in telling of his own experience with AIDS, describes how his counselor allowed him to express his feelings in a way that his lover and friends could not. Ideally, therapists allow clients with HIV disease the opportunity to transcend the physical realms of their disease by offering an openness to any issue, feeling, or concern that allows clients to freely express and explore aspects of themselves and their lives without worrying about the impact on the therapist. Alleviating distress and helping clients find meaning in their disease by focusing on healing (e.g., emotional or spiritual wholeness), rather than curing, are important roles that counselors play. Counseling also provides a critical source of social support when other supports might be shifting, as well as education, advocacy, and the means to alter attitudes and behaviors.

HIV clinical work challenges therapists in a way that few, if any, other client concerns have done. For example, sexuality and sexual practices, drug practices, declining health and overall functioning, anticipatory grief, spirituality, and death and dying are common concerns of clients who are affected by HIV disease. Although it is not unusual to work with persons who present with concerns in one or more of these areas, what is unique about HIV disease is that many of these issues need to be assessed and addressed with a degree of urgency that does not typically direct clinical work. Because of these differences between HIV disease and other client concerns, I found that the traditional ways I had used to conceptualize client issues and dynamics were often not very effective.

To illustrate, I was trained to assess the client's history and current level of functioning and to identify a presenting concern. What I found with my clients with HIV was that crises often dictated what we addressed and that past ways of responding to stressors often had little to do with current ways of responding. Disequilibrium was common in the lives of my clients, and it frequently carried over into our work. Often, just as we moved forward on an issue, something new and urgent would occur and we would have to address that issue. Many counselors working with persons with HIV (PWHIVs) tell me that they spend much of their time responding to crises, feeling pulled in many directions, thinking about how to "fix" things, or feeling overwhelmed. In other words, they are often reacting in an anxious manner to whatever momentary challenge faces them.

Yet we are trained in our clinical work to begin by developing a therapeutic alliance as we carefully assess our client's life situation, so that we are able to truly understand what is meaningful, as well as distressing, for our client. This allows us to connect empathically with what our client is experiencing. An empathic connection provides the means of gathering accurate clinical data because it allows us access to our client's subjective experience. Often, an empathic connection is difficult to develop when we are anxious about what to ask and say, are hesitant to talk about issues such as sexuality and dying, or feel unable to understand or conceptualize what is happening for our client.

Early in my work with PWHIVs, I found little in the literature to help me in assessing and understanding the enormity of what was happening to my clients and to help me connect with them so that I might intervene in more helpful ways. I began to develop and utilize a conceptual schema to guide me in this important process. My clients truly shaped my view of what was important to explore and understand and of the value of discussing difficult issues, such as stigma, loss, and dying. I then found that the literature on HIV disease fit well with my conceptual schema and this schema eventually evolved into what I refer to now as a psychosocial model of HIV disease (Hoffman, 1991b).

Chapters 3–6 present this model, or conceptual schema, that I have found invaluable in organizing the numerous and complex aspects of the client's life that should be assessed as the first step in helping the PWHIV live the best life possible. Specifically, this model provides a conceptual framework for assessing the resources the HIV-infected person has available to help adapt to or cope with HIV disease. These include material resources, such as money and health insurance; interpersonal resources, such as partners and other family members; and psychological resources, such as self-esteem and coping skills. Although the medical and neurocognitive concerns that accompany HIV disease are important and are discussed in Chapter 2, the focus of the model I have developed is on those areas in which counselors can be most helpful—the psychosocial aspects of HIV. The model has four components: (1) defining characteristics of HIV disease (e.g., stigma, progressive course of HIV), (2) social support, (3) unique life situation (e.g., changes in life roles, emotional stage of disease), and (4) personality and demographic characteristics of the client (e.g., self-efficacy, sexual orientation, race).

Assessment leads to decisions about which interventions will be most helpful in helping clients adapt to HIV disease. Interventions, discussed in Chapters 7–12, facilitate adaptation by alleviating emotional distress and optimizing coping. Although clients adapt to HIV disease in many different ways, I have grouped adaptations into six broad areas. These chapters explore how counselors can help clients enhance affective, cognitive, and behavioral adaptations to HIV disease, rethink life goals, explore spiritual and religious concerns, and prepare for death and the dying process. Empirical and clinical research about each of these areas is presented and then placed in a psychotherapeutic context through the use of clinical examples and suggested counseling interventions.

Counseling interventions for PWHIVs provide (1) a way to explore and address important HIV-related concerns, such as depression and fears about the dying process; (2) assistance with learning and maintaining self- and other-protective practices; and (3) a means of emotional and social support. Counseling interventions can be delivered through individual, group, family and systems, and community-based modalities.

Adaptations to HIV disease and the counseling interventions discussed in Chapters 7–12 are explored one area or topic at a time. For example, Chapter 12 explores the dying process. Because PWHIVs typically come to counseling with multiple concerns about various aspects of living with HIV disease, Chapter 13 presents comprehensive case examples that illustrate how to integrate assessment and intervention to address these multiple concerns.

Although there are parallels between clinical work with PWHIVs and clients with other concerns, unique challenges are often present. For example, HIV disease challenges us to rethink our views about disease, the dying process, typical therapy goals, the boundaries of the therapeutic relationship, and what constitutes a good therapeutic outcome. It challenges us to rethink what it means to "cure" or bring about therapeutic change. HIV disease also challenges us to consider the role that multicultural variables play in defining the therapeutic context.

Issues that shape and define the psychotherapeutic context are explored in Chapters 14–18. These chapters explore the counseling relationship, multicultural issues, ethical concerns, the counseling needs of formal and informal HIV caregivers, and the HIV-related training needs of counselors and other mental health providers.

The remainder of the book is devoted to prevention. Although the focus of prevention is typically on the uninfected, prevention is also an important aspect of the therapeutic work with PWHIVs. Two issues are pertinent: How did your client become infected, and how does this inform your clinical work? For example, a client who repeatedly took risks that led to acquiring HIV disease may also take risks in other aspects of his or her life. Understanding what this means for your client is important for the therapeutic work. Another goal of understanding risk factors for PWHIVs is helping them prevent the spread of the virus to others.

Prevention is discussed in Chapter 19 by exploring specific behaviors and attitudes that are associated with becoming HIV infected. Next, comprehensive models of prevention that address multiple risk variables are discussed in Chapter 20. Finally, in Chapter 21, prevention is discussed from the perspective of community-based interventions. This topic is included because it is difficult for most individuals to make and maintain HIV-related behavioral changes if their community or environment does not support these changes. Therefore, understanding and changing the individual and environmental contexts in which risky behaviors occur are important goals of prevention efforts.

I have attempted to write a book that is clinically useful for mental health professionals as well as scholarly. It is first and foremost a book inspired by the lives of my clients. They have touched and blessed me in sharing their journey with me and have taught me much about resilience, the will to live, and the indomitable nature of the human spirit. I have also been influenced by the insights of other counselors working with PWHIVs and have used our conversations to deepen my own thinking and understanding. I have carefully researched the empirical and clinical literature on psychosocial aspects of HIV, so that this book is informed by the work of others. The literature on HIV disease is truly interdisciplinary and encompasses the interface of knowledge from multiple fields. I have tried to bring this richness and complexity to what I write. Moreover, I addressed a void in the psychosocial writings on HIV disease by placing research in a clinical context through the use of case examples and counseling interventions. It is my experience that utilizing both research and clinical writings provides a multiple perspective that allows clinicians to be knowledgeable about HIV and its psychosocial consequences, while at the same time allowing them to connect with their clients through the power of empathy, compassion, and the therapeutic alliance.

CHAPTER 2

Disease Progression: Physical and Neurocognitive Changes

> I can handle death—I believe in God and heaven.
> I'm just having trouble dealing with the changes I
> have to go through to get there.
>
> —LETTY, *a 34-year-old, HIV-positive,*
> *African American heterosexual woman*

HIV disease is not simply a physical entity. Rather, the impact of this disease is reflected in many other important ways, such as in emotional responses, coping strategies, self-image, and changes in life goals. But the physical aspects of this disease often lead to the first awareness that something is amiss; then they become markers of the relentless progression of the disease. For Letty, the woman quoted above, the physical aspects of HIV disease began with fatigue and night sweats. Next came high fevers and chronic diarrhea that left her weak and embarrassed to leave her home. Eventually, painful herpes lesions covered nearly half of her body and she developed invasive cervical cancer. Surrendering to death as she lay down on the clean white sheets in the hospice, with her physical pain finally quieted, was, in her words, "the easy part." The many months leading up to this, when Letty felt tired, was in excruciating pain, and felt ashamed about the many ways in which her body was noticeably failing her, was for her the difficult part of the physical progression of HIV disease.

Understanding the physical and neurocognitive aspects of HIV disease progression for PWHIVs provides a foundation for appreciating

7

the enormity of the physical aspects of this disease and the resultant life changes that occur as they navigate the disease process. The purpose of this chapter is to lay this foundation.

HOW HIV DISEASE BEGINS

Widespread infection caused by HIV apparently began in the 1970s. The virus was first identified in 1983–1984 by Gallo and Montagnier (see Gallo & Montagnier, 1988). There has been controversy as to whether HIV is both necessary and sufficient to cause AIDS. Some researchers have argued that HIV is harmless and that AIDS is caused by factors such as illicit drug use and AZT (zidovudine [ZDV]). This point of view is typically referred to as "The Duesberg Phenomenon" after its strongest proponent, Dr. Peter Duesberg (see Cohen, 1994). However, the overwhelming number of researchers have concluded that HIV is the necessary cause of AIDS. There is still some speculation that there may be other microbiological cofactors (e.g., other viruses) that might trigger or augment the effect of HIV (Keeling, 1993).

HIV disease begins when an individual becomes infected with the human immunodeficiency virus (typically HIV-1 in the United States) and when particles of the virus bind to the outside of certain cells (e.g., CD4+ cells). HIV is a retrovirus and, as with all such viruses, works by converting ribonucleic acid (RNA) into deoxyribonucleic acid (DNA) through a process called reverse transcription (Francis & Chin, 1987; Gallo & Montagnier, 1988; Keeling, 1993; Kemeny, 1994). The HIV retrovirus selectively binds to and infects CD4+ helper/inducer T lymphocytes as well as other cells that bear the CD4 molecule on their surface (e.g., certain neurological cells).

What has puzzled researchers for years is the relatively slow net loss of CD4+ cells that results in a gradual increase in viral load and the appearance of little immune dysfunction for many years after initial infection with HIV. However, recent research has shown that the process of HIV infection can be viewed as "a titanic struggle between the virus and the immune system" (Wain-Hobson, 1995, p. 102). Two recent studies have demonstrated that there is a very rapid rate of virus production and clearance, and of CD4+ cell infection and turnover (Ho et al., 1995; Wei et al., 1995). The life span of plasma virus and of virus-producing CD4+ cells is only about 2 days. In other words, at least 30% of these cells are replaced daily. What this means is that most of the circulating plasma virus at any given time is the result of new, or recent, virus infection, replication, and turnover. Previously, circulating plasma virus was believed to come from cells that chronically produced virus or that had become activated after being latently infected (Wei et al., 1995).

One important implication of this research is that this rapid replacement of virus results in drug-resistant virus in plasma after only about 14 to 28 days of treatment with a new antiretroviral drug. Therefore, HIV makes biological changes that allow it to continue to thrive and to challenge the immune system. According to Ho et al. (1995), AIDS (resulting from HIV infection) is primarily the result of this ongoing, high-level replication of HIV-1 that leads to killing of CD4+ cells. These studies suggest that treatment strategies need to be initiated very early in the course of the infection (ideally at the time of seroconversion) and that multiple antiretroviral drugs are needed. Perhaps the most important implication of this research is the capacity of the immune system to initially produce a large number of CD4+ cells after initial treatment with a new antiretroviral drug, even late in the course of the disease. This suggests that it may be possible in the future to restore adequate immune functioning even in late stages of HIV disease progression.

MODES OF HIV TRANSMISSION

There are four major categories of HIV transmission that will be briefly described (see Chapters 9 and 18 for more information).

1. *Blood and indirect components or derivatives of blood.* Most commonly, this mode of transmission occurs as a result of sharing needles with an HIV-infected person when injecting drugs such as heroin. Transmission can also occur during needle sharing when injecting other drugs such as cocaine or steroids. Some transmission also occurs as a result of blood and blood products transfusions (e.g., for hemophiliacs, or during surgery), but this is becoming less common in the United States because of the practice of testing blood for the presence of HIV and changes in how blood derivatives or components are prepared. This latter mode of transmission accounted for about 1% of AIDS cases in 1993 (Centers for Disease Control and Prevention, 1995). Transmission also occurs infrequently during medical procedures when health care workers experience an accidental needle stick with a contaminated needle (the chance of becoming infected when this occurs is only 0.3%; Henderson, Fahey, Willy, & Schmitt, 1990). It is extremely rare to find transmission occurring from an infected health care professional to a patient.

2. *Semen and vaginal/cervical secretions during intercourse (anal, vaginal, and oral)*. Anal intercourse (most risky is receptive position) carries the highest degree of risk for HIV transmission. This is due to the greater likelihood of tears and rips in rectal tissue occurring during intercourse. Further, condoms are more likely to break and fall off during anal intercourse. For vaginal intercourse, the likelihood of transmission increases when rips or tears occur, when lesions from sexually transmitted diseases are present, and when menstrual blood is present. There is evidence of a small number of cases of transmission due to fellatio (performing oral sex on a male)—probably due to semen or pre-ejaculatory fluid. Few, if any cases, can definitively be attributed to cunnilingus (performing oral sex on a female).

3. *Mother to fetus transmission in utero*. Until recently, there was about a 25–30% chance of maternal transmission to the fetus. A recent study administering AZT (ZDV) found that the experimental protocol resulted in a transmission rate of just 8.3%, as compared with a rate of 25.5% among the placebo group (Centers for Disease Control, 1994). However, at this time most pregnant women with HIV disease do not receive AZT during their pregnancy. The possible harmful effects of AZT on the child are also unknown at this time, as AZT has been shown to be a mutagen in laboratory studies.

4. *Breast milk*. HIV has been detected in breast milk, and it is possible that transmission to an infant can occur. It is difficult to determine that transmission occurred in this manner except in cases of previously uninfected women who became infected after receiving tainted blood at delivery.

After a decade or more of studying modes of transmission, there is no evidence of other forms of transmission (Keeling, 1993). For example, there is no definitive evidence that deep (French) kissing transmits HIV disease.

PHYSICAL MARKERS OF DISEASE PROGRESSION

The current system used by the Centers for Disease Control and Prevention (which incorporates the Walter Reed system and the old Centers for Disease Control system) classifies people according to both CD4+ cell count and the type of disease symptoms (Centers for Disease Control, 1992). As can be seen in Table 1, Category 1 refers to HIV-infected people with over 500 CD4+ cells per microliter; Category 2 includes those with

CD4+ counts of 200 to 499; and Category 3 includes those with fewer than 200 cells per microliter. In terms of clinical disease symptoms, Table 2 shows that Category A refers to people who are either asymptomatic, who present with only generalized lymphadenopathy (e.g., enlarged lymph nodes), or who have an acute (primary) HIV infection with an accompanying illness; Category B includes people who are symptomatic but cannot be classified in either Category A or C (e.g., constitutional symptoms such as night sweats); and Category C refers to seropositive people presenting with AIDS-indicator conditions (e.g., Kaposi's sarcoma, *pneumocystis* pneumonia). This yields a total of nine groupings, as shown in Table 1.

In contrast, progression of HIV disease in the psychosocial literature is typically viewed in terms of stages related to symptoms, beginning with initial infection and moving from asymptomatic, to symptomatic, and finally to AIDS. These stages, corresponding closely to the current definition of disease progression given by the Centers for Disease Control and Prevention, are shown in Figure 1 and described below.

1. *Initial infection.* This is a short, seldom recognized illness that lasts for about 10–21 days following infection with the virus and before antibodies are produced (Keeling, 1993). Common symptoms mimic influenza and include fever, enlargement of the lymph nodes, fatigue, and loss of appetite. During this time the individual is very infectious and produces higher levels of the virus than perhaps at any other time in the progression of the disease. However, few newly infected people associate this illness with having acquired HIV.

TABLE 1. Centers for Disease Control Revised AIDS Surveillance Case Definition for Adolescents and Adults, 1993

	Clinical categories		
CD4+ T-cell categories	(A) Asymptomatic, or PGL or acute HIV infection	(B) Symptomatic, not (A) or (C) conditions	(C) AIDS-indicator condition
≥ 500 /μl	A1	B1	**C1**
200–499 /μl	A2	B2	**C2**
< 200 /μl	**A3**	**B3**	**C3**

Note. Categories in **boldface** type represent the expanded AIDS Surveillance Case Definition. All persons in categories A3, B3, and C1–3 are reported as AIDS cases. PGL, persistent generalized lymphadenopathy.

TABLE 2. Revised 1993 HIV Classification System for Adolescents and Adults

CD4+ T-lymphocyte categories

The three CD4+ T-lymphocyte categories are defined as follows:

- *Category 1:* ≥ 500 cells/μl
- *Category 2:* 200–499 cells/μl
- *Category 3:* < 200 cells/μl

These categories correspond to CD4+ T-lymphocyte counts per microliter of blood. The lowest accurate, but not necessarily the most recent, CD4+ T-lymphocyte count should be used for classification purposes.

Clinical categories

The clinical categories of HIV infection are defined as follows:

Category A

Category A consists of one or more of the conditions listed below in an adolescent or adult (≥ 13 years) with documented HIV infection. Conditions listed in Categories B and C must not have occurred.

- Asymptomatic HIV infection
- Persistent generalized lymphadenopathy
- Acute (primary) HIV infection with accompanying illness or history of acute HIV infection

Category B

Category B consists of symptomatic conditions in an HIV-infected adolescent or adult that are not included among conditions listed in clinical Category C and that meet at least one of the following criteria: (a) the conditions are attributed to HIV infection or are indicative of a defect in cell-mediated immunity; or (b) the conditions are considered by physicians to have a clinical course or to require management that is complicated by HIV infection. Examples include but are not limited to:

- Bacillary angiomatosis
- Candidiasis, oropharyngeal (thrush)
- Candidiasis, vulvovaginal; persistent, frequent, or poorly responsive to therapy
- Cervical dysplasia (moderate or severe)/cervical carcinoma *in situ*
- Constitutional symptoms, such as fever (38.5°C) or diarrhea lasting > 1 month
- Hairy leukoplakia, oral
- Herpes zoster (shingles), involving at least two distinct episodes or more than one dermatome
- Idiopathic thrombocytopenic purpura
- Listeriosis
- Pelvic inflammatory disease, particularly if accompanied by tubo-ovarian abscess
- Perpheral neuropathy

(continued)

TABLE 2. *cont.*

For classification purposes, Category B conditions take precedence over those in Category A. For example, someone previously treated for oral or persistent vaginal candidiasis (and who has not developed a Category C disease) but who is now asymptomatic should be classified in Category B.

Category C

Category C includes the clinical conditions listed in the AIDS Surveillance Case Definition. Once a Category C condition has occurred, the person will remain in Category C.

- Candidiasis of bronchi, trachea, or lungs
- Cervical cancer, invasive[a, b]
- Coccidioidomycosis, disseminated or extrapulmonary[b]
- Cryptococcosis, extrapulmonary
- Cryptosporidiosis, chronic intestinal (> 1 month's duration)
- Cytomegalovirus disease (other than liver, spleen, or nodes)
- Cytomegalovirus retinitis (with loss of vision)
- Encephalopathy, HIV-related
- Herpes simplex: chronic ulcer(s) (1 month's duration); or bronchitis, pneumonities, or esophagitis
- Histoplasmosis, disseminated or extrapulmonary[b]
- Isopsoriasis, chronic intestinal (> 1 month's duration)
- Kaposi's sarcoma[b]
- Lymphoma, Burkitt's (or equivalent term)[b]
- Lymphoma, immunoblastic (or equivalent term)
- Lymphoma, primary, of brain
- *Mycobacterium avium* complex or *M. Kansasii,* disseminated or extrapulmonary
- *Mycobacterium tuberculosis,* any site (pulmonary[a] or extrapulmonary[b])
- *Mycobacterium,* other species or unidentified species, disseminated or extrapulmonary[b]
- *Pneumocystis carinii* pneumonia
- Pneumonia, recurrent[a, b]
- Progressive multifocal leukoencephalopathy
- *Salmonella* septicemia, recurrent[b]
- Toxoplasmosis of brain
- Wasting syndrome due to HIV

[a]Added in the 1993 expansion of the AIDS Surveillance Case Definition.
[b]Requires positive HIV serology.

Serological diagnosis of HIV disease is based on detecting antibodies to the virus. The standard procedure is to conduct an enzyme-linked immunosorbent assay (ELISA) and, if positive, to conduct a second. This is critical because up to 70% of ELISA assays are negative on the second test, after obtaining a positive first test. If both ELISAs are positive, the more definitive (and expensive) Western Blot test is conducted. About 50–70% of cases of two positive ELISAs are confirmed by a positive Western Blot (Centers for Disease Control, 1993a). Because these tests detect the presence of antibodies to the virus rather than actual virus particles, 6 weeks or longer postinfection must usually pass before antibodies are produced. HIV antibodies are detectable in ≥ 95% of patients within 6 months of infection (Centers for Disease Control, 1993a). It is often not possible to know if an infant has HIV disease because the infected mother's antibodies are present in the child's blood until around 15 months.

2. *Chronic asymptomatic HIV disease.* The duration and course of the symptomatic and asymptomatic phases of HIV disease vary considerably. This may be due to cofactors such as mode of infection, presence or history of sexually transmitted diseases, substance abuse, nutritional status, virus strain, other microorganisms, age, and other life-style variables. Typically, the asymptomatic phase of the disease is lengthy (e.g., 7 years) and is characterized by progressive immunological deterioration which may be unnoticed. If the seropositive person is aware that he or she is HIV-positive, psychological effects often occur, such as anxiety, depression, or hypervigilance around health.

3. *Chronic symptomatic HIV disease.* This phase of the disease is characterized by the development of one or more of the following symptoms: (1) "constitutional symptoms" such as night sweats, fever, fatigue, and weight loss that may wax and wane in frequency and intensity (Keeling, 1993); (2) lymphadenopathy, where lymph nodes in various parts of the body (e.g., neck, groin) enlarge and become palpable; (3) skin and mucous membrane problems, such as herpes, shingles, thrush, canker sores, human papillomavirus, and oral hairy leukoplakia; and (4) evidence of cognitive deficits indicative of central nervous system impairment (Mapou & Law, 1994). This stage of HIV disease progression was previously called "ARC" (AIDS-related complex).

4. *AIDS.* According to the Centers for Disease Control (1992), a diagnosis of AIDS requires either being classified in CD4+ Category 3 (based on having fewer than 200 cells per microliter) or in clinical Category C (presence of an AIDS-indicator condition, such as Kaposi's sarcoma, invasive cervical carcinoma, *Pneumocystis* pneumonia, or pul-

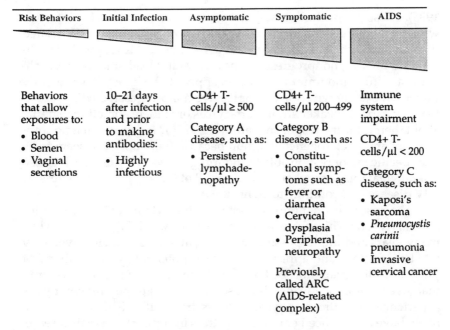

FIGURE 1. HIV disease continuum.

monary tuberculosis). How long does it take to progress to AIDS from the time of initial infection with the virus? Few people progress to AIDS in the first 2 years after seroconversion, but approximately 35% do after 7 years, and about 50% do so within 10 years (Brookmeyer, 1991). This occurs more rapidly when infection is due to a blood transfusion (50% progress to AIDS within 7 years).

A CD4+ cell count of lower than 200 per microliter is clinically meaningful because the risk of acquiring opportunistic infections becomes significant at about this level. Few deaths occur before CD4+ cell counts drop below 50 per microliter.

NONPROGRESSIVE HIV DISEASE

Presently, the ultimate outcome of HIV disease appears to be fatal for most, if not all, people who become infected. However, several recent studies have shown that about 5% of those infected appear to have nonprogressive HIV disease (Cao, Qin, Zhing, Safrit, & Ho, 1995; Kirchhoff, Greenough, Brettler, Sullivan, & Desrosiers, 1995; Pantaleo et al.,

1995). These people have 7 or more years of documented HIV infection with CD4+ counts of more than 600 per microliter, no HIV-related disease, and have had no antiretroviral treatment. Although viral replication is present, nonprogressors show low viral load, and their lymph-node structure and immune function appear to be intact. It is presently unknown exactly why some people have nonprogressive HIV disease. Do they carry a weaker strain of the virus or is there something special about their immune response (Baltimore, 1995)? It appears that nonprogressors are a heterogeneous group because there does not seem to be one specific factor responsible for nonprogressive HIV disease. It is also unknown at this time whether some or all of those with nonprogressive HIV disease will continue to be healthy.

The research on nonprogressors is important for therapists for several reasons. This means that some people with HIV disease will live many years and might possibly live a normal life span. However, they will be infectious and apparently have the potential to infect others. At present, individuals do not know that they are nonprogressors until many years after acquiring HIV disease. Although they may not have experienced significant physical effects from HIV disease, they will likely have experienced emotional distress in coping with their disease. Further, this group of PWHIVs will continue to live with ambiguity and uncertainty about the course and eventual outcome of their disease unless specific markers for nonprogression are identified. On an optimistic note, HIV disease may not represent a "death sentence" to all of those infected. Moreover, there may be specific behaviors or characteristics of nonprogressors that can inform counseling interventions and help promote greater health and longevity in others who are infected with HIV.

STRATEGIES TO ADDRESS CONSEQUENCES OF HIV DISEASE PROGRESSION

Antiretroviral Medications

Intervention with antiviral drugs typically begins when CD4+ cell counts drop below 500 per microliter. Based on a conference on state-of-the-art antiretroviral treatment sponsored by the National Institute of Allergy and Infectious Diseases in June 1993 (see *HIV Frontline*, July/August 1993a), the following guidelines were devised:

1. For asymptomatic patients with CD4+ cell counts below 500 per microliter:

- Continued clinical observation, and
- CD4+ cell counts every 6 months

2. For asymptomatic patients with CD4+ cell counts of 200 to 500 per microliter:
   - Start AZT as first-line therapy; AZT in combination with didanosine (ddI) or dideoxycitidine (ddC) may be considered; or
   - Continued clinical observation and CD4+ cell counts monitoring for clinical or laboratory evidence of deterioration, at which point antiretroviral treatment should be initiated
3. For patients with symptomatic HIV disease (regardless of CD4+ cell count):
   - Start AZT alone or in combination with ddI or ddC

These recommendations followed the reports of the Concorde AZT trials, which suggested that taking AZT did not translate into significant clinical benefit or extended longevity (Concorde Coordinating Committee, 1994). Compared with previous recommendations for antiretroviral interventions, these new guidelines offer "no treatment" as an alternative to antiretroviral treatment in asymptomatic patients with fewer than 500 CD4+ cells per microliter. Combinations of antiretroviral drugs are suggested as possible ways to initiate treatment.

Antiretroviral drugs can cause changes in cognition, emotions, and behavior (Katz, 1994). Moreover, for some PWHIVs, initiating drug treatment may intrude into their sense of well-being and cause them to focus in a negative way on their disease. Following are brief descriptions of antiretroviral drugs used to treat HIV disease, including some of their more common side effects (Katz, 1994).

1. *Zidovudine* (AZT or ZDV) is the most commonly used antiretroviral drug and is recommended as the initial treatment when CD4+ cells drop below 500 per microliter. Common side effects that occur in over half of users are headache, malaise, asthenia, insomnia, and unusually vivid dreams. Other users experience nausea, anorexia, and myalgia. These symptoms typically disappear within 6 weeks of initiating treatment.
2. *Didanosine* (ddI) is typically given to people whose CD4+ cells drop below 500 per microliter and who are intolerant to AZT or who have been on AZT at least 16 weeks, during which time signs of disease progression have occurred. The most common side effect occurring in 25% of users is insomnia.
3. *Dideoxycitidine* (ddC) is given for the same reasons as ddI and often causes headaches and dizziness. Both ddI and ddC have

more potentially serious consequences on organs of the body than does AZT. These include peripheral neuropathies and liver problems.

4. *Stavudine* (d4T) is currently available only through clinical trials and through an expanded access protocol from the company that produces this drug. It is recommended for those persons who are intolerant to AZT or ddI.

Recent Research on Viral Load and Triple Drug Combinations

Recent research has suggested that viral load (measuring viral RNA to detect latently infected CD4+ helper/inducer T lymphocytes) coupled with early initiation of treatment may provide a more effective means of slowing HIV progression (see Baker, 1994). With this approach, antiretroviral treatment would be individualized and would consist of triple combinations of drugs such as AZT, ddC, and saquinavir, or AZT, ddI, and nevirapine. This represents a potentially important treatment approach. However, it is important to note that this is at present an experimental treatment. Individualized treatment also requires that PWHIVs know their serostatus early in the disease cycle, that they are highly motivated to monitor changes in viral load and to follow more complex antiretroviral regimens, and that they have the resources to obtain cutting-edge treatment and medications. In many ways, keeping abreast of antiretroviral treatment of HIV disease is like trying to hit a moving target. For example, an experimental trial of the effectiveness of various antiretrovirals for children with HIV, including AZT as one of the treatments, recently halted the AZT treatment because it was clear that it was not as effective as the other treatments. This means that counselors need to continually keep abreast of changes in treatments by consulting with other professionals or by other means.

Deciding Whether to Initiate Antiretroviral Treatment

There are some PWHIVs who will choose not to initiate antiretroviral treatment—especially at the time that their CD4+ cell count initially drops below 500 per microliter, if they are feeling well. It is not clear what effects antiretroviral treatment has on disease progression and consequences. It does not appear to be correlated with increased longevity. However, the research in areas such as HIV-associated dementia and perinatal transmission show positive outcomes as a result of antiretroviral treatment.

Thus, quality of life may be one of the most significant outcomes of antiretroviral treatment. Nonetheless, for some PWHIVs, this type of treatment affects their quality of life adversely. This may be due to persistent side effects, intrusion into their sense of well-being, or a belief in the efficacy of other types of interventions, such as nutrition, exercise, and meditation. Others, especially African Americans, may distrust traditional medical treatments because of unethical behavior by researchers in some past government-sponsored programs, including the Tuskegee experiment where African American men with syphilis were left untreated (see Quinn, 1991, for a discussion of this issue). Other PWHIVs may believe that drugs such as AZT actually lead to death. Choosing not to initiate or maintain antiretroviral treatment should be accepted by mental health professionals as a valid choice for some PWHIVs.

Treating Opportunistic Infections

There are presently 26 clinical conditions included in the Centers for Disease Control and Prevention's definition of AIDS. These conditions, such as *Pneumocystis* pneumonia, are treated with an ever-changing array of drugs. It is important for clinicians to keep in mind that many of these drugs can cause changes in cognition, emotions, and behavior and to consider this when assessing clients with HIV disease. It is also important for clinicians to keep abreast of common treatments and side effects of these treatments.

CAUSES OF DEATH IN PERSONS WITH AIDS

Prior to the 1992 change in the definition of AIDS by the Centers for Disease Control, a significant percentage of people who apparently died from AIDS did not have AIDS listed as their cause of death. This is because the "old" definition of AIDS was not as inclusive as the current definition. For example, 70–90% of HIV-related deaths in young adult men and 61–89% in young adult women were identified previously, whereas it is expected that the new definition will capture up to 98% of HIV-related deaths (Chu et al., 1993). This is due primarily to including CD4+ count as a definition of AIDS (regardless of clinical symptoms) and, secondarily, to including symptoms such as invasive cervical cancer, so that women are more likely to become AIDS defined. In the study by Chu et al. (1993), the percentage of deaths unrelated to AIDS in PWHIVs was less than 3% and included drug abuse, injuries, suicide, homicide, and lung cancer.

WHERE AIDS DEATHS OCCUR

Where people with AIDS die has undergone a dramatic shift as increasing numbers of people die at home, in hospices, or in nursing homes. In 1983, 92% of people with AIDS died in hospitals, whereas by 1991 this percentage was down to 57% (Kelly, Chu, Buehler, & the AIDS Mortality Project Group, 1993). This trend is more evident among men, whites, and gay or bisexual men. The vast majority of PWHIVs with histories of injecting drug use as well as children infected prenatally die in hospitals (Kelly, Chu, et al., 1993). Interestingly, there are significant geographical differences, as 91% of AIDS deaths in the Northeast occur in hospitals and more deaths (27%) occur at home in the West (Kelly, Chu, et al., 1993).

MEDICAL COSTS OF HIV DISEASE

Early in the epidemic, average medical costs per person from diagnosis to death were approximately $147,000 but are now estimated to be $40,000 to $70,000 (Jonsen & Stryker, 1993). There are a number of medical and social reasons for this downshift, including greater medical familiarity with the disease, more aggressive outpatient management of traditional inpatient treatments and procedures, the availability of volunteer social service supports, and informal caregivers such as partners and parents. With shifts in the demographics of HIV disease, including increasing numbers of injecting drug users and economically impoverished people, medical support is increasingly being provided by Medicaid (Jonsen & Stryker, 1993).

EMOTIONAL ASPECTS OF DISEASE PROGRESSION

Emotional aspects of HIV disease are discussed in detail in Chapter 7, so the following is a brief overview of this issue. It is important to recognize that disease progression has emotional consequences. However, it is very difficult to assess clinically significant emotional consequences of HIV disease because (1) premorbid level of emotional functioning is often difficult to accurately assess; (2) antiretroviral medications such as AZT and other medications used to treat opportunistic infections may cause side effects including depression and anxiety; (3) complaints such as disturbances in memory can be caused by HIV-related neurological effects rather than emotional disturbance; and (4) often people with HIV disease have other major life concerns that may cause them emotional distress, such as the effects of poverty, homophobia, and racism.

NEUROCOGNITIVE EFFECTS
OF DISEASE PROGRESSION

The relationship between disease stage and neurobehavioral consequences is also complex (Mapou & Law, 1994). However, it appears that
the more severe neurobehavioral changes are most likely to occur at later
stages of the disease, when the immune system is highly compromised
(Grant & Heaton, 1990). Although PWHIVs may develop disorders of
the peripheral nervous system (e.g., peripheral neuropathies) that impair manual dexterity or walking, neuropsychological aspects of HIV,
such as impairment in cognitive functioning, are more germane to
mental health professionals (Mapou & Law, 1994). In a review of the
literature in this area, Markowitz and Perry (1992) conclude that there
is an even division between studies showing impairment at the early
stages of HIV disease and those that do not. What is compelling is that
those studies that do show impairment are relatively consistent in terms
of their findings of prevalence and symptoms. For example, these studies suggest that about 20–30% of asymptomatic PWHIVs show effects
in one or more of the following: attention, motor functions, learning,
response speed, and memory.

Once people become symptomatic, approximately 50–70% of those
with AIDS show some level of neuropsychological impairment, most
often in the areas listed above (Mapou & Law, 1994). This impairment is
often due to the direct effects of HIV on the central nervous system
(Mapou & Law, 1994). However, as will be seen later in this discussion,
the level of this impairment most often appears to be mild.

Neurocognitive effects due to HIV disease are typically placed in
one of two categories (Atkinson & Grant, 1994): HIV-associated mild
neurocognitive disorder (MND) and HIV-associated dementia (HAD).

1. *Mild neurocognitive disorder* (MND) is defined by subtle impairment in cognitive functions, such as a reduction in the speed of
   processing information, impairment in attention, and difficulties
   in learning and recalling new information. For a person to be
   classified with MND, there must be mild impairment in two or
   more cognitive areas as well as mild interference with social and
   occupational functioning. There is debate about whether this
   disorder occurs when people are symptomatic or only when
   they develop AIDS. In most cases, MND is relatively stable over
   the progression of the disease and does not appear to progress
   to HAD (Atkinson & Grant, 1994).
2. *HIV-associated dementia* (HAD) is defined by marked impairment
   in the ability to attend to, concentrate on, and process informa-

tion quickly and flexibly, marked impairment in the acquisition and recall of new information, and disturbances of language abilities such as naming and fluency. Additionally, the person may present with psychomotor slowing or affective changes. To classify a person as having HAD, he or she must show marked impairment in at least two of these cognitive areas as well as marked disruption of activities of daily living.

Early reports of the incidence of HAD were as high as 70–90% among those with AIDS, but the recent range of reported incidence is 5–35% (Mapou & Law, 1994). This decrease may be due to antiretroviral drugs such as AZT and better assessment. For example, neurocognitive concerns may be due to factors such as anxiety or other affective disorders rather than central nervous system involvement. In addition, some PWHIVs present with dual diagnoses. Therefore, an evaluation for neurocognitive concerns should include an assessment of personality and emotional functioning along with neuropsychological functioning. An adequate battery assessing neurocognitive factors would include measures of general intelligence, attention, response speed, motor functions, reasoning and problem solving, and learning/memory (see Butters et al., 1990).

Cognitive Strategies to Address Neurocognitive Changes

Mapou and Law (1994), based on their review of the literature, suggest several helpful strategies that can assist PWHIVs who are experiencing neurocognitive effects of their disease. These strategies are most helpful for clients with mild cognitive and social impairment. Therapists might teach clients cognitive compensatory strategies, such as working in a quiet environment, working on only one task at a time, and using memory aids such as lists, notebooks, and computers. Rehabilitation strategies include reducing physical demands in daily life, completing tasks at work and at home while sitting rather than standing, using time management, limiting activities to times of the day when the client feels least fatigued, and reducing work hours (Gallantino & Pizzi, 1990). Mapou and Law (1994) recommend individual and group psychotherapy as a way to help develop compensatory strategies and to gain support. Additionally, psychopharmacology can be an effective way to manage neurocognitive effects of HIV disease.

As HIV disease progresses, those diagnosed with AIDS may not be able to successfully use compensatory strategies or to structure their daily lives without the help of others (Mapou & Law, 1994).

SUMMARY

HIV disease progression involves much more than changes in CD4+ cells, viral load, or developing opportunistic infections. Rather, it also encompasses affective, psychosocial, and neurocognitive changes. For example, physical changes are often viewed as markers of disease progression and lead to affective responses such as anxiety or depression. It is also likely that personality or life-style characteristics, such as coping style or regular exercise, affect physical indices of disease progression. The types of changes due to disease progression (e.g., physical, emotional) that are most distressing for a given PWHIV will depend on many factors in that person's life. What a client views as salient or important about disease progression may also change and shift at various points.

It is helpful to assess on an ongoing basis the physical and neurocognitive changes that have occurred for a client. In what ways have these changes affected the client's quality of life? What strategies has the client tried to adapt to these changes? How effective have these adaptations been? What can be tried next?

PART I

ASSESSMENT: OVERVIEW OF THE PSYCHOSOCIAL MODEL OF HIV DISEASE

Assessing the psychosocial changes that accompany HIV disease is a critical role of the counselor and precedes implementing effective interventions. Assessment helps determine the environmental, interpersonal, and personal resources the PWHIV has to help manage the psychosocial issues that accompany this disease. Is the client able to maintain hope, achieve meaningful goals, and create a positive quality of life, or is he or she experiencing a high level of distress or despair? What social supports exist for the client? These are important questions for clinicians to ask. It is essential to realize that each client's life situation is unique, and therefore adaptations to HIV disease will reflect this uniqueness. At the same time, there are universal experiences that accompany HIV disease, as with any chronic, progressive disease.

WHEN AND HOW DOES ASSESSMENT OCCUR?

I view assessment as a dynamic, ongoing process that occurs throughout the counseling process rather than simply at the beginning. It begins from the moment the client and the therapist meet and continues as therapy unfolds. This ongoing process of refining one's view of the client is especially important in working with PWHIVs, where the physical, psychosocial, and neurocognitive consequences of the disease create an ever-shifting life situation for your client. Although it is important to learn a great deal about your client's life situation early in the clinical work, it is helpful to remember that this assessment occurs within the context of the counseling relationship and the therapeutic alliance. The way in which the counselor assesses his or her client will have a significant impact on what is learned about the client as well as creating the potential for being therapeutic and developing a strong counseling relationship. Therefore, the two primary goals of assessment are fostering a strong therapeutic alliance and developing a schema, or blueprint, for the process of the clinical work.

Formal assessment approaches, such as the Beck Depression Inventory, the Millon, and neurocognitive batteries, are also useful, but I prefer to use them as adjunctive approaches that complement the clinical interview. Two examples will illustrate why I have reached this conclusion.

Tony, a 19-year-old African American heterosexual man, completed an instrument that measured condom use at the same time that he gave blood for an HIV antibody test. On this instrument he stated that he "always used condoms" when having intercourse. I began counseling Tony when his antibody test came back positive for HIV. During this first counseling session, he admitted that he had occasionally failed to use a condom when having intercourse. As Tony and I continued to work together over a period of months, I eventually learned that he had only used a condom on a few occasions, although he always *intended* to use them. He felt so awkward and unsure of himself in sexual situations that he always drank heavily to get up the courage to have sex. Tony had an image of how he *wanted* to be in sexual situations, and this image guided his answers in the surveys he completed prior to HIV antibody testing. In contrast, Tony's low sexual self-efficacy became apparent as we developed a therapeutic alliance and he felt safe to talk about his shame and discomfort around his seuxality. Through developing a more accurate and complex view of Tony, I was able to help him develop more congruence between his self-image and his behavior, and help him practice self- and other-protective behaviors.

A second example of the problems that can occur from relying solely on formal assessment approaches involves Peter, a 22-year-old, HIV-positive, white gay man. As part of an assessment battery, Peter completed the Beck Depression Inventory and received a score well below that required for clinical depression. However, when I met with Peter, it was apparent that he was extremely distressed about some aspects of his life. He no longer had any interest in having an emotionally or sexually intimate relationship, he spoke disparagingly about his body image, and he expressed a deep sense of shame and guilt about having HIV disease. In reviewing specific items on the Beck Depression Inventory, I found that he had endorsed the items relating to these areas. Because he had endorsed very few of the other items on the inventory, his overall score was relatively low and would have led to the conclusion that Peter was not depressed. However, the items for which he received high scores represented aspects of Peter's life that were important and defining and that had been directly affected by learning that he had HIV disease.

There are several other limitations of formal assessment approaches that are worth noting. These include the cultural appropriateness of the instrument, the reading level and the physical demands needed to complete it, and the validity and relevance of the instrument for PWHIVs. These limitations and the preceding examples illustrate the importance of getting a more accurate, complete, and meaningful understanding of the client through empathic immersion in his or her subjective experience, rather than through an accumulation of facts or pieces of information that may not create an accurate picture of the client's life situation. My experience is that the counseling relationship, which can be developed in the context of individual, group, or family modalities, provides the best opportunity to develop an accurate assessment of the client. In addition, the counseling relationship offers a means of connection and social support, a way to feel understood and accepted through empthy, and an opportunity to fine tune interventions as assessment continues throughout the course of the relationship.

USING THE HIV PSYCHOSOCIAL MODEL TO GUIDE ASSESSMENT

I have developed a schema, or model, to be used as a guide in the assessment process. The psychosocial model described in the next four chapters on assessment and then utilized in the following chapters on adaptations to HIV disease and interventions to enhance adaptations has evolved from my own clinical work and research, from other models of coping (e.g., Schlossberg, 1981), and from the literature on HIV disease (see Hoffman, 1991b, for original version of the model). This model captures both the universal aspects of HIV disease as well as the unique life situation of each client. Assessment, using this schema, allows for multiple entry points for interventions by counselors, depending on the needs of the client and the setting in which services are offered.

Figure 2 shows the four components of the psychosocial model of HIV disease. These components will be described in detail in the following four chapters so they will only be discussed briefly now.

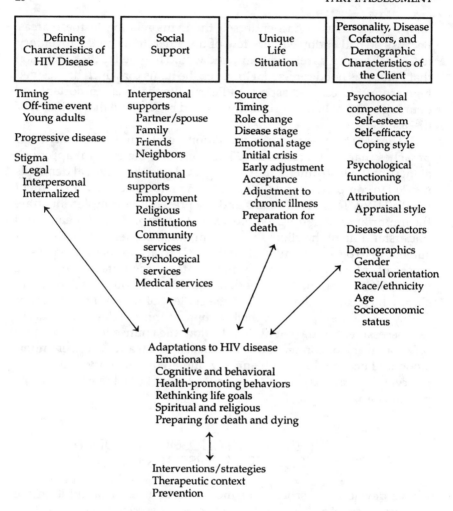

FIGURE 2. Psychosocial model of HIV disease.

Defining Characteristics of HIV Disease

Because HIV is a chronic, progressive, and debilitating disease that is highly stigmatizing due to its association with sex, drugs, and death, the first component of the model, "defining characteristics of HIV disease," is an important and essential aspect of understanding the impact of HIV on clients. This component underscores that a diagnosis of HIV disease is to some extent limiting and most likely distressing to nearly all (if not all) who receive it, and that there are some events that are experienced to some degree by nearly everyone who becomes infected. Events that affect most HIV-positive persons include the timing in one's life when HIV disease occurs (typically young adulthood, leading to premature death), progressive deterioration (e.g., physical), and social stigma.

Social Support

"Social support" represents the second component of the psychosocial model and includes the interpersonal and institutional support networks available to PWHIVs. Examples of sources of support include partners, spouses, family, friends, clergy, therapists, medical personnel, and community services. Social support has been included as a component of the psychosocial model because of the extensive literature on the moderating or buffering effects of support on psychosocial coping. In other words, social support has been shown to moderate reactions to major life events, including HIV disease.

I will discuss two broad aspects of social support, interpersonal and institutional, for several reasons. The literature is replete with clinical and empirical evidence of the importance of interpersonal social support for coping with major life events such as illness, loss, and other transitions. However, there has been less focus on the importance of institutional sources of support. These sources are particularly salient for PWHIVs who need these institutional sources to address needs that may not be met by interpersonal sources such as family and friends. These needs include access to HIV-specific psychosocial and medical care, access to psychological services such as counseling and support groups, and access to housing that is structured to meet the needs of HIV-infected individuals.

Unique Life Situation

"Unique life situation," the third component of the model, refers to the characteristics of HIV as a major life event, including the source or cause of the client's becoming infected, the timing in the client's life in the context of other psychosocial issues, role change, disease stage, and emotional adjustment to HIV disease (e.g., acceptance, preparation for death). Although characteristics of the client's life situation involve actual events (such as the onset of symptoms), the focus is also on the client's perception of these events (such as self-blame about the source or cause of becoming infected).

This component differs from the defining characteristics of HIV disease component primarily because of the range of variation in responses to HIV that persons might experience, based on their perceptions of this disease in the context of their life situation. In contrast, the defining characteristics component refers to characteristics of HIV disease that are universal or nearly so, and consequently are less indicative of the unique situation of the individual.

Personality, Disease Cofactors, and Demographic Characteristics

"Personality, disease cofactors, and demographic characteristics of the client," the final component of the model, includes variables such as psychosocial competence, psychological functioning, attributional/appraisal style, gender, race/ethnicity, and disease cofactors. These characteristics of the individual might affect disease progression as well as one's psychological responses to HIV disease. Client characteristics appear to moderate and predict responses to HIV disease and may account in part for the great variability in the psychosocial impact of HIV. Some of these characteristics can be modified through counseling interventions (e.g., attributions, life-style variables that affect immune function, such as alcohol use) and are therefore important to include in a model of clinical assessment and intervention.

SUMMARY OF HIV PSYCHOSOCIAL MODEL COMPONENTS

Clients with HIV disease typically come to counseling with multiple concerns and often with a sense of urgency to ameliorate their distress. The four components of the psychosocial model of HIV disease help therapists more systematically assess their clients. Consequently, they are able to intervene more effectively in their clients' lives. The model allows for multiple entry points for assessment and intervention, depending on the individual client as well as his or her needs at any given point in time. This model is also recursive in that aspects of one component will often influence one or more of the other components of the model. The following chapters will provide descriptions of each of the four model components, including support from the empirical and clinical literature on HIV disease, and will illustrate the components with clinical examples.

CHAPTER 3

Assessing the Defining Characteristics of HIV Disease

A disease is no absolute physical entity but
a complex intellectual construct, an amalgam
of biological state and social definition.
—ROSENBERG (1987, p. 5)

Living with HIV disease differs from living with other diseases in several important ways. I refer to these differences as the "defining characteristics" of HIV disease. These characteristics affect all, or nearly all, HIV-infected persons and create some degree of universality of experience among those affected. They include the young age at which the disease typically occurs (timing), the chronic, progressive nature of HIV disease, and the stigma that has defined this disease.

This component of the psychosocial model is similar to the concept of situational distress (i.e., a stressful event that causes distress for almost everyone in that particular situation), as described by Nichols (1986), Parkes (1971), and Weiss (1976). More than any of the other components of my model, "defining characteristics" of HIV captures those aspects of the disease that differentiate it from other serious diseases. To illustrate: Tammy, a 23-year-old white female injecting drug user is dying from AIDS. She has a 4-year-old daughter whom she will not be able to raise, and she will die before her parents. Her parents plan to tell Tammy's relatives, her daughter, and their friends in their small town that Tammy died from cancer because they are ashamed that she is an injecting drug user and that she has AIDS.

Like Tammy, the majority of persons with AIDS are young and most likely became infected in their late teens or 20s. This immediately differentiates HIV disease from other common diseases, such as cancer, which usually occur with increasing frequency as people get older. Therefore, HIV disease can be viewed as what Neugarten (1979) has referred to as an "off-time" event. This type of event is one that occurs outside an expected time frame.

The impact of such a major off-time event on the individual, the individual's support network, and on society is enormous. Not only does such an event upset the balance of life—for example, a child dying before a parent—but it is costly to society in terms of the loss of "productive years." People dying at a young age rob society of the years of contribution these persons would have made. It robs partners of their companions, children of their parents, and parents of their children.

HIV disease can also be differentiated from other major diseases in terms of the progressive, and at present typically fatal, nature of this syndrome. There is no other disease that uniformly affects persons with the slow, deadly, debilitating effects of HIV disease. When this is paired with the typical young age of onset of symptoms, HIV becomes the most devastating disease that humans struggle with today.

Finally, as illustrated by Tammy's case, HIV disease can be differentiated from other diseases in terms of the stigma that accompanies it. This stigma can occur on many levels—societal, interpersonal, and internalized by the individual. Sontag (1989) attributes these reactions to HIV's association with two major sources of stigma: an incurable and progressive disease associated with death, and transmission by already stigmatized groups. The unique aspects of HIV disease will now be discussed in depth.

TIMING

The concept of time takes on many psychosocial dimensions for people with HIV disease. Time has obvious meanings in terms of the age of the person who has HIV disease, but it also has meaning in terms of developmental issues and of compressed time in which to live one's life. Young adulthood is a time when relatively few people are coping with disability and death. PWHIVs may feel out of sync with their peers as they face vastly different issues. Some researchers have used developmental theories such as Erikson's (1950) to conceptualize the time-compressed life tasks that face PWHIVs. For example, PWHIVs often feel that they skip through typical young adulthood developmental tasks and roles (e.g., marriage/partner and career roles) to those more commonly associated with old age such as retirement and increasing physical disability.

Many life events involve transitions that are "on time" or expected milestones in life. For example, establishing a career, working in one's career for a number of years, and preparing for retirement over a period of time are expected "on-time" events. Ending one's career for health reasons, perhaps before it really got started, is clearly an off-time event, an occurrence that happens at an unexpected point in one's life—such as premature death (Neugarten, 1979). Off-time events are typically perceived as losses and may lead to a sense of grief and mourning. HIV disease can be described as such an event because it is an unexpected occurrence that often leads to compressing life events into brief time frames or missing out on certain events entirely. Both the unexpected nature of HIV disease as well as its association with early death contribute to the experience of this disease as an off-time event.

HIV, when viewed as an off-time event, has widespread and devastating implications for the individual, his or her support system, and society. To illustrate: Miguel, a 24-year-old Latino heterosexual man, had planned to help support his parents after graduating from college. Instead of being able to help his parents after their many years of sacrificing to send him to college to become an engineer, Miguel is now being taken care of by them as he dies.

The social costs to society of HIV disease are even greater than the financial costs. That is, family networks are disrupted as children die before their parents, and young people disrupt their careers to care for dying partners. HIV-infected parents die before raising their children to adulthood. Young people end careers at a time when many are at their most productive peak, with many contributions yet to be made. The impact of this epidemic on many of the more visible aspects of all of our lives, such as the arts and entertainment, is immeasurable. HIV, when viewed as an off-time event, is a metaphor for immense loss.

PROGRESSIVE NATURE OF HIV DISEASE

The psychological literature on transitions and life events has focused on how people cope and typically describes a process of adaptation followed by a return to normal functioning. Little attention is given to life events in which one is unable to regain or maintain equilibrium over an extended period of time. As Lopez and Getzel (1984) so poignantly suggest, PWHIVs often cope with one crisis but are not able to regain equilibrium before another crisis begins. Conceptualizing HIV disease as a chronic, progressive process assists counselors in understanding the difficulty clients have in achieving and maintaining a sense of equilibrium.

It is important to understand that HIV disease progression will affect nearly every aspect of the individual's life. From the perspective of the clinician, the psychological and psychosocial responses that accompany the physical progression of HIV disease provide important clinical material for the therapeutic work.

THE STIGMA OF HIV DISEASE

One of the defining characteristics of the HIV epidemic has been its ongoing association with stigma. Sontag (1989), in her book *AIDS and Its Metaphors,* writes that "plague is the principal metaphor by which the AIDS epidemic is understood" (p. 44) and "plagues are invariably regarded as judgments on society" (p. 54). HIV disease has been variously referred to as the "gay plague" (Shilts, 1987), as a "condition that is literally as well as morally contagious" (Fineberg, 1988, p. 128), and as "an epidemic of fear" (Bruhn, 1989, p. 455). To understand the complex ways in which HIV disease is associated with stigma, it is important first to understand the concept of stigma.

Goffman (1963) defines stigma as "an attribute that is deeply discrediting within a particular social interaction" (p. 3). He describes stigma as spoiling a person's identity by preventing him or her from meeting expectations—primarily those of others. For example, a young man whose parents expected him to marry and have a family may feel stigmatized by his family when he reveals that he is both gay and has acquired HIV disease through having sex with other men. He has not met his parents' expectations in two major ways: his sexual identity and the resultant implications that identity will have for assuming parentally expected marital and familial roles. This may result in his parents discrediting who he actually is because he is not who they expected him to be.

Two major aspects of HIV disease create stigma: the fact that it is a progressive and infectious disease associated with death, and the view that it is transmitted by already stigmatized groups—gay men and injecting drug users (Herek & Capitanio, 1993; Herek & Glunt, 1988). HIV disease has always been associated with private sexual behaviors, but as the epidemic shifts, HIV is increasingly associated with marginalized groups (e.g., economically impoverished people of color). Thus, stigma is perhaps the primary filter through which society views HIV disease. Stigma is often translated into discrimination, isolation, and indifference toward those affected. In his detailed and compelling book chronicling the beginnings of the AIDS epidemic, Shilts (1987) suggested that stigma delayed political, medical, and compassionate societal responses to the crisis.

> Acquired Immune Deficiency Syndrome had seemed a comfortable distant threat to most of those who had heard of it before, the misfortune of people who fit into rather distinct classes of outcasts and social pariahs. But suddenly, in the summer of 1985, when a movie star was diagnosed with the disease, and the newspapers couldn't stop talking about it, the AIDS epidemic became palpable and the threat loomed everywhere. (p. xxi)

More recently, Herek (1990) described stigma as representing the intersection of psychological processes with the cultural construction of HIV disease. He listed five areas of analysis related to stigma:

1. The biomedical perspective (e.g., lack of information vs. accurate and sufficient information; biomedical history of the disease in terms of who is infected and how they became infected).
2. The cultural construction of HIV disease and AIDS (e.g., its association with death, marginalized groups, "blamable victims," association with semen and blood).
3. Reactions of the nonstigmatized (e.g., moralism, fear of contagion, attitudes toward gays and other groups disproportionately affected by HIV disease).
4. The experience of AIDS-related stigma (effect on self-esteem or self-concept of those infected; others' suspicions or condemnation of private behaviors related to HIV transmission).
5. Managing social interactions between those who are infected and nonstigmatized others (e.g., disclosing infection status, social consequences of disclosure).

Herek's (1990) complex view of stigma acknowledges the multiple forces that converge to create HIV-related stigma: biomedical, cultural, interpersonal, and individual (the PWHIV's internalized view of him- or herself). As therapists, we are often most aware of how the "uninfected" perceive those who are seropositive. We may be less aware of how stigma affects the self-image of the PWHIV and the many ways in which HIV-positive clients may experience and anticipate stigma. Stigma can occur on many levels, but it is helpful to conceptualize three broad levels when understanding its impact on HIV disease: legal, interpersonal, and internalized stigma.

Legal Sources of Stigma

Legal sources of stigma and discrimination have traditionally evolved from conflicts between the rights of those with HIV disease versus the protection of the public at large ("Constitutional Rights," 1986). Debate has occurred over mandatory or compulsory testing (Herek & Glunt, 1988), confidentiality of test results versus mandatory reporting of test results, job and employment protection or discrimination, and discrimination in health insurance. In other words, HIV disease has repeatedly raised the dilemma of the individual's rights and equal protection under the law versus the role of the government in protecting the larger society.

Legal debate has occurred over the confidentiality of test results versus mandatory reporting of results as well as mandatory testing for pregnant women. Many fear that mandatory reporting of HIV test results might result in fewer people getting tested. This concern is especially relevant to whether testing should be anonymous or confidential. Other legal issues include contact tracing or partner notification, and employment, housing, school, and health insurance discrimination.

A number of studies have examined whether PWHIVs encounter discrimination when they seek medical or dental services. For example, one study surveyed gay and bisexual men to see whether they believed that they had been refused medical or dental treatment (Kass, Faden, Fox, & Dudley, 1992). Men with AIDS were significantly more likely to report having been refused treatment than were men who were seropositive or seronegative. A study of the influence of the AIDS epidemic on medical students' career choices provides some insight into why some health care providers might be reluctant or unwilling to provide care for PWHIVs (Loring & Kelen, 1990). Few medical students (19%) reported that they found HIV care challenging and enjoyable, and a substantial minority reported that the AIDS epidemic had influenced their choice of subspeciality field and geographical areas in which to practice. Perhaps the most important finding of this study was that 30% of the medical students believed that their risk of acquiring HIV through their work was considerable. Both the reported experiences of PWHIVs and the concerns of medical students suggest that stigmatization, possibly involving anxiety about aspects of HIV disease such as becoming infected, can take the form of discriminatory behaviors.

Discrimination in the workplace resulting from HIV-related stigma is an extremely important issue because employment provides not only income but access to health and other types of personal insurance (Nussbaum, 1991). Often, PWHIVs will experience subtle discrimination, reflected in an inhospitable work environment. The Americans with Disabilities Act of 1990 (which became law on July 26, 1991) will likely have major implications regarding discrimination in the workplace that may result from stigmatization of PWHIVs.

Interpersonal Stigma

HIV disease has at times been compared to cancer. At one time cancer was a highly feared and stigmatized disease. However, there are several important distinctions between these diseases: (1) the present fatality rate of HIV, (2) the modes of transmission (e.g., sex and injecting drugs), (3) the belief that acquiring HIV disease is typically the person's own fault and often due to engaging in "unacceptable" behaviors, and (4) the current association of HIV disease with frequently stigmatized groups—gay/bisexual men and injecting drug users and their partners.

Few studies have empirically examined the relationship of stigma to HIV disease. Those that have done so have primarily used paper-and-pencil measures or an analogue methodology to examine others' perceptions of PWHIVs. For example, in a study comparing perceptions of AIDS patients to those of cancer patients, university students rated both groups on 12 semantic differential bipolar scales (Walkey, Taylor, & Green, 1990). AIDS patients were perceived as more dangerous, dirty, foolish, and worthless than cancer patients. Similar results demonstrating stigmatizing attitudes toward PWHIVs have been found in other studies (Katz et al., 1987; St. Lawrence, Husfeldt, Kelly, Hood, & Smith, 1990).

One reason why PWHIVs may be viewed in stigmatizing ways is because they are often seen as being responsible for becoming HIV positive. This conclusion is supported by the results of a study by Westbrook and Nordhom (1986) that showed that PWHIVs were held personally responsible and blamed for the onset of their disease because of their behavior, which was viewed as controllable (e.g., sexual behavior, drug use).

More recently, Trezza (1994) surveyed both undergraduates as well as counseling and clinical psychologists to examine their stigmatization of PWHIVs. Undergraduates expressed moderately nonstigmatizing views of PWHIVs, but were more stigmatizing than were psychologists. For both groups, homophobia was related to AIDS stigma, and women were significantly more positive toward PWHIVs than were men. Interestingly, many of the psychologists were uncertain as to whether they would knowingly eat in a restaurant where an HIV-infected person worked. This response reflects a more subtle and insidious form of misinformation and stigma among this group of psychologists. Another interesting aspect of this study was that the psychologists, although fairly positive toward PWHIVs, viewed the rights of the public at large as superseding the rights of PWHIVs. This is noteworthy because in most situations, therapists consider the rights of their clients as being central. Although this study did not look at therapists' responses to clients, it is likely that this concern about the rights of HIV-positive clients versus the public creates discomfort for many therapists.

PWHIVs also often report instances of feeling stigmatized. These feelings affect interpersonal comfort across a variety of situations, from work to intimate relationships. For example, in discussing reactions of members of a support group for HIV-positive men, Cadwell (1991) noted that all described how difficult it was to disclose their HIV status publicly due to fears of being stigmatized. My own research has also supported this fear of interpersonal stigma. Using an open-ended question asking respondents to describe stigmatization they had experienced as a result of their HIV status, we found that many had either experienced stigmatization or were worried about experiencing stigmatization (Hoffman & Driscoll, 1993). To illustrate, of a sample of 50 men (primarily African American) receiving HIV treatment in an inner-city clinic, approximately 55% had told no one of their HIV-positive status, and 40% had told only one or two people (typically their partner, their mother, or a sibling). Many of these respondents stated that the reason they had told few, if any, people about their HIV status was that they expected to experience stigmatization.

Other PWHIVs that we interviewed for our research described experiencing the greatest stigmatization from potential lovers or partners. James, a 35-year-old white gay man described how potential partners initially denied having any difficulty with his HIV status, but as the relationship moved toward physical intimacy, he sensed the tension and withdrawal in their bodies. He felt as if he were "contagious" and "toxic" and felt that his partners would only feel safe to be around him if he were completely enveloped in a body condom. James's metaphor of the body condom powerfully describes the social stigma he felt—the feeling that he was contagious and dangerous to touch.

In contrast, the majority of the interviewed PWHIVs who were in committed relationships at the time they learned of their HIV-positive status reported experiencing continued acceptance and support by their partner. Many of these PWHIVs reported feeling closer to their spouse or partner as a result of their situation.

What these studies suggest is that the expectation and experience of interpersonal stigmatization is common. Blaming the PWHIV for his or her situation, homophobia, and fearing negative consequences through association with the PWHIV seem to be common causes of interpersonal stigma. Interpersonal stigma seems to occur more often when there is not a strong bond with the PWHIV prior to learning of the person's seropositive status.

Internalized Stigma

What I refer to as "internalized stigma" is also important to consider in clinical work with HIV-infected clients. These are stigmatic views that are internalized and that negatively affect one's self-esteem or discredit one's self-concept. Winston, a 28-year-old, HIV-positive, white gay man, had prepared from childhood to enter his family's successful business, which had been in the family for five generations. When he found out he had HIV disease, he felt ashamed and despondent both because his family would learn about his long-kept secret, that he was gay, and because he would not live long enough to take over the family business. Worse yet, he would not produce the expected son to be the sixth generation. To use Goffman's (1963) notion, Winston's internalized stigma about being gay "spoiled" his identity by preventing him from meeting self-expectations.

The importance of internalized stigma becomes clear when one considers the modes of transmission of HIV disease: exposure to bodily fluids such as semen, vaginal secretions, and blood. This exposure typically occurs within the context of private, highly intimate behaviors. Often the riskiest behaviors for HIV transmission—sharing injecting drug needles and anal intercourse—are associated with groups of already stigmatized individuals. It is helpful to remember that all people develop within the context of a cultural milieu and internalize many of the values and norms of that culture. Despite the process of individuating from one's family of origin and developing an adolescent and young adult identity, the imprint of one's childhood cultural experience becomes internalized in many ways.

An example will illustrate this concept. Many gay men, such as Winston, have been raised in families or cultures that espouse homophobic attitudes and values. The young man may eventually achieve a positive gay identity as he matures and become comfortable with and proud of his sexuality. However, if he becomes HIV infected, he may be surprised to experience internalized homophobia because of the mode of transmission of HIV disease and its resultant association with having sex with another man.

Although it makes intuitive sense that PWHIVs internalize stigma based on their socialization in their families and communities, this important area has not been examined in depth in the literature. Eric, a 32-year-old, HIV-positive, white gay man I interviewed as part of a study, illustrates how PWHIVs often expect to experience stigmatization by others and may also suffer from internalized stigma. Although Eric estimates that he has had sex with over 1000 men (often anonymous, unprotected oral and anal intercourse), he attributes his HIV status to a single episode of sharing a needle when injecting cocaine. Because of his conservative Baptist background and his parents' expectations that he will marry and provide them with grandchildren, he has been unable to successfully integrate a view of himself as a gay man into his self-concept—especially a gay man who almost certainly contracted HIV disease through sex with other men. Although his CD4+ count is below 200 per microliter, he is losing his vision, and he cannot work, Eric has told no one that he is HIV-positive.

HIV disease may also bring about a recurrence of internalized stigma. For example, a gay man who believed he had successfully navigated the coming-out process may find that he must once again come to terms with his gay identity given its new association with a stigmatizing disease. Some have likened this process to the initial coming-out process and have referred to it as "coming out with AIDS" (Nichols, 1986). Others may face multiple sources of stigma in addition to the stigma of being gay. For example, Steve, a 20-year-old African American gay man had positive feelings about being gay prior to learning he had HIV disease. Following his diagnosis, he tried to dissociate himself from an overt gay identity. He believed that if others thought he was gay, they would assume he had AIDS. He also felt that the African American community could not accept him as a gay man and that the gay community did not embrace him because of his race.

Steve was reexperiencing a sense of internalized stigma regarding his homosexuality. He had connected being gay with getting HIV disease and expected others to make a similar connection. Steve also struggled with his African American community's view of homosexuality, as well as what it means to be a young African American man today. These multiple sources of societal stigma had been internalized in Steve's identity and frequently surfaced as he came to terms with HIV disease.

SUMMARY

The defining characteristics of HIV disease—the timing in the PWHIV's life when it typically occurs, its progressive nature, and the associated stigma—have many implications that make coping with this disease unique. These issues frequently define the clinical work and can arise in many different contexts. Several areas should be explored: (1) Who, if anyone, has your client told about his or her HIV status? (2) Has your client experienced discrimination or stigmatization because of telling? Has your client not revealed his or her HIV status because of concerns about stigma or discrimination? (3) Are there "off-time" aspects of HIV affecting your client? (4) Is your client experiencing psychological or psychosocial consequences of disease progression?

These defining characteristics often set the stage for understanding the clinical significance of the other three components of the psychosocial model. To illustrate, being developmentally out of synchrony with one's contemporaries because HIV disease is an off-time event may have an impact on one's support network. Or, fearing stigmatization if others learn of one's HIV status may lead to avoiding social interactions. Both of these examples show how aspects of this component of the model often provide the clinical filter through which the other psychosocial aspects of HIV disease must be viewed.

CHAPTER 4

Assessing
the Social Support
of Clients with HIV Disease

> For those of you with friends with AIDS, please
> remember that this is no time for an "out of sight,
> out of mind" philosophy. When your friends are
> too ill to participate in your life as they did before,
> don't just forget them. Remember, this is when
> they need you the most. . . .
>
> —Ferrara (1984, p. 1285)

Social support often acts as a buffer when people are in distress and positively affects psychosocial adjustment, perceptions of health status, and overall well-being (Green, 1993; Zich & Temoshok, 1987). As expressed by Ferrara in the quotation above, friends and family are most important during times of stress. This is true for PWHIVs as well as for individuals experiencing other illnesses and stressful life transitions (Schlossberg, 1981). There are many definitions of social support (Tardy, 1985), with most focusing on both the quantity and the quality of support available. Quantity refers to the number of sources of support available to an individual and quality refers to whether these supports are accessible and satisfying. It is helpful to conceptualize two broad categories of social support when assessing support systems for clients with HIV disease: interpersonal and institutional support systems.

INTERPERSONAL SUPPORT SYSTEMS

Interpersonal support represents the core of a social system and represents those individuals that one is most likely to turn to for help (Kahn & Antonucci, 1980). These supports include spouses, partners, family, friends, colleagues, and neighbors. Interpersonal supports need to be viewed as both available and helpful. Research has shown a relationship between HIV-infected persons' perceptions of social support and their reporting physical and psychological symptoms (e.g., Namir, Alumbaugh, Fawzy, & Wolcott, 1989; Ostrow et al., 1989; Zick & Temoshok, 1987). Similar conclusions have been drawn by others based on clinical interviews with PWHIVs (e.g., Christ & Wiener, 1985; Dilley, Ochitill, Perl, & Volberding, 1985; Martin, 1989; Price, Omizo, & Hammett, 1986). Findings from both clinical observations and empirical research on interpersonal social support will be discussed.

Clinical Data on Interpersonal Support

What are the interpersonal support systems like for PWHIVs? Do they change as a result of HIV? How does social support relate to physical and psychological well-being? Clinicians have often noted the isolation and alienation that many HIV-infected persons report (Christ & Wiener, 1985; Dilley et al., 1985; Martin, 1989; Price et al., 1986). Fears of rejection, abandonment, and loss of connectedness to others are commonly expressed by PWHIVs (Beckett & Rutan, 1990; Christ & Wiener, 1985; Gambe & Getzel, 1989; Martin, 1989). Some PWHIVs report feeling that others view them as "toxic" or "contagious"—as if they pose a risk to anyone who gets close to them (Beckett & Rutan, 1990; Gambe & Getzel, 1989).

Others with HIV worry that they will infect others and consequently may avoid relationships. Some fear rejection, and these fears are sometimes confirmed when they inform potential partners of their status and the relationship is immediately ended (Martin, 1989). In the words of one 33-year-old white gay man whom my colleagues and I interviewed, "others don't tend to want to get to know me if they don't think we're going to have sex—and once they find out I have HIV they fear having sexual contact."

Seropositive persons may also emotionally and physically distance themselves from family, friends, and colleagues as a way of keeping their status secret (Christ & Wiener, 1985; Martin, 1989). For instance, my colleagues and I have interviewed a number of PWHIVs who report that they avoid or have become emotionally distant from people from whom they had previously sought social support because they are afraid to tell them that they have HIV disease. Why do people express loneliness and a strong desire for support and connection on the one hand, and on the other hand appear to avoid the very relationships that may have the greatest potential to satisfy these needs? There are a number of reasons for this paradox.

For example, some PWHIVs may avoid seeking HIV-related support as a way of holding on, for as long as possible, to their present support network. Ed, a 23-year-old African American man who became HIV infected from having sex with women, lives in a semirural area where "everyone knows everyone and everyone talks about everybody's business and people don't keep secrets." This is the essence of the social support system of his community. Ed has decided not to tell any of his close-knit family members about his situation because of the very nature of this support system. For instance, his mother seeks support for all things that concern her from her own sisters. Ed cannot imagine telling his mother and expecting her to cope without going to her sisters. Although Ed would gain some support from telling, he believes that overall he would lose a greater amount of acceptance and support. For example, he fears that well-intentioned family members would worry that he would transmit the virus to his nieces and nephews through casual contact. Ed feels that he has already lost his future dream of getting married and having his own children. Losing the pleasures of enjoying his nieces and nephews would add to the sadness he feels over his serostatus.

Other PWHIVs may fear losing social support because they are not fulfilling the expectations of their families or significant others. James, a 33-year-old white man, has not told his parents that he is gay. He is their only child, and "my parents are still waiting for me to bring home a wife and a grandchild." Despite having full-blown AIDS, James cannot imagine his parents providing emotional support for him and overcoming their disapproval and disappointment in him for being gay. For many, revealing that one has HIV disease involves revealing an aspect of one's self that has been kept hidden.

It is important to note that many PWHIVs maintain a high level of support after disclosing their HIV status to significant others. Others may actually increase their level of social support. Increasing or maintaining support may be a function of factors such as coping style, intimacy of relationships prior to becoming seropositive, and one's community's acceptance of HIV disease. For instance, gay men with strong ties to the gay community may maintain higher levels of support because HIV disease is more openly acknowledged and less stigmatized in this community than in others. To illustrate: Ray, a 35-year-old white gay man, found that after he disclosed his HIV-positive status to several friends, he began to be more open and disclosing about other aspects of his life. This led to a level of closeness and support that he had not previously experienced.

Empirical Data on Interpersonal Support

A number of empirical studies have examined correlates of social support in HIV-positive gay men, but few have examined social support in other populations (Green, 1993). Some of these studies have examined the link between social support and psychological well-being, and others have looked at the link with physical aspects of HIV disease, such as disease progression.

In an attempt to determine if social support per se is related to lower distress, or, if social support has a differential (or buffering) effect on individuals experiencing higher perceived threat, respondents were grouped into three categories of threat (those with HIV disease, those who chose not to be tested, and those who had tested negative; Britton, Zarski, & Hobfoll, 1993). Results showed that the amount of social support was not significantly related to distress, but that social support showed a buffering effect for those experiencing high threat (being HIV-positive). In other words, seropositive gay men with lower levels of social support reported high distress, whereas those with higher levels of social support reported low distress. For the other two groups of men (HIV status unknown or known to be seronegative), level of social support did not differentially affect reported level of distress. This study is useful for counselors because it suggests that when there is a greater need for social support (e.g., being HIV-positive), people may be more receptive to support and may experience greater distress when support is unavailable.

A number of studies have found a relationship between social support and both psychological and physical concerns in seropositive persons. For example, Ostrow et al. (1989) found that gay HIV-positive men who had no one to "talk to about serious problems" were significantly more depressed than those who had a support system. It is especially interesting that the depressed men also reported more HIV-related symptoms, regardless of whether symptoms (e.g., swollen glands, fungal infections) were detectable during a physical examination. In another study looking at both psychological and physical variables, satisfaction with social support was associated with higher scores on a quality of life index, less physical pain, and a higher global health estimate (Namir et al., 1989). Zich and Temoshok's (1987) respondents with HIV reported an increase in physical distress and feelings of helplessness and depression when perceptions of available support declined.

More recently, Turner, Hays, and Coates (1993) found that acceptance of one's gay identity and talking to family members about having HIV were positively associated with social support in a sample of seropositive gay men. Additionally, depression was negatively related to total social support, and the number of HIV symptoms was associated with negative changes in social support over time. The researchers concluded that those men most in need of social support (i.e., depressed and/or symptomatic) were the least satisfied with the support they received.

These studies all show a link between social support and psychological and physical well-being. They suggest that as HIV-related symptoms and psychological distress increase, social support often decreases. However, it was not possible to determine which occurs first. Do seropositive men withdraw from support due to depression and/or disease progression? Do others withdraw from the PWHIV because he or she is depressed and/or has HIV? Or does social withdrawal occur first and then result in depression or an increase in physical symptoms? It is likely that all of the above are possible outcomes and are important to explore with seropositive clients who report having little social support. At the very least, HIV disease often affects social interactions and functioning.

HIV Disease and Social Functioning

How does HIV disease affect social functioning, which in turn may affect social support? In part this can be understood from a clinical perspective by thinking about the developmental stage, young adulthood, of most PWHIVs. One of the developmental tasks of young adulthood is to form enduring intimate relationships and friendships (Christ & Wiener, 1985). However, a diagnosis of HIV disease might affect both the continuation of current relationships as well as the development of new ones. In a study asking participants to evaluate global, nonspecific changes in social functioning, 54% of the sample of asymptomatic gay men reported that being HIV-positive had a negative effect on their social functioning, 14% reported no change, and 32% reported a positive change (Kaisch & Anton-Culver, 1989). Although the majority of men reported a negative effect, it is noteworthy that a sizable number reported positive changes, such as feeling closer to significant others. HIV, like other major life crises, provides an opportunity to reexamine the role of relationships and support in one's life.

However, disease progression does appear to result in diminished social interactions. For instance, Donlou, Wolcott, Gottleib, and Landsverk (1985) found that gay men with a confirmed diagnosis of AIDS reported fewer social interactions since the onset of illness. Perceived sources of social support were also examined in this study. Participants reported mothers and close friends to be the most important sources of support. Fathers and partner/lover were reported much less frequently. Perhaps many of these men did not have a partner when they learned of their infection, or lost relationships because of the progression of their disease or the death of their partner. In another study examining sources of social support in men with AIDS, 62% of respondents had no contact or minimal contact with their family of origin, and 73% reported living alone. Only half said that they had friends and neighbors who could assist them, and the other half reported having no one (Christ & Wiener, 1985).

These studies suggest that as HIV progresses, the energy and motivation required to seek and maintain social support may diminish. This means that many PWHIVs may experience a loss of social support. For PWHIVs who do not have a strong preexisting support system, this may mean that they find themselves increasingly isolated.

Forming New Relationships

HIV serostatus also affects forming new primary relationship bonds in gay male communities, according to a San Francisco study (Colleen, Hoff, & McKusick, 1992). Whereas the vast majority of seronegative (83%) and untested men (74%) preferred uninfected partners for romantic relationships, 68% of seropositive men reported that antibody status did not matter. Seropositive men were also less likely to report serostatus preferences for friendships. This study suggests that HIV-positive gay men may have a more difficult time finding new friendships and romantic relationships than do seronegative men.

The studies that have been reviewed show an important link between social support and physical and psychological well-being. However, it is not clear whether social support leads to psychological well-being and consequently to better health, or if better psychological and physical well-being lead to higher levels of social support. For example, some of these studies suggest that many men experience a diminishment in social functioning as their disease progresses. Perhaps this loss of social support is due in part to the physical aspects of the disease. The Colleen et al., (1992) study also illustrates how uninfected gay men perceive infected gay men to be less desirable as potential romantic partners. Thus, physical symptoms and psychological distress, as well as the simple fact of being seropositive, appear to negatively affect social support.

HIV-Related Bereavement

Some PWHIVs may also experience a loss of social support because of AIDS-related bereavement. For instance, often more than one member of a support system dies from AIDS. This phenomenon is especially well documented in the literature on gay men. Examining this phenomenon in New York City, one of the early epicenters of the epidemic, 27% of the sample of gay men reported the loss of a lover or close friend to AIDS (Martin, 1988). Even though this study was conducted early in the epidemic, many respondents reported multiple bereavements. A positive relationship was found between number of bereavements and use of psychological services, sleep problems, sedative use, recreational drug use, demoralization, and traumatic stress responses. In a more recent study following this same cohort of gay men, Martin and Dean (1993) found that an even greater proportion of their sample had experienced recurring losses due to HIV disease.

Men with more losses due to AIDS also report a greater preoccupation with thinking about deceased partners and friends than did men with fewer losses (Neugebauer et al., 1992). Not only does death affect support networks, but the symptoms described by many of these men also negatively affect their ability to maintain and expand social supports. People may avoid forming new, intimate relationships because they may not want to reexperience loss if their new friend or partner were to also die. For many HIV-infected gay men, the focus of close relationships has shifted from living to saying good-bye (Beckett & Rutan, 1990).

AIDS-related bereavement for gay men is also important because research has shown that social support networks of this population are relatively small when compared to other samples. For example, Namir et al. (1989) found that the average network size of their gay sample was 7.8, with an average of 6.5 people who would "provide help." The majority of the support members were friends, with 52% of respondents reporting "one or no family members" in their support network. These findings are similar to those found by other researchers (e.g., Wolcott, Namir, Fawzy, Gottlieb, & Mitsuyasu, 1986). Consequently, the support networks of gay men may be more vulnerable to shrinkage given the composition of their networks and the effects of bereavement.

Support Networks of Other Populations of PWHIVs

Much less is known about the support networks of other groups of PWHIVs. In a study of injecting drug users, the majority of respondents "hung around" with other injecting drug users, lived with members of this group, and were satisfied with the support received (Stowe, Ross, Wodak, Thomas, & Larson, 1993). For this group, similar to gay men, friends were a more important source of social support than were family of origin members. Perhaps injecting drug users, especially in HIV epicenters, experience network shrinkage due to AIDS much as have gay men. For example, in some large cities, as many as 50–70% of injecting drug users are HIV-positive. Most injecting drug users are heterosexual and may have a partner or spouse with HIV as well as children, which results in significant network disruption and shrinkage. Injecting drug users also report relatively small social support networks, with few family members offering accessible, ongoing support. This is often because the former's "using" has led to estrangement from their families.

Very little is known about the social support systems of women with HIV. Because many HIV-infected women are mothers (Cochran & Mays, 1989), they often must contend with being the primary source of support for young, dependent children at the same time that they need support from others (Zuckerman & Gordon, 1988). Additionally, many of these women are injecting drug users or recovering users, and they may be isolated or alienated from traditional sources of support, such as their family of origin. The challenge of receiving social support while needing to provide support to dependent children is immense (Hansell, Budin, & Russo, 1994).

INSTITUTIONAL SOURCES OF SOCIAL SUPPORT

Institutional sources of support represent the least stable source of social support (Kahn & Antonucci, 1980). They include religious institutions, health and mental health clinics, schools, and places of employment. These relationships are typically role specific. That is, if roles change (such as leaving a job), relationships with other people associated with that particular institution often do not continue or continue with less frequency of contact. Institutional supports are critical in the lives of PWHIVs because of the importance of feeling connected to one's community and its resources. Resources can run the gamut from jobs to spiritual nourishment to recreation to HIV-specific services that address psychosocial as well as medical needs.

Employment

Work provides an important component of one's identity as well as providing financial remuneration. Additionally, work provides ongoing and regular access to coworkers, who are often an important part of a social support network. By examining employment patterns of PWHIVs as they move from asymptomatic to full-blown AIDS, it is apparent that employment status dramatically changes (Massagli, Weissman, Seage, & Epstein, 1994). Unemployment for PWHIVs is usually associated with financial difficulties and lack of insurance. What is often overlooked is the role that employment plays in providing social support, structure, and a sense of contributing to one's community. Employment is discussed in greater depth in Chapter 10.

Religious and Spiritual Support

The role of religious and spiritual support has often been examined in the literature on other potentially terminal illnesses, such as cancer. To date, few studies have addressed this issue for PWHIVs, and none of these studies have specifically examined the role that religious institutions may play as a source of support. Anecdotally, many gay and bisexual PWHIVs who were raised within religions that denounce homosexuality view organized religion as a source of rejection rather than as a source of institutional support. For other PWHIVs, religious institutions might be an important source of support. My colleagues and I found in our interviews with African American women with HIV that the vast majority identified religion and religious activities (e.g., praying, attending church services) as one of their major sources of support (Hoffman & Driscoll, 1993). For most of these women, religion did not provide HIV-specific support (often ministers and church members did not know of the women's seropositive status) so much as providing a place for spiritual nourishment that gave them hope and strength to cope with their disease.

Medical, Psychological, and Community Sources of Support

Examples of community, medical, and psychological services that can serve as sources of social support include support groups, buddy programs, housing programs, hospice care, AIDS hotlines, and legal assistance. HIV support groups have become one of the most important sources of institutional support available for many PWHIVs. Being in a group with others who face the same life-threatening disease can provide a sense of community and ameliorates a sense of isolation (Spiegel, Bloom, & Yalom, 1981). These factors are very important to many PWHIVs, who face a life-threatening and stigmatizing illness that isolates them from others, frequently presents new obstacles to overcome, and often robs them of opportunities to feel useful and helpful to others.

Communities vary widely in the availability of support services for those with HIV disease. Large urban areas with many cases of HIV have typically offered the greatest range of services (e.g., New York City, San Francisco, Washington, D.C.). However, most of the community interventions have been used by white gay men; few have been designed specifically for minority gay or bisexual men (Peterson & Marin, 1988) or for heterosexual men and women.

SUMMARY

It is important to note that the research examining social support in PWHIVs is based almost entirely on gay men (Green, 1993). Based on his review of this literature, Green concluded that few studies included HIV-negative controls or considered socioeconomic, cultural, or gender variables. This is important because others, such as Ostrow et al. (1989), have found racial differences in the correlates of social support. For white gay men, they found a positive association between social support and mental health, whereas the opposite was true for black men. They concluded that these differences were due to fundamental differences in the structure and composition of the support networks for these two groups of men. Clearly, more research needs to be done on other groups affected by HIV. The body of research also shows little consistency in how to conceptualize or measure social support, making it difficult to compare the results of different studies.

What is known from this body of research is that there is a link between social support and psychological well-being for white gay men with HIV disease (Green, 1993). The exact nature of that link is less clear. Similarly, the relationship between social support and physical health status is also unclear. For example, many men report a marked decrease in social relationships that is especially apparent as the disease progresses and they become symptomatic. What is not known is if adequate social support promotes longevity or better health, or if those whose disease progresses more quickly find that social support decreases due to diminishing social interactions. It is likely that some persons actually develop more physical and psychological symptoms when they are lonely and isolated, whereas others become more vigilant and self-focused when they have no supportive others with whom to relate. It is also important to have opportunities to give support to others as well as to receive support. This reciprocity is at the center of intimacy and is important to address in clinical work with clients with HIV disease.

Assessing and discussing social support is an important aspect of counseling PWHIVs. Several areas should be explored: (1) What were the support networks of the client like prior to becoming HIV positive? What are they like now? (2) If the client's support network has changed, what are the reasons? (3) How did the client seek social support in the past? Is this an effective way to seek support now? (4) Is the client knowledgeable about accessing commmunity resources? Is he or she using them? If not, why not?

Helping people seek positive sources of support can take many forms. For some, it will mean reexamining patterns of relating to others and changing self-defeating behaviors. For others, it will mean reconciling and reconnecting with those from whom they have been estranged. For other clients, it may mean learning how to access community and institutional sources of support.

CHAPTER 5

Assessing the Unique Life Situation of Clients with HIV Disease

What life role will I have to give up on because of
AIDS?—the baby part, I wanted to have my own
kids, I love them. Now that will have to change.
—DARYL, *a 25-year-old African American man
with HIV disease*

Living with HIV disease creates a unique life situation for each individual who contends with this illness. Aspects of the individual's life situation, the third component of the HIV psychosocial model, include the source (or cause) of becoming HIV-positive, timing, role changes, and where the individual is in terms of the physical and emotional stages of HIV disease. Schlossberg (1981), in her model of adult transitions, recognized the importance of variables such as these defining the individual's life situation. Although these aspects of the individual's life often involve or are triggered by actual events (e.g., the onset of symptoms), most importantly they include the client's perception of his or her situation.

Daryl, the young man quoted above, viewed the loss of the hoped-for role of becoming a father as a painful aspect of being HIV-positive and one that defined for him what it meant to live with HIV disease. In contrast, another PWHIV's life situation might be defined by his or her stage of emotional acceptance of HIV or by the loss of other roles. Through assessment, you will find great variability in how clients live with HIV disease, based in part on their unique life situation. In contrast, the defining characteristics component of the model addresses aspects of HIV disease that are more universal and that affect nearly everyone.

SOURCE OF INFECTION

Often PWHIVs express a need to understand how or why they contracted HIV disease (Weiss, 1988). They might wonder, "Who gave this to me?" "When did this happen to me?" "Why is this happening to me?" Attributions about the source or cause of infection can lead clients to blame themselves, to blame others, to blame God, or to view becoming infected as inevitable or as bad luck. According to Heider (1958), whose research serves as the foundation for attribution theories, attributions of causality help people make sense of the world and of their lives and help them manage what would otherwise be overwhelming information. There is a large body of literature on diseases such as cancer, diabetes, and heart disease that examines how causal attributions give meaning to illnesses and how these attributions affect adjustment and longevity (Lowery, Jacobsen, & McCauley, 1987). Some studies have suggested that self-blame is predictive of successful coping (e.g., Bulman & Wortman, 1977; Westbrook & Nordholm, 1986). However, self-blame seems to be more helpful for coping with diseases such as heart attacks or strokes, with high life-style involvement (where there are behaviors that you can easily change, such as weight or smoking) as opposed to diseases such as cancer and arthritus, with low life-style involvement (Westbrook & Nordholm, 1986). This may be because self-blame often leads to positive behavior changes, when these changes can make a difference in the eventual course of the disease.

However, there is a paucity of this type of research in the HIV literature. Because HIV acquisition typically involves high life-style involvement (e.g., engaging in risky behaviors such as unprotected sex) and occurs in the context of private, potentially stigmatizing behaviors, self-blame often occurs. For example, viewing HIV disease as retribution for past behaviors is a common reaction (Dilley et al., 1985). However, it is my experience that little is to be gained through blaming oneself for becoming seropositive. Blaming oneself or someone else cannot reverse the course of HIV disease. It is more useful to explore the context in which infection occurred and to use this exploration to make changes, if needed and desired, in the client's life.

For example, Margaret, a 28-year-old white woman who was addicted to crack cocaine, traded sex for drugs and became HIV-positive from unprotected sex. What was most important to her in understanding how and why she became HIV-positive was the way in which her addiction dominated her life and prevented her from being concerned about long-range consequences. In contrast, Jackie, a 30-year-old Latina woman, had only been involved with one man—her husband, James. She had been married to him for over 10 years and had been with him since she was 16 years old. Learning that she was HIV-positive meant experiencing betrayal because James had not been monogamous. Betrayal and trust about the source of Jackie's infection became central themes of her work in counseling.

TIMING

HIV disease as an off-time event has already been discussed in Chapter 3. Because of the long latency period from initial infection to becoming symptomatic, timing takes on other meanings for many people with HIV. That is, many PWHIVs become aware of their HIV-positive serostatus some time after making a significant change in their lives—for example, after falling in love, having a child, or completing substance abuse treatment. Now they are in a different phase of their life than when they became infected. "Paying" for something that seems, at least psychologically, a part of their distant past is painful and intrudes dramatically in their current life situation.

Illustrating this point is the case of Sarah, a 23-year-old white woman who ran away from home when she was 15 and supported herself and her drug habit by prostituting herself. At age 18 she entered a job training program, got off drugs, completed her GED, and then began a full-time job. She fell in love, got married, and discovered when she became pregnant that she was HIV-positive. She described feeling as if she had escaped from her past only to find that it had caught up with her and pulled her back to "pay" for her past behavior.

PWHIVs may also describe feeling that they are moving through life and life stages in "fast-forward," or at an accelerated rate. They may feel that they move quickly through or entirely skip some developmental phases (e.g., establishing and building a career). For example, 22-year-old Ed, who acquired HIV disease from sex with women, often described feeling "old" and acting more like his parents than his peers. Whenever a young woman appeared interested in Ed, he would lecture her about the dangers of getting sexually involved. His peers had difficulty relating to his seriousness and his cautions to them about risk taking. This was especially true because they didn't understand where he was "coming from," as he could not imagine telling his peers about his HIV. It is apparent that many of the psychosocial and physical concerns with which Ed contends represent developmental or life stage issues that differ from his contemporaries. For example, most persons in their 20s and 30s are building careers and relationships, whereas seropositive persons may be thinking of ending a career and saying good-bye to significant others or to relationships they had hoped to have.

ROLE CHANGE

All persons have multiple roles, such as partner, spouse, parent, son /daughter, brother /sister, friend, and employee. Most people find it challenging and difficult to balance the demands and commitments of their many roles. Often role changes occur with a diagnosis of HIV disease or as the disease progresses. This may result in the loss of achieved or hoped-for life roles. The change from employed to unemployed or retired person, the change from providing care or being self-sufficient to needing and receiving care, or the change from being sexually active to being afraid to have sex for fear of infecting someone else can be extremely difficult. For instance, Steve, a successful and ambitious lawyer, defined his primary role and source of identity as "being a lawyer." When he retired for reasons of health, he felt as if a major part of who he was ceased to be.

Positive role changes also occur. Viewing life from a time-limited perspective can bring certain roles into focus. For example, a person who has neglected interpersonal connections because of a career might find new energy and commitment in roles such as partner, mother, or friend. Gene, a 40-year-old ex-banker, retired because of HIV-related symptoms. Although he was initially devastated about giving up what he loved best, his work, he soon found that he was able for the first time to develop a deep level of intimacy with his partner. He had been so distracted by the demands of his career that he had never given sufficient attention to the interpersonal aspects of his life.

Perhaps what is most difficult for people with HIV disease is losing roles that are at the center of their identity and that are developmentally appropriate. For example, deciding not to become a parent because one has HIV disease takes away a hoped-for and highly valued role. This may also serve to isolate one from friends and contemporaries who are committing most of their time and energies to being a parent.

PERCEPTIONS OF DISEASE PROGRESSION

Chapter 2 discussed disease progression from a medical perspective. Disease progression has a psychological component as well because the course of HIV is often unpredictable, leading to great uncertainty (Dilley et al., 1985). Some research suggests that persons with symptomatic HIV (but not AIDS) experience significantly more psychological distress than do persons with AIDS (Tross & Hirsch, 1988). This may be due to the uncertainty of their status or to not knowing if and when the onset of AIDS might occur.

Frequently, PWHIVs become hypervigilant—watching closely for signs of disease progression. One of the characteristics of HIV that makes hypervigilance so common is that many of the symptoms, such as swollen lymph nodes, coughs, and fatigue, occur frequently with other physical problems, such as colds and flu. As a result, PWHIVs often worry that they are becoming symptomatic. For example, John, a 30-year-old gay lawyer, became depressed and highly anxious whenever he had a cold. He felt his neck for swollen glands and counted the days the cold symptoms persisted to assess the strength of his immune system.

Hypervigilance is often heightened in people who are knowledgeable about the symptoms and progression of HIV. For example, research suggests that life expectancy may be shortened in people who view their disease with realistic acceptance (e.g., "prepare myself for the worst"; Reed, Kemeny, Taylor, Wang, & Visscher, 1994, p. 302). Perceptions of the disease process can also intrude and affect a client's sense of well-being even when he or she is relatively healthy. Devins et al. (1990) referred to this concept as illness intrusiveness.

As the disease progresses, HIV-infected persons experience physical changes, such as chronic lymphadenopathy, lesions, and fungal infections that affect self-image as well as energy (Beckett & Rutan, 1990). HIV-associated dementia may make it difficult to perform cognitive tasks, and they may become apathetic toward work and social activities (Hall, 1988; Mapou & Law, 1994). Becoming symptomatic often leads to an acute sense of loss—physical, intellectual, and interpersonal. Ferrara (1984), in relating his own experience of having AIDS, described the pain of realizing he could no longer maintain the level of physical fitness he had worked so hard to achieve. Changes in health status may affect work, energy level, the confidence needed to interact socially, and body image. These changes typically occur at a time in life when one's contemporaries are not experiencing similar changes. This differs from the normal experience of aging when one's contemporaries are also experiencing declines in physical health and stamina.

Some persons report a sense of relief, mixed with sadness, when they finally have a clear diagnosis of AIDS. This anecdotal material is supported by a study in which gay men with ARC (symptomatic HIV disease) had the highest incidence of adjustment disorders (78%), as compared with 56% of those with AIDS, and 39% of the asymptomatic men (Dilley et al., 1985). These findings may seem paradoxical to the clinician who underestimates the effects of uncertainty and ambiguity in a threatening situation.

EMOTIONAL STAGES OF HIV DISEASE

Some writers describe the emotional reactions of PWHIVs in terms of stages. Nichols (1983, 1986) modified earlier situational distress models such as Parkes's (1971) and Weiss's (1976) to arrive at a situational distress model for AIDS. Nichols' model has four stages: initial crisis, early adjustment, acceptance, and preparation for death. The initial crisis corresponds to the intense negative emotions, such as despair and anxiety, that many PWHIVs experience around the time that they receive a positive antibody test. Early adjustment refers to attempts to manage labile emotions and to achieve a sense of equilibrium. Acceptance refers to emotionally accepting that one has a progressive, and likely fatal, disease.

Because of earlier detection and the potential for advances in medical treatments as well as the possible role of health-promoting behaviors in increasing longevity, I suggest that another stage be added to his model—"adjusting to chronic illness." Chronic illnesses, even when not causing current physical disruptions, require a psychosocial adaptation, such as making alterations in life-style to increase immune function. In addition, one needs to incorporate one's "view" of the disease into one's self-concept. This requires integration and acceptance of oneself as one now is, not as one used to be, a process that often involves letting go or grieving for aspects of past, hoped-for definitions of one's self and one's life. Although this situational distress model has not been empirically tested, it may be a useful way to assess and understand changes in the client's coping and adaptation as he or she moves through the progression of the disease.

SUMMARY

Each person's life situation is unique, and because of this, PWHIVs vary considerably in how well they live with HIV disease. Finding ways to maintain valued roles like caring for children or remaining in a job contributes to the PWHIV's unique life situation.

Several areas should be explored when assessing a client's unique life situation: (1) Does the client seem distressed by how he or she acquired HIV disease? How can self- or other-blame be explored or reframed to become emotionally protective for the client? (2) How does the client view the timing of HIV in his or her life? Is HIV viewed as "retribution" for past behaviors? Does the client worry that he or she will not be able to do the things that were looked forward to in life? (3) What role changes has the client experienced? What hoped for roles appear to be threatened? What meaningful new roles can the client seek? (4) How does the client view disease progression? What aspects of disease progression are feared and why? Is the client so hypervigilant that enjoying life in the here and now is compromised? (5) Where is the client in the process of emotional acceptance of having HIV disease? Helping the client find ways to achieve a meaningful and satisfying life situation is an important therapeutic task. Assessing what has changed the most in the client's life as a result of HIV disease and understanding the changes that are most distressing allow the therapist to help the client make changes that can enhance his or her life situation.

CHAPTER 6

Assessing Personality, Disease Cofactors, and Demographic Characteristics of Clients with HIV Disease

> Whatever happens, I just try to keep on going. I sometimes think I'm like one of those bobo dolls I learned about in my psychology class. I keep getting knocked down by this disease, but I just bounce right back up.
>
> —KEVIN, *a 25-year-old, HIV-positive, white gay man*

Personality, disease cofactors, and demographic characteristics of PWHIVs often affect their psychosocial adaptation to HIV disease. Characteristics such as psychosocial competence, psychological functioning, cognitive appraisal, attributions, disease cofactors, and demographics such as gender, age, and race/ethnicity may affect both quality of life and disease progression. For example, Kevin, the young man quoted above, shows great resilience in living with HIV disease. He has high self-esteem, is able to see setbacks as challenges, and has taken a number of steps to develop a healthy life-style through exercise and nutrition. Assessing these characteristics, which in many ways define the very core of each client, is important in helping therapists understand the personal resources the client has to help him or her live with HIV disease.

PSYCHOSOCIAL COMPETENCE

Psychosocial competence refers broadly to personality variables that help explain an individual's success or failure in handling life events. These variables include self-esteem, self-efficacy, and coping style.

Self-Esteem

Low self-esteem may be a factor in being exposed to HIV as well as a consequence of being infected with HIV. For instance, drops in self-esteem may occur as a result of HIV disease (Price et al., 1986), due to guilt, self-blame, and self-condemnation (Coates, Temoshok, & Mandel, 1984). In one study examining the self-esteem of 21 symptomatic gay men, 7 reported low self-esteem. It was not possible to determine if self-esteem dropped as a result of HIV infection and its consequences or if it was already low prior to becoming infected. It seems intuitive that common aspects of HIV disease, such as experiencing stigmatization and guilt or physical changes leading to a loss of positive body image, might lead to a drop in self-esteem for some persons. However, there is little empirical data on this variable. It is also possible that higher preexisting levels of self-esteem might predict more adaptive responses to HIV.

My clinical experience suggests that many PWHIVs experience a loss of self-esteem when a centrally defining aspect of themselves changes. For example, John, an HIV-positive teenager, dropped out of a clinical trial for a new retroviral drug when he began to experience hair loss. This noticeable change led to a drop in self-esteem about an aspect of himself in which he had formerly taken pride. Additionally, this hair loss led to ridicule from his peers. In his words, "I'd rather die looking good, than be alive looking bad."

Self-Efficacy

Self-efficacy refers to the belief that one can exert control over one's motives and behaviors and the social environment. Beliefs about capabilities affect effort, choices, perseverance, thought patterns, depression, and stress (Bandura, 1990). Research on risk behaviors and prevention have often linked self-efficacy to health-promoting and -impairing behaviors. For example, in a study of heterosexually active college students, self-efficacy was related to condom use (Wulfert & Wan, 1993). It is important to note that self-efficacy is viewed as situation specific. For example, a person may have high self-efficacy as a litigation attorney, but may have low sexual self-efficacy. In other words, he or she may feel embarrassed and uncomfortable asking sexual partners to use condoms or practice other safer sex behaviors. Therefore, it is important to assess self-efficacy in areas that are relevant to HIV disease.

It is likely that many PWHIVs have low self-efficacy in some aspects of their lives that directly contributed to them acquiring HIV disease. For example, they may feel uncomfortable or powerless in sexual situations, they may have difficulty with emotional intimacy, or they may feel helpless in the face of a drug addiction.

Coping Style

Coping is another promising variable that predicts variability in both responses and adaptations to HIV disease. Coping is generally defined as the cognitive and behavioral effort made to tolerate, reduce, or master demands that challenge or exceed a person's resources (Pearlin & Schooler, 1978). There is considerable controversy about whether coping is consistent across situations or if individuals employ specific approaches to manage different problems (Kessler, Price, & Wortman, 1985). Most schemas of coping agree that there are three common coping approaches: altering the problem directly, changing one's way of viewing the problem, and managing emotional distress created by the problem (Pearlin & Schooler, 1978). For example, trying drugs such as AZT might be an example of trying to alter the problem (i.e., limit or stop the spread of the virus to new cells). However, the primary focus of counseling PWHIVs will be on the latter two coping approaches. For instance, changing the way one views HIV might include finding new meaning in being HIV-positive such as viewing it as an opportunity to influence others to make behavioral changes. Managing emotional distress might be achieved through attending a support group, taking antidepressants, or practicing yoga.

In assessing PWHIVs, which coping strategies are most adaptive? Research in this area has primarily examined whether different strategies are associated with different outcomes in adjustment and health. For example, active behavioral coping (altering the problem directly) was related to lower mood disturbance and higher self-esteem in recently diagnosed gay men, whereas avoidance coping was negatively correlated with self-esteem and positively correlated with depression (Namir, Wolcott, Fawzy, & Alumbaugh, 1987).

My clinical experience suggests that active cognitive-behavioral coping, paired with an ability to "turn off" thinking about having HIV at times, is quite adaptive. Tony, a 25-year-old African American gay man, viewed getting HIV as a "wake up call" to pay attention to aspects of his life that needed changing. He would identify an area of change, such as promoting health through diet and exercise, and develop an active, cognitive-behavioral plan to address this issue. Tony also had a remarkable ability to enjoy the moment. That is, he was able to push HIV to the "back burner" when he chose to, instead of always allowing it to intrude on the moment.

Overall, clinical observations as well as empirical studies on coping show that there are vast differences between persons in both the amount and the effect of the stress they experience as a result of HIV. It is possible that differences in premorbid coping styles might account for some of this variability. Another important issue is whether and how coping strategies change as individuals progress through the disease process. If we broaden successful coping to encompass "living well with HIV," rather than simply long-term survival, what coping mechanisms assist in this process? This issue will be addressed Chapter 10.

PSYCHOLOGICAL FUNCTIONING
(INCLUDING DSM-IV DISORDERS)

Many PWHIVs show poor psychological functioning, including meeting DSM-IV criteria for adjustment disorders, dysthymic disorder, major depression, or substance abuse disorders. However, it is often difficult to determine whether HIV caused these disorders or exacerbated preexisting disorders, or if these disorders existed premorbidly. Often, the disorders will be more distressing to the client than is having HIV disease. Because substance abuse is a factor in over half of the cases of HIV disease in the United States, substance abuse disorders may need to be managed before the PWHIV is able to address concerns related to HIV disease. For example, PWHIVs who are addicted to crack cocaine are rarely able to worry about infecting others or making other health-protective changes while they are controlled by their addiction. This issue will be discussed again in Chapter 7. Whatever the cause of these disorders, it is important to consider them when assessing clients with HIV disease.

COGNITIVE APPRAISAL

The way in which a person construes an event shapes his or her behavioral and emotional responses to that event (Lazarus & Folkman, 1984).

Although a diagnosis of HIV is often viewed as a catastrophic event (Gambe & Getzel, 1989; Nichols, 1986), there is great variability in terms of attributions of causality, appraisal of future threat (losses that have not yet occurred), and challenge (potential for growth or deterioration). Appraisals about stressful events include three components: harm/loss, threat, and challenge (Lazarus & Folkman, 1984). Clearly, learning that one has HIV disease represents an injury or loss. Progression of the disease represents the threat of anticipated future losses. Challenge, or the PWHIV's perception of the potential for gain or growth, will determine which coping mechanisms are mobilized.

Assessing a client's appraisal of what it means to be seropositive right now and what it might mean in the future is an important aspect of the counseling progress. For many PWHIVs, their disease dominates all other aspects of their lives. For others, it may be secondary to issues such as poverty, homelessness, and addictions. Because it is not yet possible to dramatically alter the physical course of the disease, most counseling will focus on aspects of the disease process that are amenable to change, such as the client's cognitive appraisal of what HIV means in the context of his or her life. For example, the challenge of living "well" (as defined by the PWHIV) might replace the challenge of living "long." Cognitive appraisal is one of the most potent ways available for PWHIVs to experience a sense of control over their situation.

ATTRIBUTIONS

Somewhat similar to cognitive appraisal, attribution theories posit that people form hypotheses about the causes and meanings of important things that happen to them, and that these attributions have an important impact on emotional responses to events. Attributions can assist in adjustment to illnesses if they are emotionally protective and create a sense of understanding and control. The opposite can also be true. For example, Moulton, Sweet, Temoshok, and Mandel (1987) found that for gay respondents, self-attributions of responsibility for their infection had a negative effect on emotions, whereas external attributions such as bad luck were emotionally protective. In terms of self-attributions, the belief that one could influence health status through positive life-style changes was associated with less distress (Mandel, 1986). These findings fit well with studies about the effect of self-attributions on situations that can be modified (e.g., health practices, managing emotions) versus those than cannot (e.g., having already acquired HIV disease).

Other research suggests that having a sense of personal responsibility for one's health and the belief that one can influence health outcomes is related to longevity (e.g., Solomon, Temoshok, O'Leary, & Zich, 1987). However, feeling responsible for health outcomes is different from feeling responsible for disease *acquisition*. For example, a person may assign responsibility to him- or herself for becoming HIV-positive, which could represent a negative attribution. Nevertheless, this same person may feel responsible or in control of some positive aspects of disease progression (such as exercising, initiating antiretroviral treatment), which represents a positive attribution.

DISEASE COFACTORS

The relationship of disease cofactors to immune functioning and disease acquisition and progression is one of the most promising areas for both research and counseling interventions. Life-style factors have been linked to immune functioning in PWHIVs (Kiecolt-Glaser & Glaser, 1987, 1988) as well as to host vulnerability (Martin & Vance, 1984).

Several disease and life-style factors have consistently been linked with immunosuppression, including use of illicit drugs (e.g., cocaine), alcohol, cigarettes, repeated infections with sexually transmitted diseases (STDs), repeated infections with common viruses (Burns et al., 1991; Martin & Vance, 1984; Penkower et al., 1991; Siegel, 1986), and a range of behavioral and psychosocial factors, such as level of stress, nutrition, health habits, social supports, and coping behaviors (Martin & Vance, 1984).

Additionally, alcohol and drug use are often paired with sexual activity. This is one important reason why noncompliance with safer sex practices often occurs when people are "high" (Coates et al., 1987; Leigh & Stall, 1993; Siegel, 1986). It is apparent that cofactors such as substance use and abuse play a role in (1) vulnerability to HIV disease, (2) engaging in high-risk behaviors, (3) the transmission of the virus to others, and (4) the maintenance of one's health status. These cofactors will be discussed in depth in Chapters 9 and 18.

DEMOGRAPHIC VARIABLES

Demographic variables, including gender, age, sexual orientation, race/ ethnicity, and socioeconomic status will be discussed extensively within the context of multiculturalism and diversity in Chapter 15. What follows is a brief overview of these important client variables.

Gender and Sexual Orientation

Gay/Bisexual Men

Gender and sexual orientation have been major variables in defining HIV disease in the United States. The majority of cases (59%) in the United States involve gay or bisexual men (Centers for Disease Control and Prevention, 1995). Most of these men became infected as a result of sexual behaviors (only 6% also reported injecting drugs as a risk factor). Because of the association of "having sex with men" with "acquiring HIV disease," many gay men contend with homophobic reactions from others as well as their own internalized homophobia. Issues that they believed had been resolved about sexual orientation and sexuality are often recapitulated as they resurface as a result of HIV status.

HIV disease has been a highly salient issue in the gay community because of the large number of gay men who have died from AIDS or who presently have HIV disease. To support PWHIVs, the gay community, especially in major cities, has launched a highly effective political and activist approach that has provided access to medical and psychosocial services. Thus, a variety of supports are available for many HIV-positive gay men. This is especially true for gay white men.

Heterosexual Men

There is a dearth of research on heterosexual seropositive males (3% of AIDS cases among men), other than from the perspective of being an injecting drug user or a hemophiliac. The ways in which being HIV-positive impacts one's view of being a heterosexual male is not addressed in the literature. Heterosexual men often mourn the loss of expected or hoped-for roles, such as having a long marriage or becoming a father. Based on my clinical work with this group of men, most report feeling isolated because they do not know any other HIV-infected persons. They frequently express concern that they will be labeled as "gay" or as "injecting drug users" if others discover their HIV status. They may be reluctant to seek support services that are oriented to gay men, such as support groups. Additionally, men of color are disproportionately represented in this group, which suggests that research and interventions are needed that address the needs of these men.

Women

Women, as a group, represent the fastest growing category of new HIV cases in this country. Until recently, the majority of these women became infected through injecting drug use. Recently, the proportion infected through heterosexual contact has increased dramatically. It is difficult to talk about what HIV-infected women face without also examining the impact of race, socioeconomic status, and poverty. For example, the majority of HIV-infected women (about 75%) in the United States are African American or Latina (Centers for Disease Control and Prevention, 1995). Nearly 90% of these women have dependent children (Levine & Dubler, 1990), and in many cases they are single parents. Most of these women are also struggling with issues of poverty, so they may have difficulty addressing their HIV-related needs within the context of caring for dependent children and having limited resources.

Women may also face greater difficulties than men in obtaining and maintaining medical treatment and support services. For example, often clinics do not offer support services such as childcare to facilitate women's access to medical and psychological services, support groups for women, and housing for persons with dependent children. Unlike the literature on gay men, there is a paucity of research on the impact of HIV disease on the woman herself. Rather, the literature focuses more on the woman's role in disease transmission to children and to men.

Race/Ethnicity

Race has become a defining theme in the demographics of HIV disease in the United States as African Americans and Latinos are overrepresented in all transmission categories: among gay/bisexual men, among injecting drug users, among women, and among children (Centers for Disease Control and Prevention, 1995). For example, African Americans and Latinos comprise 46% of AIDS cases in men and 75% in women (Centers for Disease Control and Prevention, 1995). Many African Americans and Latinos with HIV disease also live in poverty. Moreover, because of limited resources and other more immediately pressing everyday problems associated with poverty, such as unemployment and lack of housing, it is possible that these PWHIVs may not view their disease as the most important problem in the context of their overall life situation.

In contrast, little is known about groups of persons underrepresented in both HIV statistics and in the literature such as Asians and Native Americans. There are few HIV-related services that specifically address the needs of these groups of people.

Socioeconomic Status

HIV disease in the United States is increasingly becoming identified with lower socioeconomic, inner-city populations. As fewer infected persons have the financial resources or health insurance to cover their care, the medical costs of HIV disease are increasingly being covered by Medicaid. However, few studies have looked specifically at the impact of socioeconomic status on HIV antibody status, on access to HIV-specific services, or on responses to HIV disease. One study that found an association between low income and HIV infection in men linked this finding to other research that has uncovered a relationship between poverty and poor health (Krueger, Wood, Diehr, & Maxwell, 1990).

Quality of health care in general is linked to socioeconomic status (Ginzberg, 1991). Higher income typically correlates with having adequate health insurance as well as access to health care. Poverty may also lead to people feeling disenfranchised from the health care system and from psychosocial services such as counseling. For these reasons, socioeconomic status, and specifically poverty, will play a major defining role in both HIV acquisition and in responses to this epidemic.

SUMMARY

Personality characteristics such as self-efficacy and coping style, and disease cofactors such as substance use are amenable to change and can be directly addressed through counseling interventions. Although demographic characteristics such as gender and race cannot be changed, it is important for counselors to be aware of how these characteristics often play a significant role in what it means to live with HIV disease and the resources available to manage one's disease.

Several questions should be asked when assessing the personality, disease cofactors, and demographic characteristics of a client: (1) How is the client handling living with HIV disease? How has he or she managed past crises? (2) Does the client show evidence of an adjustment, mood, or substance abuse disorder? When did this begin? (3) Did disease or life-style cofactors contribute to acquiring HIV disease? Are these currently affecting the client's health or increasing the risk of spreading the disease to others? (4) How does the client self-identify in terms of demographic factors? How does this primary identification affect his or her coping with HIV disease? For example, an African American gay man may primarily identify with his African American community rather than with the gay community. Therefore, his own resources, the acceptance of HIV in his community, and the HIV-specific resources available for him in his community may differ from the experience and resources of a white gay man.

PART II

INTERVENTIONS TO FACILITATE ADAPTATION TO HIV DISEASE

Assessing clients using the psychosocial model helps the counselor understand how his or her client is adaptating to HIV disease. Adaptations represent the PWHIV's affective, cognitive, and behavioral efforts to live with this disease. Not all adaptions will be positive or effective. This is especially true at the beginning of counseling, when clients often utilize ineffective and even destructive ways to manage anxiety and to cope. For instance, I have seen HIV-positive persons fall apart and turn their volatile emotions into self- and other-destructive behaviors. I have also seen PWHIVs "pull together" and channel their anger, hurt, and fear into achieving a quality of life and living that surpassed many aspects of what they had achieved in the past.

Counseling and psychotherapy seek to ameliorate distress and to help clients adapt through affective, cognitive, and behavioral change. Although research has described many ways that people adapt to HIV disease, I have selected those that I view as most important and useful for counseling interventions. Each chapter first presents empirical and clinical literature about a particular response or adaptation to HIV disease and then describes counseling interventions to address this concern.

Counseling interventions are increasingly recognized as one of the most valuable tools in managing HIV disease—both in terms of the quality of life for the PWHIV and in preventing transmission of the virus to others. Counseling interventions for PWHIVs provide (1) a means of

assessing emotional, cognitive, behavioral, and neurocognitive functioning; (2) a way to explore and address important HIV-related concerns, such as depression and fears about the dying process; (3) assistance with learning and maintaining self- and other-protective practices;
and (4) a means of emotional and social support. A strong therapeutic
relationship allows important issues and fears to emerge. Yet the importance of the therapeutic relationship has been ignored in many counseling interventions for PWHIVs (Grace, 1994).

In addition to individual psychotherapy, counseling interventions
include group interventions, such as support and therapy groups; peer
interventions including peer counseling, hot lines, and buddy programs;
and family or systems interventions. All of these counseling modalities
can provide social support, promote effective coping, support other
positive life-style behaviors, and, most importantly, provide a connection to others. The following brief overview defines some of the salient
characteristics of counseling modalities, other than individual therapy,
that are helpful in clinical work with PWHIVs.

GROUP INTERVENTIONS

In my view, groups are the single most effective intervention for many
PWHIVs. A number of other writers also view group interventions as
an important and powerful way to provide services for PWHIVs (Baiss,
1989; Beckett & Rutan, 1990; Coleman & Harris, 1989; Gambe & Getzel,
1989; Lopez & Getzel, 1984; Tunnell, 1991). Group interventions have
several advantages over individual counseling strategies: Group members can serve as role models for each other as they share solutions to
common dilemmas; members benefit from helping one another; and
being in a group with others who face the same life-threatening disease
provides a sense of community and ameliorates a sense of isolation
(Spiegel et al., 1981). Additionally, group interventions are cost efficient
and allow more PWHIVs to receive counseling services. These factors
are very important to many PWHIVs, who face a life-threatening and
stigmatizing illness that isolates them from others, frequently presents
new obstacles to overcome, and often robs them of opportunities to feel
useful and helpful to others. Because group members are coping with
the same disease, they may have an impact in a way that an unafflicted
therapist cannot (Beckett & Rutan, 1990).

Many of the descriptions of group interventions describe group
members who are homogeneous on one or more dimensions. For example, there are groups for gay men, women with HIV, injecting drug users,
those who are newly diagnosed, those who are asymptomatic, and those
who are symptomatic. Often counselors report that groups that are

homogeneous on the dimension most central to the identity of the PWHIV (e.g., being an injecting drug user) seem to be more effective than mixed groups.

Certain themes are also common in support groups for PWHIVs. Support groups for gay PWHIVs described by Norsworthy and Horne (1994) and by Stewart and Gregory (in press) showed many similarities in the types of issues that emerged. Themes included medical and health concerns, existential and meaning-of-life issues, stigma and marginality, and issues around sexuality and sexual identity.

How should groups be structured to allow these themes to emerge? The literature in this area suggests that there are important components to include in group interventions for PWHIVs. A group should ideally include the following:

1. An educational component that allows for sharing HIV-specific information,
2. An opportunity to express intense, often labile emotions,
3. An opportunity to observe how others (effectively and ineffectively) cope with the crises that occur with HIV,
4. An opportunity to experience the therapeutic value of both receiving help from group members and giving help to others,
5. An opportunity to discuss how one will tell others of one's diagnosis and/or about other aspects of one's life,
6. An opportunity to come to terms with one's diagnosis, and
7. An opportunity to discuss "dreaded issues," or difficult issues such anticipatory grief and death.

Finally, support or therapy groups for PWHIVs need to be structured differently than many other types of groups. For example, attrition and absenteeism will be more common as group members become ill or die; there may be sessions when there is not a "critical mass" of group members because of illness or death (Stewart & Gregory, in press); themes or issues may be discussed multiple times as they become salient for new members or as members experience changes in their lives; and members and group leaders need to cope with the loss of fellow group members and the anxiety and piercing of denial that such loss often engenders.

PEER INTERVENTIONS, SUCH AS BUDDY PROGRAMS

There are many ways in which peers can serve as informal sources of counseling or supports. Buddy programs are an excellent example of this type of support and will be described to illustrate this category. As Weiss (1988) writes, "The buddy is an extraordinary invention. Buddies are, in a way, big brothers or big sisters to adults who, because of their illnesses, have extraordinary needs" (p. 21).

Volunteer buddies assist PWHIVs with daily-living activities as well as providing emotional support. Buddy programs have evolved from organizations and clinics offering an array of support services. Buddies, unlike spouses, partners, friends, and family members, enter a relationship with a PWHIV knowing that he or she has HIV, knowing the person as he or she is at this moment in time, and knowing what the disease progression might entail.

FAMILY OR SYSTEMS INTERVENTIONS

Systemic therapy deals with intimate networks of people—typically the family. The family can be defined as either the family of origin or the family of choice (Bor, Miller, & Goldman, 1993). Similarly, an ecosystemic family approach helps the client by mobilizing natural support systems and formally conceptualizing the family as the unit of care (Walker, 1991).

Systemic approaches help create or enhance a natural, available, and ongoing source of support for the PWHIV. It not only strengthens the family by healing conflictual relationships and engaging family members in a beneficial process of giving and receiving, but it is cost efficient compared to approaches using support systems outside the family system.

SUMMARY

Counseling interventions help PWHIVs reduce distress amd enhance adaptation through affective, cognitive, and behavioral means. A number of modalities, including individual, group, and peer, are effective ways to deliver counseling interventions. These counseling modalities share the goals of providing support, helping alleviate the PWHIV's sense of powerlessness and isolation, inspiring hope, and facilitating opportunities to adapt to HIV disease in order to enhance quality of life.

CHAPTER 7

Interventions to Facilitate Emotional Adaptation to HIV Disease

Sometimes knowing that I have AIDS just pops up—
it breaks my serenity. I'll go from feeling good to
hitting a real low. It feels like a slap in the face.

—DARREN, *a 39-year-old African American man
who became HIV-positive from injecting drug use*

Emotional distress is common when people learn that they have HIV disease. Although many PWHIVs achieve some level of emotional equilibrium while they are asymptomatic, many again experience distress when they become symptomatic or when they develop an AIDS-defining condition. Other occurrences related to HIV disease, such as experiencing stigmatization or rejection or losing social support, can also create a sense of emotional disequilibrium. Sometimes, as Darren describes above, the enormity of what it means to have HIV disease suddenly breaks through the surface of awareness and creates distress. It may not even be clear what has triggered this intense and powerful awareness. Thus, one of the hallmarks of HIV disease is this experience of disequilibrium.

This emotional roller coaster often begins with a positive antibody test, which is initially often viewed as a death sentence (Martin, 1989). The emotional upheaval that typically accompanies a positive test has been referred to as "life after diagnosis (life A.D.)" (Haney, 1988). It is truly difficult for anyone who is not HIV-positive to grasp the enormity of what this diagnosis may mean. Nearly every aspect of one's life has the potential to change—health, life roles, interpersonal relationships, career.

73

Unlike most life events where there is the possibility to move forward or to return to the status quo, there is not at present the possibility to return completely to "life as usual" or to what may be perceived by the PWHIV as a "better" life. Therefore, HIV disease is typically viewed by the PWHIV as an event that significantly alters one's life path.

STAGES OF EMOTIONAL REACTIONS

Many writers have drawn parallels between the emotions that persons report when dealing with HIV disease and the stages that Kübler-Ross (1969) described for dying persons: denial, anger, bargaining, depression, and acceptance (Barret, 1989; Nichols, 1983). Although Nichols (1983) described emotional stages of HIV disease similar to those described by Kübler-Ross (1969) as reactions to death and dying, he noted that emotional reactions to HIV appear to be more intense and labile than what Kübler-Ross described. The words of James, an HIV-positive gay priest in his 40s whom I interviewed, illustrate how emotions are ever shifting because of HIV. "I see the world as a beautiful place—full of color, vibrancy, and possibilities—when I wake up in the morning feeling good. I'm full of ideas and plans about what I want to accomplish and how I see my value to others. But when I wake up after a terrible night of sweating, nausea, and night terrors, I feel discouraged, guilty, and questioning of my relationship with God, my purpose in living and dying, and of what lies ahead for me."

Although the notion of stages of emotional adjustment to HIV disease is intuitively appealing, empirical literature could not be found to support these phases. From the clinical literature and my own clinical experience, it does seem that emotional reactions vary considerably from person to person and that PWHIVs often "recycle" through an array of feelings as their disease progresses and they react to new experiences. Nevertheless, there do seem to be some "emotional markers," or points in the disease continuum where most PWHIVs find that they have a powerful emotional reaction. Examples of these emotional markers, discussed in detail below, include deciding to get tested for HIV, getting one's test results, and points of significant disease progression, such as learning one has an AIDS-defining illness.

Reactions to Being Tested and Obtaining Results

A number of studies have found that serologically untested persons who view themselves as at risk for HIV experience emotional distress—even before taking an antibody test (Faulstich, 1987; Ostrow et al., 1989). This pretest level of distress appears to be similar for those who test seropositive and those who test seronegative (Perry, Fishman, Jacobsberg, Young, & Frances, 1991). In other words, the person's perception that he or she is at risk for HIV seems to lead to a higher level of distress at the time of testing.

What effect does actual testing have on distress levels? This question was addressed in a study of adults who, prior to testing, believed they were at risk for HIV disease (Perry et al., 1991). Those participants who were found to be seropositive and who were assigned to only a pre- and posttest counseling intervention did not, on the average, suffer increased distress after learning of their positive test results (Perry et al., 1991). Seronegative participants assigned to the same intervention showed marked reductions in distress following counseling interventions. The researchers suggest that the adverse emotional impact of voluntary testing can be reduced by a brief counseling intervention. In other words, pre- and posttest counseling can minimize distress in those who learn they are HIV-positive.

It is important to note that participants in this study were volunteers specifically recruited because of high-risk behaviors such as having unprotected sex with multiple partners, being a former injecting drug user, and so on. Their initial pretest anxiety level and perhaps their responses to the counseling interventions might in part be explained by their belief that they were at risk for HIV and, consequently, by their lack of denial about the possibility that they were seropositive. In contrast, other people get tested expecting to reassure themselves that they are HIV-negative. For example, Jeff, who voluntarily got tested on a regular basis during the time he was an injecting drug user, began to feel invulnerable after getting seronegative results time after time. After he had completed treatment for his drug use, he got tested again and was shocked and devastated to get a positive result. Although Jeff had repeatedly been tested, he had expected to get confirmation that he was HIV-negative and had never truly accepted the possibility that he could become HIV-positive.

Perhaps reactions to taking the HIV antibody test and obtaining a positive result are in large part based on one's expectations. Exploring with the client (1) reasons for taking an antibody test, (2) expectations about whether or not the antibody test is likely to be positive, and (3) what a positive antibody test will mean are important issues to examine before the test. Clients who expect a positive result and who have already experienced distress prior to getting tested may not experience significantly greater distress when they learn they are seropositive. Others may even experience a sense of relief to be able to finally "name" and begin to cope with what they believed to be true. In contrast, clients who learn through routine antibody testing (e.g., joining the military, joining Job Corps, prior to surgery, or as part of routine prenatal care) often do not expect to have positive antibody results and may react to this news quite differently. Those who do not perceive themselves to be at risk, for whatever reasons, may experience the greatest distress. For example, getting an unexpected positive result may lead to feeling betrayed by a partner they believed to be monogamous or HIV-negative. Or they may feel that their past behavior has "caught up" with them after making changes in behaviors that put them at risk.

Reactions to Initial Diagnosis of HIV Disease

A number of researchers have examined initial reactions to a diagnosis of HIV disease. In my clinical experience, reactions to initial diagnosis run the gamut from stoic acceptance to shock, anger, and fear, often in the same person in a matter of minutes. Mary, on learning she was infected, clutched me as she cried out, "Am I going to die? Am I going to die?" Sean ran out of the room in anger to confront the woman he thought had infected him. A few minutes later he returned to the room sobbing in despair. Others appear stunned, as if they have retreated to a distant space within themselves. One of the most difficult aspects of learning one is HIV-positive is contending with feeling threatened and overwhelmed at the same time one is being asked to make immediate, and perhaps major, changes in behaviors to protect both self and others (Christ & Wiener, 1985). Suffice it to say, I cannot think of another situation about which clinicians report feeling so torn between helping their client deal with painful, intense emotions while at the same time providing direct and concrete information about what an HIV diagnosis means and the ways the client can protect him- or herself and others.

The impact of a seropositive diagnosis on significant others, including sexual partners, also needs to be considered and addressed. Troy, a 22-year-old white bisexual man, felt so distressed, overwhelmed, and guilty about testing HIV-positive that he immediately disclosed his bisexuality and his HIV status to his long-term girlfriend. She felt betrayed about his bisexuality, was convinced that she too was HIV-positive, and attempted suicide. This case underscores the importance of considering the impact of a positive antibody test on significant others, helping the client find the best way to tell others, and assisting significant others with finding some type of psychological support.

Reactions to Living with HIV Disease

Once a PWHIV gets past the initial upheaval of a seropositive diagnosis, he or she begins the process of learning to live with HIV disease. It is common for clinicians to see great variability in how different clients adapt to living with HIV. For some, life almost goes back to normal. For others, a high level of emotional distress continues. When a PWHIV does come to counseling with emotional difficulties, it is very difficult to ascertain the source of distress. Is it HIV and the resultant difficulties of living with this disease? Are emotional reactions due to substance abuse? Are HIV-related organic factors involved, causing depression or anxiety? Or is it a combination of these factors? Finally, how did this person function prior to acquiring or learning of his or her seropositive status?

One problem with the research on emotional reactions to HIV disease is the limited information available on premorbid level of functioning. To address this concern, Perry et al. (1990) gave DSM-III-R diagnoses to asymptomatic adults (both male and female) seeking antibody testing. These participants were at risk for HIV disease (due to behaviors relevant to transmission) but were unaware of their antibody status. The researchers found higher lifetime and current rates of mood disorders and substance dependence as compared to a community sample. However, it is important to note that this sample consisted of "at-risk" individuals who may have believed they were HIV-positive and may have been feeling the distress of this expectation. Or, it is possible that their lifetime history of mood disorders and substance abuse made them more vulnerable to becoming HIV infected. This illustrates the difficulties many counselors encounter in understanding the relationship between emotional distress and HIV disease. This is especially true if a client comes for counseling after learning that he or she has HIV disease, so that the therapist has less information about how the client previously functioned.

Earlier studies examining the link between DSM Axis I disorders and HIV disease concluded that HIV led to mood disorders in many individuals. For example, responses of participants in one study ranged from viewing HIV as causing "no emotional difficulties" to "it has consumed the rest of my life." Other respondents described feelings of depression, guilt, and loneliness (Donlou et al., 1985). Based on their samples of hospitalized AIDS patients, both Dilley et al. (1985) and Woo (1988) concluded that "adjustment disorder with depressed mood" was the most common diagnosis for this group, as it occurred in between 50–90% of the sample.

In contrast, more recent studies using gay men as participants have suggested that this population has a high level of premorbid disorders such as major depression and alcohol abuse and that these levels may not differ significantly between seronegative and seropositive men (Atkinson & Grant, 1994; Perkins et al., 1994). For example, gay men in general show rates of major depression of 25–35% (as compared with 3% in the general community) and alcohol disorders of 25–40% (as compared with 15% in the general community), according to Atkinson and Grant (1994). These high rates are often attributed to the effects of oppression and homophobia. It is also likely that the specter of HIV disease, especially in AIDS epicenters, affects the emotional well-being of seronegative men because of multiple bereavements and the fear that they will become HIV infected.

Despite these relatively high rates of Axis I disorders in gay men in general, it does appear that symptomatic anxiety, lasting anywhere from days to months, may occur more often in gay men with HIV disease than in seronegative men (Atkinson & Grant, 1994). Moreover, men who experienced anxiety prior to an HIV diagnosis may also experience relapses at various points, such as becoming symptomatic, during the course of their disease (Fernandez & Levy, 1994).

The studies cited so far present equivocal findings about the emotional impact of HIV disease. They suggest that an assessment of premorbid functioning is essential (1) in understanding the PWHIV's vulnerability to emotional distress throughout the course of his or her disease and (2) in differentiating distress created by the disease versus that created by other factors. Results of these studies may also differ because respondents were surveyed at different points in the disease process. For example, a study of HIV-positive persons, comprised primarily of gay men and lesbian women, found a positive relationship between depression and number of HIV symptoms and a negative relationship between depression and time since learning of serostatus (Kelly, Murphy, Sikkema, & Kalichman, 1993). This supports my clinical experience that levels of depression and anxiety may differ at different points in disease progression and that these emotional reactions are often HIV situation-specific.

In summary, the emotional distress that a client may experience due to living with HIV disease may vary for several reasons: (1) premorbid level of functioning, (2) stage of disease, and (3) time since being diagnosed or since significant disease progression (e.g., becoming symptomatic). Most of the studies examining emotional distress have studied gay men, so it is possible that other populations of clients might react differently to living with HIV disease. Finally, it is important to consider multiple hypotheses about why a client with HIV disease might be experiencing emotional distress. In addition to distress caused specifically by the disease, clients might also be experiencing substance abuse, neurocognitive changes due to HIV, side effects from medications, or other life stressors, such as homophobia, racism, or poverty.

EFFECT OF EMOTIONS ON DISEASE PROGRESSION

Several studies have examined the relationship between symptoms of depression and HIV disease progression. These studies specifically address the question of whether emotional state hastens or lessens the physical progression of HIV disease. In a study of 1809 homosexual men from the Baltimore area, 21.3% were classified as depressed, using the Center for Epidemiologic Studies—Depression Scale (CES-D) (Lyketsos et al., 1993). Depressive symptoms did not accelerate the progression of HIV disease based on when the men developed full-blown AIDS. However, depressed participants had lower CD4+ counts and more symptoms related to AIDS, such as fatigue, fever, rash, diarrhea, thrush, and weight loss.

In a similar study of men in San Francisco, patients diagnosed as depressed showed a decline in CD4+ cells at a 38% greater rate and also reported more symptoms than did nondepressed respondents (Burack et al., 1993). As in the Lyketsos et al. study, there was no significant difference in terms of when the depressed and nondepressed men died.

Several things are noteworthy about these studies and are important for counselors to consider. First, clinical depression affected only between 20% and 30% of the men, meaning that the majority of the men were not clinically depressed. However, it is not possible to know what percentage of these men were depressed prior to acquiring HIV. Next, it is helpful to know that depression does not appear to hasten the progression of HIV. Nevertheless, it is well known to mental health professionals that quality of life is affected by depression, and these studies support that conclusion. Depressed men reported significantly more HIV-related symptoms that likely affected their comfort, appearance, and self-esteem. Thus, longevity should be viewed as only one index of successful management of HIV disease. Since a cure has not been found, I believe it is important and meaningful to focus on quality of life rather than simply on length of life. Because enhancing the quality of life is often a goal of psychotherapy that can be achieved through the efforts of the PWHIV, this focus offers a hopeful and valuable approach to managing emotional reactions to HIV.

INTERVENTIONS TO EXPRESS AND STABILIZE EMOTIONAL REACTIONS TO HIV

Although little empirical research has examined the effectiveness of various counseling strategies to manage emotional reactions to HIV disease, several writers have suggested interventions based on their clinical work (Allers & Katrin, 1988; M. A. Cohen, 1990; Lomax & Sandler, 1988; Miller, 1988; Nichols, 1986; Selwyn, 1986). The thrust of these suggested strategies has been to assist the PWHIV in expressing and working through negative emotions so that positive goals and activities can be initiated and pursued.

HIV disease, especially at the time of initial diagnosis and at times when disease progression is marked, often evokes intense and labile emotions. It is important for clients to have an opportunity to safely explore and ventilate these feelings. It is also helpful for counselors to validate the intensity of the client's feelings without the client feeling that intensity is necessarily negative. As one PWHIV said, "my counselor . . . understands that being depressed is not so bad, but rather a normal mental experience. She also understands when I am not 'up,' as so many of my friends, my lover, expect me to be at their slightest urging" (Ferrara, 1984, p. 1285). Friends and family members are likely contending with their own intense emotions and anticipatory grief and may not be able to stand back and allow the PWHIV to freely express his or her own feelings.

PWHIVs need a place to express feelings without having to take care of the feelings of others. It is important for the counselor, or support group members, to be able to provide this setting and to endure intense emotions such as anger and despair. This allows the client the opportunity to vent as well as to realize that dealing with feelings will not result in being swallowed up and overwhelmed by those feelings. For example, my client Antonio spent nearly half of every session raging at his family, his friends, at things that happened during the week, and at me. During the week he often felt out of control and fearful of "using up" those who were close to him, and it was a relief to be able to safely express his feelings in therapy. When his anger subsided midway through our sessions, Antonio was able to move ahead and focus on the more controllable aspects of his life.

USE OF EMOTIONS BY PWHIVs
TO MANAGE HIV-RELATED DISTRESS

Some common emotions often serve as a way for clients to moderate or defend against stressful events of all kinds; this is also true for clients with HIV disease. Emotions such as denial, hope, and anticipatory grief allow clients to manage the threat that HIV poses to their selves, their lives, and their future. When these emotions are used to take the "edge" off the intensity of the experience, they can be very adaptive, as they allow the PWHIV to examine in a manageable way the enormity of what it means to have HIV. When the emotions significantly alter or distort what it means to have HIV disease, they may negatively affect adaptation to living with HIV.

Denial

What role does denial have in managing HIV? When is denial adaptive and when is it potentially dangerous and harmful to the PWHIV and others? Denial has been viewed in an array of ways: as a healthy psychological defense, as a primitive defense mechanism, as an avoidance of active coping, as a dangerous avoidance of reality, as an aspect of depression, and as an important and essential ingredient of hope (Reiss, 1994). Denial can be a coping mechanism that is consciously and selectively chosen, or it can be an unconscious mechanism. Much of the research on denial has examined perceptions of personal risk of people who are uninfected with HIV or who do not know their serostatus (e.g., Bauman & Siegel, 1987). Other research has focused on denial in terms of condom use (e.g., Aronson, Fried, & Stone, 1991). There is little research on the role of denial in terms of behavior and disease progression in PWHIVs. Some research examining long-term survivors suggests that the absence of denial is associated with positive outcomes, such as satisfaction with one's life and psychological resilience (Rabkin, Remien, Katoff, & Williams, 1993; Remien, Rabkin, & Williams, 1992). However, other research has suggested that realistic acceptance of one's HIV disease, or being fully aware of the likely outcome of the disease, is related to quicker disease progression (Reed et al., 1994).

Clinical wisdom supports the view that denial serves as an essential filter for pain and anxiety. I have often seen denial play a critical role in managing feelings of hopelessness and despair when a person first receives a positive HIV antibody test. For example, my client Sharon wanted to get a second test to confirm the first. Allowing herself the possibility that the first test was wrong provided her with some much-needed time to prepare for what it might mean to be seropositive. Denial in this case is often very protective. Where that denial could shift to becoming a mechanism of dangerous avoidance would be if a client never took the second test, or never got the results, and then convinced him- or herself that the first test was wrong and failed to get medical care or continued to engage in unsafe behaviors.

Perhaps it is most important for clinicians to explore what denial allows the client to do or feel and how it affects the client's emotional and behavioral response to HIV. Several therapeutic considerations might be explored: Is denial representative of a primitive defense mechanism that allows the client to completely deny that he or she has HIV, so that it blocks the client from protecting self or others? Is denial interfering with the client exploring issues of grief and loss? Or does some degree of denial about the expected course of the disease serve a positive function by acknowledging the information that the client has HIV and allowing the client to make needed changes in behaviors, yet enabling him or her to focus on living? Odets makes the important and astute observation that "most denial is a low-level manic rally against depression. The alternative is depression, and people fear that, it can be very destructive" (*HIV Frontline*, July/August 1994a, p. 5).

Hope

Hope may at times be closely linked with the positive aspects of denial. PWHIVs who are completely stripped of the healthy aspects of denial that allow them to be optimistic about the future have difficulty maintaining the flame of hope. Clinicians and others working with PWHIVs often fear giving false hope or optimism. Why is this? It may have to do with fearing that hope (and denial) will lead PWHIVs to take risks with their own health and with that of others, or the therapist may believe that his or her client should address death and dying issues on some sort of timeline. However, hope is essential to achieving a quality of life, to the belief that making plans and setting goals is important, and to pulling together one's resources to move forward. Without hope, the most basic aspects of survival become threatened, including protecting oneself and others. Because HIV disease is apparently terminal, many therapists may struggle with a way to convey hope that is not embedded in an expectation of *cure*. I am struck by the parallel that most people make between a good and satisfying life and a long life. Therapists may first need to rethink this issue. If therapists can help PWHIVs reframe what is meant by a rewarding and satisfying life, then it will be possible to help the PWHIV find many aspects of his or her life that can nurture hope.

This reframing can be illustrated by the situation of Barbara, a 45-year-old white woman, who became HIV-positive following a blood transfusion during surgery 10 years ago. Barbara's own mother had abandoned her when she was several years old. This abandonment had made Barbara establish her most important life goal: to be a good and available mother for her own children. Initially, when Barbara learned she was seropositive, she was most upset about "abandoning" her three children. She was eventually able to reframe what it meant to raise her children and to change her goal to living until the youngest one finished high school and went off to college. Although she is sad about the many events in her children's lives that she will miss, she believes that she has been able to fulfill her mothering role when they most needed her. Now that they are young adults they are mature enough to carry her love for them and her mothering of them forever in their hearts.

What is hoped for may also shift and change as HIV progresses. Fortunato (1993) noted that there are stages of hope that occur when counseling PWHIVs. Specifically, he believes that the domain over which hope occurs becomes smaller as the disease progresses and changes in life roles and relationships occur. Over time, the PWHIV's world becomes smaller and smaller, and his or her attention may eventually focus on an important source of hope that is rarely discussed—eschatological hope, or, in other words, the hope that something does happen to people when they die, in the sense of moving on to an "other-worldly" place. Fortunato suggests that many seropositive persons shift from a "this-worldly" locus of hope to the hopefulness of an "other-worldly" focus. The important role of spirituality is discussed in Chapter 11.

Anticipatory Grief

Another useful way to view emotional responses to HIV disease is by using the concept of anticipatory grief. PWHIVs are confronted from the day of diagnosis with the anticipation of major, unplanned changes— with the loss of health, the loss of certain opportunities, and with the expectation of an earlier death. Anticipatory grief can be viewed as a cycle of feelings of loss and anguish over the expectation of these events. This process often begins at the time of diagnosis of a life-threatening illness, even before significant changes have occurred (Welch, 1992). Anticipatory grief may recur at each significant stage of disease progression.

Anticipatory grief may focus on the loss of oneself as one once was or on the loss of physical fitness, vitality, sensuality, and dreams of a long future. At the same time that the client is experiencing anticipatory grief, family and friends may be going through this same process and may not be able to soothe the PWHIV. For example, Sara's mother would burst into tears every time Sara would try to talk to her about how she felt or about her latest medical information. Rather than feeling supported, Sara felt that her own needs to grieve were superseded by the intensity of her mother's grief. She ended up taking care of her mother and felt that her own emotions were put on the back burner.

Often, significant others' grief may not mesh or synchronize with the client's grieving process (Ryan, 1988). For instance, at end-stage HIV disease, significant others are saying good-bye just to the person with AIDS, whereas the PWHIV is anticipating saying good-bye to many persons, as well as to important aspects and expectations about his or her life. Each change in health status, each death of a significant other from AIDS, each change in a major life role can trigger anticipatory grief. Greg, watching his partner, Ted, die from AIDS, described feeling as if he were in a time capsule—watching himself several years down the road. He wondered, "How will I die?"; "Who will hold my hand and cry for me?"; "Will I die alone?" Greg grieved in anticipation of Ted's death and the loss that would entail, and he also grieved in anticipation of his own death from HIV disease.

Because of the difficulties significant others may experience in offering consistent and helpful emotional support, counseling interventions may be important and essential in assisting clients with this grieving process.

Interventions to Address Anticipatory Grief

One intervention that addresses anticipatory grief is life review (M. A. Cohen, 1990; Pickrel, 1989). Life review allows the client to review the past and to bring unresolved issues to the forefront so that these issues can be grieved for, or achieved, if possible. Accomplishments and gains are also an important part of this review. The participation of significant others in this process is helpful, although this may be difficult for them initially. For example, parents typically experience great difficulty handling the death of a child before their own death. It may be extremely painful for them to help their son or daughter think in terms of life review and bringing closure to important issues.

Often significant others (and therapists) fear that they will be expressing pessimism about the PWHIV's future if they openly grieve about what is happening or review accomplishments or unresolved issues. In other words, therapists may also feel uncomfortable discussing finitude. However, therapists, significant others, and support group members are extremely helpful in this process of life review as they provide support and a sense of connection to the future.

SUICIDAL THOUGHTS AND SUICIDE

Some PWHIVs may feel so despairing about their situation that they contemplate suicide. Others may view suicide as a way to be in control of their pain and deterioration and to achieve a dignified death. Rates of suicide have been reported to be higher in PWHIVs as compared to the general population. Marzuk et al. (1988) investigated the rate of suicide in New York City in 1985, early in the epidemic. They concluded that the relative risk of suicide in men with AIDS ages 20 to 59 was 36.3 times that of men in that same age group without this diagnosis. Using a sample of men with AIDS living in California, Kizer, Green, and Perkins (1988) found that the suicide rate was slightly less than that reported by Marzuk et al. (1988), but was still much higher than that found in the population at large.

More recently, research suggests that suicide rates in PWHIVs may be decreasing as compared with the early years of the epidemic (Cote, Biggar, & Dannenberg, 1992). Based on a review of death certificates across the United States that listed both suicide and AIDS, men with HIV disease were 7.4 times more likely than seronegative men to commit suicide (all but one of the sample committing suicide were men). Of those committing suicide, 87% were white and 35% died as a result of drug poisoning. There were also regional differences, as 30% of the suicides occurred in California. Additionally, the rate of suicide decreased significantly from 1987 to 1989. It is important to note that this study only included persons whose death certificates listed both suicide and AIDS. Death certificates typically report the cause of death rather than listing all comorbidities. Further, some people die of drug overdoses that may not be viewed by others as intentional and therefore are not reported as suicides. For these reasons, it is difficult to accurately assess the frequency of suicide among PWHIVs.

Perhaps it is more useful for clinicians to focus on the notion that many people with HIV disease have suicidal wishes at various times over the course of the disease. For example, results of a review of the literature examining suicidal thinking, suicide attempts, and suicide suggested that people with HIV disease do appear to be at increased risk in these areas (Beckett & Shenson, 1993). However, the authors concluded that the number of those who actually commit suicide is low and that a number of factors, such as social support, are important in reducing the likelihood of suicide.

Although relatively few PWHIVs act on suicidal wishes, depression and suicidality clearly affect quality of life. Because mood disorders in this population are not always a result of HIV disease, an array of factors should be assessed and considered: situational factors, substance abuse, side effects of medications, and organic damage to the brain (Baker, 1993). Additionally, dispositional factors (premorbidity) should be explored (Treisman et al., 1993). Often, clinical depression can be managed by counseling, by antidepressant medication, or by additions or changes in other medications. Contemplating suicide may also represent a way for the PWHIV to take control of his or her life. Reframing other ways in which the client can take control of his or her life may be helpful.

Rational Suicide

As persons with AIDS come closer to death, some consider rational suicide. This comes at a point when quality of life, from their perspective, becomes intolerable. Rational suicide is the informed and well-planned decision to end one's life (Jones & Dilley, 1993; Werth, 1992). It is not known how many persons with AIDS commit rational suicide (Quill, 1991). However, the American Hospital Association estimates that as many as 6000 daily deaths (not just people with HIV disease) in the United States are in some way planned or assisted by patients and significant others, including physicians (*New York Times*, June 14, 1990). From the clinician's perspective, there is an important distinction between a client who is considering suicide before exploring the causes of his or her depression and before making viable attempts to ameliorate the depression versus one who is considering rational suicide near the end of a terminal illness. This issue is discussed in Chapter 12.

Interventions to Monitor Suicidality

It is important first to assess and monitor the client's emotional reactions to determine if other interventions are needed (e.g., more frequent therapeutic contact, joining a support group, neuropsychological assessment, evaluation for antidepressant medication, or even short-term inpatient care). Because suicidal thoughts and behaviors often occur in PWHIVs, it is important to assess for suicide potential by making a direct and thorough evaluation of symptoms and thoughts that are associated with depression and suicidal ideation (Miller, 1988). Being aware of the types of issues that serve as emotional triggers for your client is also helpful. For example, do changes in physical markers, such as drops in CD4+ cells or the development of HIV symptoms, cause extreme distress? Or do changes in roles or rejection in interpersonal relationships cause emotional distress? What role does substance use or abuse have, both in terms of addictions and in terms of self-medication? Assisting clients in managing issues and emotions in positive ways before they become overwhelming is important. This includes identifying and using ways of managing emotions through means other than illicit drugs or other self-destructive behaviors, reframing aspects of the disease that allow the client a greater sense of control, or helping the client view his or her life as still having a significant and meaningful quality.

What are the signs of emotional distress? As clinicians we are trained to recognize common signs of depression and anxiety, such as sleep disturbances, fatigue or loss of energy, feelings of worthlessness, and feelings of hopelessness. But not all clients express their emotionality in this way. Some self-medicate with prescribed and illicit drugs, while others soothe themselves through behaviors such as sexual activity. It is not possible to monitor and assist the client in managing emotions if the clinician is not extremely tuned in to the ways in which a particular client expresses emotional distress.

INTERVENTIONS TO MANAGE DEPRESSION THROUGH ANTIDEPRESSANTS

Antidepressant medications may be another way to assist PWHIVs in managing emotions. They are especially useful as an adjunct to various counseling interventions. However, it is often difficult to assess whether antidepressant medication will be useful, because it is difficult to determine both the prevalence of psychiatric disorders as well as a pattern or typical diagnosis (Bialer, Wallack, & Snyder, 1991). For example, clinicians often find it difficult to distinguish nonorganic disorders from organic disorders (Bialer et al., 1991). Others also note the difficulty distinguishing the classifications of psychiatric disorders due to variables such as substance abuse, dementia, and personality style (Treisman et al., 1993). For example, major depression may have an organic cause, may reflect premorbid functioning, or may be due to aspects of the client's present life situation, including HIV disease.

Given the complexities of HIV disease, which are often superimposed on existing problems such as addictions, personality disorders, and poverty, accurate assessment is critical in deciding on an effective course of action. Even when a careful assessment is made, the effectiveness of antidepressants for PWHIVs may not be as great as with other populations. Some studies have shown that PWHIVs experience more side effects and less improvement than seronegative persons (Atkinson & Grant, 1994; Fernandez & Levy, 1994); this is especially true for persons with AIDS. In contrast, Treisman et al. (1993) report that after making a correct diagnosis, responses to antidepressants in a population of PWHIVs suffering from major depression was 85%, with 50% making a complete recovery from their depression.

These studies suggest that a number of factors, in addition to the issues presented by HIV, must be considered in optimal treatment with antidepressant medications. Antidepressant medications are effective when appropriately prescribed following a thorough and accurate clinical assessment. Antidepressants are likely to be more effective when used along with other psychosocial interventions such as counseling.

SUMMARY

Although therapists often describe the emotional distress that many PWHIVs experience, it is difficult to assess clinically significant emotional consequences of HIV disease for several reasons: (1) Premorbid level of emotional functioning is often difficult to accurately assess; (2) complaints such as memory disturbances can be caused by HIV-related neurological effects rather than emotional disturbance; (3) antiretroviral medications such as AZT and other medications to treat opportunistic infections may cause side effects, including depression and anxiety; (4) emotions are often labile and therefore may vary considerably from day to day or week to week; and (5) people with HIV disease often have other major life concerns that may cause them emotional distress, such as the effects of poverty, homophobia, and racism.

Despite the challenges of accurately assessing the cause of emotional distress and psychiatric disorders in PWHIVs, it does appear that anxiety disorders lasting one to several months are common and often coincide with significant markers in disease progression, such as initial diagnosis or becoming symptomatic. Rates of current depression in HIV populations may be double those found in healthy community populations and are similar to rates found for other chronic illnesses (e.g., 5 to 8%) (Atkinson & Grant, 1994). Anxiety and depression, even when not clinically significant, can interfere with one's overall quality of life and with setting goals and looking forward to the future. Denial, while often emotionally protective, can also interfere with adjustment to HIV disease. For these reasons, it is an important focus of counseling to address emotional responses to HIV so that the client can live as well as possible with HIV disease.

CHAPTER 8

Interventions to Facilitate Cognitive and Behavioral Adaptation to HIV Disease

> It's so hard not to use when I get really down. I been using coke, crack, and anything else I can get my hands on for so many years to help me get by. Now that I got AIDS, I know I have to be good, but sometimes it's just so hard—I pray, I talk to Mom, I take a walk but sometimes I feel so helpless and like I just don't have it in me to get me through all this AIDS stuff I gotta get through.
>
> —LaVonda, *a 31-one-year old, HIV-positive, African American woman*

A unique aspect of HIV disease is that it frequently prevents sustained and consistent problem solving on the part of the client (Lopez & Getzel, 1984), in part because of the erratic and unpredictable course of the disease. As described by LaVonda, above, the psychosocial and physical effects of the disease can challenge and overwhelm the coping strategies of PWHIVs. The ways a client coped in the past may no longer be effective, or coping approaches such as substance abuse may be destructive. Helping clients learn effective coping responses can minimize many of the negative consequences of HIV disease and can enhance their quality of life. Coping can be defined as "constantly changing cognitive and behavioral efforts to manage specific external and/or internal demands that are appraised as taxing or exceeding the resources of the person" (Lazarus & Folkman, 1984, p. 141).

Stress and a number of other factors, such as exhaustion, nutrition, social supports, and coping mechanisms have been related to immune functioning (Kiecolt-Glaser & Glaser, 1987; Martin & Vance, 1984; Monat & Lazarus, 1985). Greater distress is associated with poorer immune function (Kiecolt-Glaser & Glaser, 1987). Therefore, teaching HIV-positive clients effective coping strategies for day-to-day living may reduce stress levels, provide emotional benefits, and promote health. Research on cancer has supported the link between coping style and health status and found that active coping and a sense of control are associated with improved adjustment and perhaps longer survival (Bloom, 1982; Weisman & Sobel, 1979). Similar effects may also be true for PWHIVs (Coates et al., 1984; Namir et al., 1987).

Coping with a diagnosis of HIV disease may involve continued attempts to master the changing demands created by the disease. PWHIVs may not be able to depend on a restoration of equilibrium allowing for a stage of reintegration to take place following each crisis (Gambe & Getzel, 1989). This is especially true after becoming symptomatic. Research has also linked major and minor stressful events to immune function changes (Kiecolt-Glaser & Glaser, 1987, 1988). Thus, HIV disease challenges the coping strategies that a person may have previously used and makes meeting the demands of day-to-day living more difficult.

The literature has consistently pointed out the high incidence of adjustment disorders and mood disorders in PWHIVs, especially those who are symptomatic. Although these disorders may be the result of a variety of factors ranging from premorbid functioning to HIV-related dementia, it is likely that the capacity to cope is diminished for many PWHIVs as a result of the physical, neurocognitive, and psychological demands of HIV as well as other stressors in their lives. In contrast, other literature describes PWHIVs who are successful at maintaining a relatively high quality of life throughout much of the course of their disease. What factors account for differences in coping?

There are a number of internal as well as social resources that PWHIVs draw on for managing various aspects of their disease, including psychological distress. Resources include aspects of the individual's personality, such as hardiness (Kobasa, 1979), that are related to effective coping. Kobasa describes persons high in hardiness as having a stronger commitment to self, a sense of meaningfulness about their life, and an internal locus of control. Coping styles and social support represent other types of coping resources.

The literature on coping has distinguished two broad types of coping efforts: efforts at problem solving and efforts at emotional regulation (Lazarus & Folkman, 1984; Pearlin & Schooler, 1978). Appraising one's disease to be threatening or challenging leads to the initiation of coping efforts or strategies (Lazarus & Folkman, 1984).

THE ROLE OF APPRAISAL IN COPING EFFORTS

How an individual construes an event may shape the emotional and behavioral reactions to that event (Lazarus, DeLongis, Folkman, & Gruen, 1985; Lazarus & Folkman, 1984). Cognitive appraisal is often what sets the stage for how a person will cope with a specific event in his or her life. The evaluative meaning or significance that PWHIVs give to their disease may account, in part, for how well they cope with HIV. This process of appraisal may explain the variations in response among individuals under comparable conditions. To illustrate, a client with hemophilia who became HIV-positive as a result of tainted blood products may attach a very different meaning to having this disease than does a client who believes that he or she acquired HIV disease due to retribution for "sinful" behavior. "Cognitive appraisal can be most readily understood as the process of categorizing an encounter, and its various facets, with respect to its significance for well-being" (Lazarus & Folkman, 1984, p. 31). Primary appraisal is the evaluation of what is at stake in a particular situation and secondary appraisal is the evaluation of what coping options exist to reduce a perceived threat or harm.

According to Lazarus and Folkman (1984), appraisals about stressful events include three components: harm/loss, threat, and challenge. In the harm/loss component, some injury or loss has occurred (e.g., becoming seropositive, or progressing from asymptomatic to symptomatic) for the individual. This injury may result in a loss of commitments or the choices, values, and/or goals that are most meaningful to the individual. In the case of a client with HIV disease, these losses might include the belief that one may never have a lifelong, committed relationship with a partner; that one may never have children or may not have the family size one had wished; or that one will lose physical fitness and other abilities, independence, or sexual freedom. Haney (1988) refers to these losses as disconnections: for example, as disconnections in the ways one had defined one's self.

Threat, the second component of cognitive appraisal, refers to losses or harms that have not taken place yet but are anticipated as likely to occur in the future. Because of the debilitating and progressive nature of HIV disease, threat is a constant feature of clinical work. A person may get through one crisis, medically, psychologically, or interpersonally, only to be blindsided by the next crisis or to face uncertainty about the future. Many clients become so anxious and hypervigilant about what lies ahead that they lose their capacity to enjoy the moment.

The third component of appraisal, challenge, is similar to threat in that it requires a mobilization of coping responses. Unlike threat, challenge focuses on the potential for gain or growth as a result of HIV disease. An example to illustrate this process involves Janet, a 24-year-old white woman whose estranged husband was an injecting drug user. Janet discovered that she was HIV-positive when she became pregnant. This discovery represented the harm/loss aspect of cognitive appraisal. Initially, Janet felt that she had lost her opportunity to have a long life and to raise her unborn child. In terms of threat, during the pregnancy Janet became ill with HIV-related symptoms and became convinced that she would transmit the virus to her unborn child. She anticipated that her child would be born sick and would not survive infancy. She also wondered who would take care of her child if she died, because her family had severed contact with her several years previously because of her husband's drug use.

Because of the precariousness of her situation, Janet reassessed her estrangement from her parents and siblings and decided to challenge herself and seek a reconciliation. This went surprisingly well. When Janet learned that her daughter was seronegative, this reconnection with her family provided her and her daughter with essential social support and security. In contrast to Janet, many clients are painfully aware of the threat and potential losses that accompany HIV disease, but have great difficulty seeing the potential for gain or growth. Motivating clients to set goals and challenging them to achieve a meaningful quality of life is an extremely important aspect of counseling PWHIVs. The therapist must first believe that there is "life after HIV," and this belief in the client's future needs to be conveyed to the client in a manner that instills hope and fosters motivation.

Interventions to Change Clients' Appraisals about HIV

Although a counselor cannot change a client's perception that harm/loss has occurred as a result of having HIV disease, it is possible to help clients reframe their sense of loss and harm. It is helpful to begin by exploring with the client what the greatest losses are that he or she has experienced because of HIV disease. These losses can then be reframed. For example, through exploration a client may learn that a commitment to life per se may not be as important to him or her as a commitment to quality-of-life issues, such as fulfilling life goals, con-necting emotionally with significant others, or making a lasting contri-bution. Counseling interventions can then assist the client in selecting the most important goal(s) and finding a way to achieve that goal.

Research has also shown that the stronger a commitment to a goal or a value, the more vulnerable a person is to psychological distress in that area (Lazarus & Folkman, 1984). Thus, a client who is highly committed to affiliation may be most vulnerable if that aspect of his or her life changes. In contrast, a person who is highly committed to achievement may experience the greatest sense of loss over leaving his or her career. Therefore, recognizing and exploring losses in areas that are important to your client is the first step in understanding what these losses might mean to him or her.

Perhaps the most challenging aspect of the cognitive appraisal process to address with PWHIVs is the perception of anticipated threat. There is a very real aspect to the threat of HIV disease progression as compared to many other life events people face. For example, one does not "get over" or "work through" HIV disease in the ways that are possible for most other life transitions. The course of HIV disease is also unpredictable and uncertain. Moos and Tsu (1977), in their comprehen-sive review of studies examining how people cope with the stresses of serious physical illnesses, state that dealing with uncertainty is a major adaptive task. Uncertainty is highly stressful, in part because it affects one's sense of control.

In the case of HIV, the client is dealing with multiple sources of uncertainty. Who gave this to me? Why did I get this? What will happen to me? Can anyone or anything help me? Will there be a cure in time to help me? Will anyone want to be close to me? Will I lose my job? Will I be helpless and dependent? Will anyone be with me when I die? PWHIVs also contend with temporal uncertainty—not knowing when an event (e.g., symptoms, AIDS, death) may occur. There is little research to guide the clinician in designing interventions to address the threat component of cognitive appraisal. Yet the HIV literature is replete with examples of how infected persons are vigilant (and often hypervigilant) in anticipation of new symptoms or signs that signal disease progression. How can counselors help clients manage uncer-tainty? Cognitive therapy techniques such as reattribution, thought stopping, self-talk, and active problem solving (Coates et al., 1987) might be helpful in shifting the client's focus away from appraisals of harm.

To illustrate: Bill was not afraid to die, but he was terrified of the dying process. He had seen elderly relatives in excruciating pain for months on end being kept alive through medical interventions despite begging to be allowed to die. As he became sicker and stopped enjoying his life, Bill decided to sign an advance directive so he would have some control over being helpless and uninvolved in his own treatment. Additionally, he obtained pills so that he could opt for rational suicide if he so chose. Through active problem solving, Bill reduced the most threatening aspects of the dying process.

Challenge, the third kind of stress appraisal, may offer many opportunities for clinical intervention because it affords the client the opportunity to mobilize coping efforts that can lead to growth and gain. For example, Moulton et al. (1987) found that the individual's belief that he or she could positively influence his or her health status through health-related life-style changes was associated with less distress. Clients can be helped to focus their appraisal of HIV on the potential for gain as well as the potential for loss. This will be best achieved by acknowledging that loss is also occurring, rather than negating that experience. To illustrate: Daryl was in his sophomore year in college when he learned he was HIV-positive. He initially felt it was pointless to "waste time" finishing college when he might not have that many years to work, so he dropped out of school. Eventually, Daryl returned to college because he realized he really enjoyed school and it would still be a meaningful accomplishment (and gain) to be the first in his family to graduate from college.

COPING STYLES OF PWHIVs

There is an extensive body of literature on coping styles, although relatively few studies have examined this variable for PWHIVs. Research on coping styles in other populations suggests that there is at most only moderate consistency of coping styles across situations for a given individual (Folkman, Lazarus, Gruen, & DeLongis, 1986). In general, research on problem-focused coping shows that it is strongly influenced by the situational context, whereas positive-reappraisal (e.g., reframing an event in a positive manner) coping showed moderately strong correlations across situations. This suggests that reappraisal may be strongly influenced by personality factors.

Predicting how a person might cope with HIV may be a function of both premorbid appraisal style and of the specific situational factors related to HIV with which the individual is contending. This seems to be supported in part by the results of a multisite study of PWHIVs that examined the relationship of coping to depressive symptoms. A factor analysis of 16 coping behaviors revealed three factors: Positive Coping,

Seeking Social Support, and Avoidance Coping (Fleishman & Fogel, 1994). Positive coping was related to decreases in depression.

This study was unique in that the coping behaviors of gay and bisexual men were compared to those of injecting drug users. Injecting drug users had higher scores for Avoidance Coping and lower scores for Positive Coping than did gay men. Avoidance Coping was also more prevalent among members of disadvantaged groups such as injecting drug users, women, and those with lower incomes. This suggests that coping behaviors might differ between different populations of HIV-positive persons.

Other studies (e.g., Namir et al., 1987) have also shown the positive effects associated with active behavioral coping and the negative outcomes associated with avoidance coping. For example, active behavioral coping, or strategies that dealt directly with HIV disease and used reliance on others for emotional, instrumental, and informational support, were related to higher self-esteem, lower mood disturbance, and higher levels of social support (Namir et al., 1987). The opposite was true for the avoidance coping style.

These studies show that some styles of coping are more effective than others and that different groups of people may employ different coping methods. For example, people with few financial resources might cope differently than people with many resources. Thus, a person who is homeless might focus more on day-to-day survival than a person who has a home and a job. From a clinical perspective, it is important to explore how the client is coping and to determine if that coping method is effective.

Although all coping methods represent attempts by the individual to reduce anxiety and distress, it is apparent that some may help in the moment but may ultimately create distress (e.g., heavy alcohol and drug use to self-medicate). Lucy, a recovering injecting drug user, often lapsed and turned to drugs when she was feeling overwhelmed. She would initially feel wonderful and confident while she was high, and then would feel remorseful and ashamed of herself when she came down. Overall, she felt worse about herself, and the things she did while high, each time she lapsed.

This overview of the literature on coping styles and strategies in response to HIV disease shows that there is great variation between people. Coping responses appear to be a promising research direction and may account for some differences in responses to HIV disease. As Zich and Temoshok (1987) concluded, coping style may be the first line of defense when stressors occur in an individual's life. Therefore, it is important for counselors to explore the coping styles of their clients and determine whether the clients might benefit from learning more effective coping skills.

Interventions to Increase Coping Skills

Monat and Lazarus (1985) grouped coping techniques into three categories: (1) alterations of the environment and/or life-style; (2) alterations of personality and/or perceptions; and, (3) alterations of biological responses to stress.

These three broad areas are helpful when designing interventions to assist HIV-positive clients. Because life-style changes will be discussed in the next chapter, interventions will be described that focus on altering perceptions and physical/biological responses to stress. Three broad areas will be discussed: (1) stress management interventions, (2) aerobic exercise interventions, and (3) coping effectiveness training.

Stress Management

The Center for the Biopsychosocial Study of AIDS at the University of Miami has conducted a series of studies examining interventions to help HIV-positive persons cope through stress management and aerobic exercise. For example, using a cognitive-behavioral intervention to manage stress, 47 asymptomatic gay men were assigned to a stress management condition or an assessment-only control group 5 weeks before being notified of their positive antibody status (Antoni et al., 1991). Participants assigned to the cognitive-behavioral stress management (CBSM) group met twice weekly for 10 weeks in groups of 4 to 6, led by two cotherapists. They also received an additional session per week of training in progressive muscle relaxation, including an imagery component. The CBSM group members met for 5 of the 10 weeks prior to being informed of their positive antibody status. The assessment-only control group only participated in the assessment aspect of the study. The CBSM group did not show significant pre–post changes in depression, but showed significant increases in CD4+ cells, whereas the control group showed significant increases in depression pre- to postnotification of serostatus. This means that the CBSM intervention lessened the effects of getting a positive HIV diagnosis as compared with the control treatment.

Although this intervention was used to moderate the effects of learning of one's positive antibody status, the components of this cognitive-behavioral intervention might be useful in assisting PWHIVs to cope with other aspects of their disease. The components of CBSM are progressive muscle relaxation, behavioral role playing, and cognitive restructuring. However, analyses suggested that many of the positive effects of the CBSM treatment were due to the relaxation skills that were learned.

Aerobic Exercise

This same group of researchers has also investigated the role of aerobic exercise as a means of coping with HIV (Antoni et al., 1991; LaPerriere et al., 1994). Asymptomatic HIV-positive, as well as HIV-negative, gay men participated in aerobic exercise (riding a stationary bike) for 45 minutes, three times a week for 10 weeks. Both psychological and immunological benefits were found for both groups of men. However, HIV-positive men experienced fewer immunological benefits than did seronegative men, suggesting that HIV interfered with obtaining optimal benefits.

A survey of the limited number of studies on the benefits of exercise for PWHIVs suggests that exercise may have an effect on immune responsiveness (Eichner & Calabrese, 1994), possibly due to the psychological benefits of exercise that lead to a reduction in stress, anxiety, and depression. Reducing stress and depression will have a positive effect on the client's quality of life, and can also provide the client with an important sense of control over his or her life, can provide structure, and can provide opportunities for socializing.

Coping Effectiveness Training

Coping effectiveness training (CET) emphasizes "fitting" the chosen coping strategy to the characteristics of the stressful situation (Chesney & Folkman, 1994). In other words, participants learn to use coping strategies that have the greatest chance of being effective for a given situation. This means that PWHIVs can be taught strategies that are effective in reducing distress and enhancing overall quality of life.

CET consists of ten 2-hour weekly sessions, including a daylong retreat between the fourth and fifth sessions. To maintain changes, participants meet as a group every 2 months for the remainder of the year. The following elements are included in CET: (1) appraisal of stressful situations, (2) cognitive-behavioral approaches to problem- and emotion-focused coping, (3) appraisal–coping fit, (4) the use of social support, and (5) self-efficacy and maintenance training. This approach has been used successfully to help HIV-positive persons cope more effectively. CET is very promising because counselors can help their clients learn coping approaches that have the greatest likelihood of success with a particular stressor in the client's life.

COPING WITH AIDS-RELATED BEREAVEMENT

Another stressor that is unique to this crisis and that challenges coping skills for many individuals with HIV is AIDS-related bereavement. AIDS often hits more than once in an interpersonal network, leaving that network more fragile. This phenomenon has been well-documented in the literature on gay men, but it also occurs in the networks of injecting drug users and in families where more than one family member is infected (e.g., when a mother transmits the virus to her child; or a husband to his wife).

Several researchers have examined the effect of AIDS-related bereavement on coping. Martin (1988) found a positive relationship between the number of bereavements and the symptoms of traumatic stress response, recreational drug use, and sedative use, as well as use of psychological services. However, Martin did not differentiate between seropositive and seronegative bereaved men. In a study that examined the relationship of antibody status to bereavement, 50% of the chronically bereaved group were seropositive as compared with 42% of the intermittently bereaved and 28% of the not bereaved (Dean, Hall, & Martin, 1988).

This same cohort of gay men was followed through 1991 (Martin & Dean, 1993). Over this time frame, significant effects of bereavement were found in each year, although the intensity and duration of these bereavement effects diminished over time. However, men who were both bereaved and HIV-positive reported the highest level of distress in every year when compared with the other groups of men. This finding is important for counselors because it means that men who are grieving the loss of significant others as well as anticipating the losses they themselves may experience as a result of being HIV-positive report the highest level of distress.

Interventions to Address AIDS-Related Bereavement

Many of the coping strategies that have been discussed in this chapter would be helpful in addressing recurrent AIDS-related bereavement. For example, stress management techniques and exercise would be useful in reducing some of the distress. In addition, grief counseling with a specific focus on grieving the loss or losses of partners, family members, and friends represents an important strategy. Further, losing significant others to HIV disease may trigger anticipatory grief in PWHIVs, as they see what might lie ahead for them. Because bereavement results in a shrinking of support networks, strategies to find new sources of social support or to reconnect with former sources of support are another important strategy.

SUMMARY

Cognitive and behavioral ways to adapt such as the ones described in this chapter, are similar to what Namir et al. (1987) called "active–positive coping." Namir (1986) found that individuals who actively cope with HIV fare better than those who do not; she referred to this as a "fighting spirit." Siegel (1988) referred to such coping as embodying the mind. This type of adaptation includes cognitive and/or behavioral components. These strategies provide clients with an attributional framework that is emotionally protective in reframing their disease, give clients a sense of control over aspects of their disease that are controllable, provide structure and opportunities to interact with other people, and help promote a higher quality of life.

CHAPTER 9

Interventions to Facilitate
Health-Promoting Behaviors
and Attitudes

> Ya know, if I tell the ladies I have AIDS, no one
> will ever want to make love to me again. They
> won't even want to deal with me.
>
> —DANTE, *an 18-year-old, HIV-positive,*
> *African American heterosexual male*

Adopting or increasing health-promoting behaviors that benefit the
seropositive client as well as lessen the likelihood of transmission of HIV
to others is an important and desired adaptation to HIV disease. Yet this
is often quite difficult for many PWHIVs, for a number of reasons.
Education and exhortations to make changes are rarely sufficient because risky behaviors are often pleasurable or involve successfully
negotiating with others. Dante, the young man quoted above, could not
imagine telling a woman he had just met that he had HIV disease. He
had virtually no experience developing emotional intimacy before becoming physically intimate. He felt that revealing his HIV status, or
insisting on using a condom, would lead to rejection. Exploring Dante's
concerns represents an important counseling issue that needs to be
addressed in helping him reduce risky behaviors.

Health-promoting behaviors can be grouped into two broad categories: HIV risk-reduction practices and health-promoting life-style

changes. Risk-reduction practices include practicing safer sex and safer drug practices, eliminating or reducing drug and alcohol use, and informing sexual partners of antibody status to increase the likelihood of consistently practicing safer sex. Health-promoting life-style changes include increasing health-protective attitudes; increasing health-protective behaviors such as good nutrition, vitamins, and exercise; and reducing or eliminating substance use and cigarettes. The benefits of risk-reduction practices in reducing the spread of HIV to others are obvious. In contrast, the benefits of health-promoting behaviors for the PWHIV are less clear. Although some health-promotion strategies may contribute to slowing the progression of the disease, perhaps equally important is the role that these interventions play in increasing the well-being of PWHIVs and involving them actively in their own health care (Jewett & Hecht, 1993).

HIV RISK-REDUCTION PRACTICES

Sexual Behaviors

Practicing Safer Sex

Does knowledge of HIV disease lead to reductions in risky sexual behaviors and drug practices? Research is equivocal in this area. Several studies have shown a significant reduction in risky behavior after learning of one's seropositive status. For example, in a sample of gay men in California, Coates, Stall, and Hoff (1988) found that only 5% of seropositive men in their sample practiced unprotected anal intercourse, as compared to 18% of those who tested negative. Results from a Baltimore–Washington sample of gay men were less impressive. HIV-positive respondents decreased their incidence of unprotected anal receptive intercourse to 42% of baseline as compared to 62% for the seronegative group (Fox, Ostrow, Valdiserri, VanRaden, & Polk, 1987).

Research on risk reduction in injecting drug users has also shown equivocal findings, with most cities studied reporting a significant reduction in risky drug practices (Des Jarlais & Friedman, 1988). To a lesser extent, reductions in unsafe sex practices have also been shown with this population.

In a more recent study with a sample comprised primarily of gay and lesbian seropositive persons, 29% of respondents reported engaging in unprotected intercourse in the past 3 months (Kelly, Murphy, et al., 1993). In examining what variables predicted unsafe sexual practices, recreational drug use was the best predictor, followed by level of depression. It is easy to understand why pairing substances with sex interferes with one's motivation and/or ability to practice safer sex. The linkage between depression and unsafe sex is less clear. One could speculate that people who are depressed are feeling hopeless, overwhelmed, and not in control. This might lead to difficulties in sexual self-efficacy, or substances and sexual contact may be a way to feel less depressed. To illustrate: Sally, a 30-year-old white woman with HIV and a history of injecting drug use, reported that she had great difficulty managing depression without using substances and sex. Because she typically paired substance use with sexual activity, she often practiced unsafe sex. For Sally, learning other ways to manage depression and life stresses was necessary before she could consistently practice safer sex.

Although some studies show significant decreases in unsafe practices when people are aware of their seropositive status, it appears that many persons do not alter their behavior (e.g., McCusker, Stoddard, Zapka, Zorn, & Mayer, 1989), or practice safer behaviors inconsistently. Others who are seropositive (up to half in many studies) do not even return after antibody testing to get their results. It is also important to consider that estimates of risk reduction are typically based on self-report. Self-report is naturally susceptible to bias—especially where major normative changes in the social desirability of various practices have occurred (Catania, Gibson, Chitwood, & Coates, 1990). Although gay men may be one of the few groups of persons to have made significant changes in sexual practices, recent studies show a significant decrease in safer sex practices among this group. This is especially true for younger gay men (e.g., Osmond et al., 1994). It also appears to be the norm, rather than the exception, that people lapse and do not consistently practice safer sex. These important findings highlight the difficulties many people experience in both changing and maintaining sexual practices. Counselors need to explore and help clients understand barriers to practicing and maintaining safer sex practices and view lapses and relapses as an integral part of behavioral and attitudinal change.

Informing Sexual Partners of HIV Serostatus

Although one can practice safer sex without informing partners that one is seropositive, discomfort about telling others or unwillingness to do so may reflect a lack of efficacy about safer sex practices. It may also put the burden of safer sex on the seropositive individual if his or her partner challenges or questions the need to do so. How frequently do seropositive persons inform their sexual partners of their status? Several studies have addressed this issue by asking respondents who already know that they have HIV disease whether they have disclosed their status to sexual partners. In a sample of seropositive men (most of whom were gay or bisexual) being treated at a public HIV clinic located in a predominantly Latino section of Los Angeles, 76% had disclosed their status to an intimate lover and 83% had told their spouse or partner (Marks et al., 1992).

In a similar sample comprised predominantly of Latino men, results showed that the greater the number of sexual partners, the less the likelihood of status disclosure (Marks, Richardson, & Maldonado, 1991). Of the men with only one sexual partner since diagnosis, 69% had disclosed their serostatus, whereas only 18% of the men with five or more partners had disclosed to at least one of these partners. Nearly half of the sexually active men had participated in unprotected anal intercourse without disclosing their status to their partner. These rates of disclosure to partners are considerably lower than those found in other studies. For example, a sample of gay, non-Latino white men in San Francisco reported a disclosure rate of 98% to lovers (Hays, McKusick, Plooack, & Hilliard, 1991). High disclosure rates as well as significant reductions in risk behaviors have been shown for heterosexual couples where one member of the couple is HIV-infected (Higgins et al., 1991).

These studies on disclosure of seropositive status are extremely important for counselors because they show that many people have difficulty informing partners about their HIV status and that a number of important factors may influence this process. Having one partner or spouse seems related to a relatively high level of disclosure whereas having multiple partners does not. Some people in this latter group may be engaging in anonymous sex where there may be no emotional investment in their partner. Others may fear that insisting on safer sex practices will make others suspicious of their HIV status. Or, like the teen-ager quoted at the beginning of this chapter, PWHIVs may fear that no one will ever want to kiss, hug, or have sexual relations with them if their status is known. Others may not disclose their HIV status because of their culture's negative view of homosexuality or bisexuality. For a variety of reasons, many PWHIVs have difficulty disclosing their status to some or many of their partners and continue to engage in unsafe sexual activity at least part of the time. Unlike other health-promoting behaviors where occasional lapses may be of little consequence, difficulties practicing safer sex consistently may have disastrous consequences in terms of transmitting HIV. Lapses also create guilt and shame for many clients and ethical and clinical dilemmas for counselors.

Injecting Drug Behaviors

Efforts to reduce the risk of HIV transmission from injecting drug practices has met with some success. Many of these interventions have focused on community outreach programs that educate about the dangers of sharing needles, teach behavioral skills for needle cleaning, exchange dirty needles for clean ones, and offer greater access to substance abuse treatment (e.g., Des Jarlais & Friedman, 1994). There are other reasons, in addition to the spread of HIV, for eliminating injecting drug use. Continued injecting drug use has been associated with an increased risk of HIV disease progression (see Jewett & Hecht, 1993). Injecting drug use in PWHIVs also decreases the likelihood of practicing safer sex.

Interventions to Increase
HIV Risk-Reduction Behaviors

Research has consistently shown that education alone is rarely sufficient to change self- and other-destructive HIV-related behaviors (Selwyn, 1986). Therefore, interventions promoting positive, health-protective behaviors should both educate the client about needed changes as well as assist the client in making these changes. Interventions should also address how changes will be maintained over time and how lapses will be managed. Herein is one of the critical roles that an ongoing counseling relationship can play. Behavior that is harmful to the client may also be harmful to others by increasing the possibility of HIV transmission. However, I have found that it is more helpful in building a therapeutic alliance and bringing about change to focus on the ways in which a client can protect his or her own health, rather than initially focusing on the importance of protecting others.

If the client consistently engages in behaviors that are health promoting, risk to others will be greatly minimized and the locus of the therapy remains on the client. Risk-reduction behaviors can be grouped into two broad categories: teaching clients safer sex and drug practices and instructing clients in specific life-style changes that can enhance quality of life and that might promote longevity.

Teaching Safer Sex and Drug Practices

Teaching clients about safer sex and drug practices requires that the therapist understand HIV transmission and strategies to reduce transmission. HIV disease is transmitted through sexual contact involving exposure to semen, vaginal secretions, and/or blood, exposure to blood through sharing needles or receiving contaminated blood transfusions or blood products, through perinatal transmission, and during breast feeding. The exact risk of infection from a single sexual encounter is unknown. However, it is important to note that a single sexual encounter with an infected partner is sufficient in some situations for infection to occur. The most effective means of sexual transmission is receptive anal intercourse with an infected person (Francis & Chin, 1987).

There are a number of cofactors that make transmission more likely, so each incidence of unprotected intercourse, for example, will likely not carry the same risk. Examples of cofactors include a history of sexually transmitted disease, which may leave lesions that allow for easier entry of HIV when a person is exposed. Sexual practices that lead to bleeding or tearing also make transmission of the virus more likely (e.g., receptive anal intercourse, fisting, rough vaginal intercourse that leads to bleeding and tearing, or using sex toys such as dildos in a manner that leads to bleeding or tearing).

Studies have consistently shown that some HIV-positive persons continue to engage in unsafe sex, at least part of the time. This seems to be especially true when both partners are seropositive (Kline & Van Landingham, 1992). Research has also shown that the best predictor of post-antibody test sexual practices are sexual practices prior to testing (McCusker et al., 1989). In other words, men who engaged in unprotected receptive anal intercourse prior to learning of their HIV-positive status are more likely to continue this practice (at least some of the time) posttesting. It is also helpful for PWHIVs to avoid additional exposures through unprotected sex because they may be exposed to other viruses (e.g., herpes, cytomegalovirus) to which many persons with compromised immune systems are susceptible. Therefore, it is critical that both the therapist and the client understand what safer sex means and why it is important for both self- and other-protection. Safer sex requires an understanding of the risk of transmission associated with various sexual practices and accurate information about how to use condoms.

Sexual Practices and Risk of HIV Transmission. Table 3 shows sexual practices and the risk of transmission of HIV. Some practices are considered "safe" in that they convey no risk of virus transmission. They include practices such as massage, hugging, cuddling, and mutual masturbation. Other behaviors are considered "unsafe" and carry a risk of HIV transmission. They include vaginal intercourse without a condom, anal intercourse without a condom, and contact with blood, including menstrual blood. Activities that are "safer" include vaginal intercourse with a condom, anal intercourse with a condom, and cunnilingus with a dental dam or some other barrier. Clearly, the most challenging counseling issues will center around those activities that are "unsafe."

However, counselors may also experience discomfort about some safer sex activities. For example, they may feel a conflict between supporting and understanding a client's desire for intercourse (with a condom) and their concerns that the condom may break or may be used improperly, exposing the client's partner to risk. This might especially be true in situations where the client is practicing safer sex but is not informing a partner of his or her HIV status, so that the partner does not have the opportunity to decide whether or not to accept any degree of risk of exposure.

For injecting drug users, transmission can occur as a result of sharing needles, or "works," or through the same sexual practices listed in Table 3. It is not unusual for seropositive injecting drug users to focus on practicing safer drug practices while at the same time ignoring safer sexual practices.

Condom Effectiveness in Preventing HIV Disease. Studies have shown that latex condoms are not permeated by the HIV virus, unlike condoms made of animal skin/intestines. Additionally, *in vitro* studies have shown that spermicides containing nonoxynol-9 kill HIV (Kelly & St. Lawrence, 1988). It is important to note that condoms, even when used correctly and consistently, occasionally slip or break (see "How Reliable

TABLE 3. Sexual Practices and Risk of HIV

Safe
  Massage, hugging, cuddling
  Mutual masturbation
  Social kissing (dry)
  Body-to-body rubbing (frottage)
  Voyeurism, exhibitionism, fantasy

Probably safe
  Tongue kissing

Possibly safe
  Vaginal intercourse with condom
  Anal intercourse with condom
  Cunnilingus[a] (with a dental dam)
  Fellatio with condom
  Fellatio without condom, stopping before climax[a]

Unsafe
  Vaginal intercourse without condom
  Anal intercourse without condom
  Blood contact (including menstrual blood)
  Fellatio without condom; semen or urine in mouth
  Anilingus ("rimming")
  Hand in rectum ("fisting")
  Sharing sex toys that have contact with body fluids

Note. Source: San Francisco AIDS Foundation. (Available from San Francisco AIDS Foundation, P.O. Box 42682, San Francisco, CA 94142-6182.)
[a]Also considered *possibly unsafe* or *unsafe*.

are Condoms," 1995, for a rating of the most effective condom brands and the estimated failure rates). Research also suggests that "practice almost makes perfect," in that gay men engaging in protected receptive anal intercourse more than 10 times a year reported a condom failure rate of below 1% (Thompson, Yager, & Martin, 1993). In contrast, condom failure rate was 15% for men who used a condom for receptive anal intercourse only once in the previous year.

Studies have also examined HIV transmission rate in serodiscordant couples. In one study, 2% of the 171 partners who used condoms consistently seroconverted (Saracco, Musicco, & Nicolosi, 1993). In comparison, 15% of the 55 partners who used condoms inconsistently became HIV-positive. This sample was comprised of seropositive men and their seronegative female partners.

Studies on condom failure rates and efficacy suggest that correct and consistent use provide a relatively high level of protection from HIV transmission. Therefore, instructing clients in using condoms should include opportunities for practice (e.g., using bananas, plastic models) until they become expert. Barriers to consistent condom use should also be examined.

In summary, only those behaviors in the "safe" category can truly be considered safe. "Safer sex" refers to sexual practices that are probably safe when practiced correctly and consistently.

How to Use a Condom Effectively. Clients should be instructed in the following steps on correct condom use as described by the United States Department of Health and Human Services.

- Use a new latex condom for every act of intercourse.
- If the penis is uncircumcised, pull the foreskin back before putting on the condom.
- Put the condom on after the penis is erect and before any contact is made between the penis and the partner's body.
- If using a spermicide, put some inside the condom tip.
- If the condom has a reservoir tip, first squeeze out the air. If there is no reservoir tip, pinch the tip enough to leave a half-inch space for semen to collect.
- While pinching the half-inch space, place the condom over penis and unroll it all the way to the base. Put more spermicide or lubricant on the outside, but use only water-based products.
- If you feel a condom break while you are having sex, stop immediately and carefully pull out.
- After ejaculation and before the penis gets soft, grip the condom rim and carefully withdraw from your partner.

Preparing Clients to Practice Safer Sex

It is one thing to educate a client in the necessary information to practice safer sex. It is quite another thing for many clients to make the desired changes in their sexual behaviors and to consistently maintain those changes. One way this might occur is through increasing self-efficacy (Bandura, 1989). According to Bandura, to effect change people must not only be educated as to why they need to alter risky behavior, but they need to be provided with the means and resources to do so.

Perceived sexual self-efficacy can be achieved by teaching clients to talk frankly about sexual matters, to develop a set of internal standards about conduct, to use motivating self-incentives, to avoid social situations that might involve risk, and to learn to extricate themselves from potentially troublesome situations (Bandura, 1987). Although these steps sound reasonable and possible, they involve the acquisition of new skills and shifts in attitudes, as well as the cooperation of one's partner. This model of risk reduction, as well as others, are discussed in Chapter 19.

Risk-reduction strategies based on self-efficacy or other models must be directed at both substance use and sexual behaviors. For injecting drug users, the emphasis on drug behaviors is apparent. However, it is important to remember the frequency with which alcohol and recreational drugs are paired with sexual activities for many people. Additionally, many injecting drug users trade sex for drugs or drugs for sex. Self-protective and other-protective skills can be taught through the following four steps: (1) dispensing detailed, correct information about sexual practices; (2) providing social modeling (including skills to practice creative, fulfilling safer sex); (3) increasing the client's perception of his or her ability to make the needed changes; and (4) allowing opportunities to practice the new behaviors so they can be used consistently under difficult circumstances (e.g., role playing, practicing putting on condoms).

Preparing Injecting Drug Users to Practice Safer Behaviors

Educating injecting drug users about safer drug practices is again the first step in bringing about change, but other goals are also important. For example, a desired goal of counseling for injecting drug users is helping them to begin the process of recovery, which often involves making a referral for substance abuse treatment. Many injecting drug users will experience lapses and relapse as they go through the recovery process. Others may decide that they do not want to stop their drug use. Therefore, counselors need to educate injecting drug users about the risks of sharing needles or works (includes needles and cookers) and the importance of using sterile works (Des Jarlais & Friedman, 1988). Specific instructions should be given on how to sterilize needles and how to obtain clean ones.

Bandura's (1989) self-efficacy model is also useful as a guide for dispensing information, demonstrating social modeling, increasing clients' beliefs that they can make the necessary changes, and allowing opportunities to practice new behaviors. Some states allow the distribution of free, sterile needles and bleach, thus providing the means to assist the client in developing self-efficacious behavior (Des Jarlais & Friedman, 1988). Interventions should also be directed toward teaching safer sex practices.

HEALTH-PROMOTING LIFE-STYLE CHANGES

A number of behaviors, such as smoking, have been shown to negatively impact immune functioning. In contrast, other behaviors, such as exercising, have been linked to enhancing immune function.

Alcohol, Drug, and Cigarette Use

Alcohol and drugs are viewed as cofactors in HIV acquisition because of their frequent pairing with sexual activity. They often lower inhibitions and impair judgment, and may also reduce the likelihood of an individual's practicing safer sex (Room, 1985; Stall, Coates, & Hoff, 1988). Additionally, alcohol and drugs suppress the immune system and make an individual more vulnerable to acquiring HIV when exposed (Molgaard, Nakamura, Hovell, & Elder, 1988; Penkower et al., 1991; Siegel, 1986). Cigarette use may also alter immune response to HIV disease (Burns et al., 1991) and appears to correspond with more rapid depletion of CD4+ cells (Royce & Winklestein, 1990). Thus, the elimination or reduction of these behaviors is an important health-promoting response to HIV disease.

However, many people use these types of behaviors as ways to manage stress and to be more comfortable in interpersonal situations. Therefore, it is not surprising that the literature shows substance use increasing for some people and decreasing for others when they learn they are HIV-positive or when the disease markedly progresses. In a study of symptomatic gay men, Kaisch and Anton-Culver (1989) found that alcohol, recreational drugs, and tobacco were often used as coping behaviors. After being diagnosed, use of these increased in a sizable minority. Although the researchers concluded that the trend of changes was toward more healthful behaviors, the majority of respondents either did not change or actually increased their unhealthful, immune system-impairing behaviors. This research suggests that counselors need to explore the client's reasons for substance use, explain the effect of these behaviors on immune functioning, and explore the possible link of alcohol and recreational drug use with unsafe sexual practices.

Although there is agreement that health-promoting behaviors are important, empirical data suggest that at least a sizable minority of people do not respond to HIV disease by adopting these behaviors or that they do so inconsistently. In part this may be because HIV-related health-protective behaviors often involve negotiating with others, which requires a high level of interpersonal skill as well as cooperation from one's partner. However, an adequate understanding of why it is so difficult to change sexual behaviors and then maintain these changes over time is not fully known.

Health-Protective Attitudes

Health-protective attitudes are believed to lead to health-protective behaviors. There are a number of models or theories that attempt to explain why some people make and maintain self- and other-protective behaviors. One such model that will be briefly described to illustrate this concept is the health belief model, which has been used to explain why people knowingly jeopardize their health through practices like smoking (Hayes, 1991; Janz & Becker, 1984; Maiman & Becker, 1974). This model includes five predictors of health-risk behavior: perceived susceptibility, perceived severity of consequences, perceived benefits of changes, perceived barriers to change and perceived self-efficacy.

Applying this model, a PWHIV may not perceive that continued exposure to HIV (or other sexually transmitted diseases such as herpes and genital warts) may make him or her more susceptible to increased immunosuppression. The seropositive person may believe that once he or she is exposed, reexposure is not a problem. Perceived severity could be viewed in several ways. For example, the PWHIV may believe that a cure or medical treatments can remove the severity of the consequences of having HIV. Alternatively, other problems in the PWHIV's life, such as addictions or homelessness, may make a relatively slow-progressing disease seem less severe and consequently reduce his or her motivation to make behavior changes. In terms of benefits, the PWHIV may not believe that condoms and other health-promoting practices really work or make a difference.

Barriers to change include physical barriers, such as access to condoms, sterile needles, nutritious food, or AZT. Barriers might also be cultural or gender based. For example, the PWHIV may be economically dependent or believe that women should not be assertive in sexual situations. Finally, barriers can be attitudinal, such as believing that condoms interfere with pleasure, interrupt the mood of sex, or will make others suspicious that one has HIV disease. Self-efficacy, the last component of the health belief model, may be a factor if the PWHIV feels powerless in sexual situations, has difficulty negotiating health-protective behaviors or setting limits, or does not know how to use a condom or sterilize a needle.

Models of risk reduction, including the health belief model, are discussed in Chapter 19. Although the PWHIV has already acquired HIV, many aspects of these models are useful in supporting self- and other-protective behaviors and attitudes. However, most models of risk reduction are based on rational, cognitive views of behavior which often ignore important variables in HIV transmission.

Role of Vitamins and Diet in Promoting Health

What role can vitamins have in slowing disease progression? Several studies have shown that PWHIVs often lack one or more essential nutrients (e.g., Drolet, Reaidi, Taggart, & Reidy, 1993). It is difficult to determine if this is due to disease progression or in part due to the effects of poor diet or factors such as injecting drug use. Some studies have suggested that these deficiencies occur relatively early in the course of HIV disease and that higher than standard doses of vitamins are necessary to maintain adequate blood nutrient level (e.g., Baum, Cassetti, Bonvehi, Shor-Posner, Lu, & Sauberlich, 1994; Baum et al., 1992).

To illustrate the possible role of vitamins on disease progression, a recent study suggested that moderate-to-large doses of certain vitamins may slow the onset of full-blown AIDS in seropositive men (Graham & Tang, 1993). Results showed that 71% of the men who were given a daily intake of more than 715 milligrams of vitamin C remained AIDS-free during the course of the study, compared with 58% of men who took 715 milligrams or less. Of men who took more than 61 milligrams of niacin per day, 74% stayed AIDS free, whereas of those who took 61 milligrams or less, only 57% stayed AIDS free. The researchers concluded that vitamin intake needed to be sustained for at least 2 years and started early in the course of HIV disease. There is very little research to date in this area, and there do not seem to be consistent findings that could be used to guide PWHIVs in a vitamin supplement regimen. However, this may be a promising area in the future.

Although empirical data could not be found showing a link between diet and HIV progression, many PWHIVs report physical and psychological benefits from improving their diets. For example, Carson (1993) found that PWHIVs who engaged in "health-promoting activities" (special diets, exercise, and vitamins) scored higher on a measure of hardiness. Hardy people are those who moderate the effects of stress through positive coping (Kobasa, 1979).

Interventions to Help Clients Make Life-Style Changes

Life-style changes include assisting the client in eliminating or reducing the use of alcohol, recreational drugs, and tobacco. All of these substances have immunosuppressant effects (Siegel, 1986). Some clients may need to be referred to inpatient or outpatient substance abuse treatment as well as to Alcoholics Anonymous or Narcotics Anonymous.

Proper nutrition, rest, and exercise may also assist the client's health (Katoff & Dunne, 1988; Ryan, 1988). The possible role of certain vitamins in slowing disease progression was noted above. In addition to the health benefits these behaviors may promote, they also provide clients with a sense of positive control through the process of active behavioral coping. In addition, they may reduce stress, diminish depression, and enhance energy. Other coping strategies, such as exercise, were discussed in the previous chapter.

SUMMARY

Health-promoting behaviors represent controllable aspects of HIV that have multiple benefits, such as enhancing one's own health, reducing or eliminating the spread of HIV to others, and enhancing psychological well-being through a sense of control and a reduction in stress.

However, compared to other areas of living where self- and other-protective skills might be used most of the time and still offer a high degree of protection, the danger of even occasional lapses can have devastating consequences in terms of HIV disease. It is extremely important for the counselor to recognize how difficult it is for many clients to make these changes and to maintain them consistently. Therefore, it is essential to explore barriers to making health-protective and other-protective changes and barriers to maintaining these changes. Counselors should be prepared to help their clients understand and manage lapses so they do not give up trying to make positive behavior changes.

CHAPTER 10

Interventions to Facilitate Adaptation to Changes in Life Goals and Roles

> The hardest part about all of this so far is retiring.
> I never thought I would have to stop so soon after
> I got started. My dad hasn't even retired yet. All
> those years I went to school, then to law school,
> working constantly, making partner. . . . I feel like
> a useless, old man—I just don't get it.
>
> —TODD, *a 32-year-old, HIV-positive, white gay man*

Life goals provide excitement, a sense of meaning, and structure to life. HIV disease often means that goals are disrupted, and this can result in a sense of profound loss for the PWHIV. It is important for therapists to explore these issues of loss around important and defining life goals. Because goals and life roles are often viewed in terms of developmental stages, the orderly progression of psychosocial development is disrupted with a diagnosis of HIV disease. PWHIVs often wonder, "Am I going to die?"; "When?"; "How should I live my life?"

Young adulthood is a time "to choose an occupation, establish a career, form enduring intimate relationships, solidify one's sense of identity, and establish and refine an adult life pattern" (Christ & Wiener, 1985, p. 278). A life-threatening, progressive disease can severely hamper the achievement of these goals and makes it imperative to rethink life goals and life's meaning (Grant & Anns, 1988). Todd, the young man quoted above, spent many years preparing for a career as an attorney. This involved focusing his time, financial resources, and energies on a goal that he expected to shape his life for many years. Learning that he was HIV-positive left Todd wondering why he had sacrificed so much for what seemed to be so little. He also wondered what he should do about the future.

Western culture operates with a strong future orientation and with the belief that people will live to be old. HIV disease is an event that challenges a future orientation. In our culture, we often deny the end of life and base our present on the sense that the end is very far away. A diagnosis of HIV disease prematurely pierces that important denial and leaves the client vulnerable to existential despair (Beckett & Rutan, 1990). Clients not only have to reorder goals and priorities, but may need to give up hopes, fantasies, aspirations, and goals they have spent much time working toward.

It is important for therapists to explore how changes in life goals might result in the loss of actual roles or the anticipated loss of valued or hoped-for life roles such as becoming a parent, having a long-term committed relationship, or distinguishing oneself in a career. It is also important for therapists to help PWHIVs continue the process of making life goals because goals fuel motivation and provide excitement and hope about the present and the future. Moreover, many PWHIVs will have good health and live for a number of years following a diagnosis of HIV disease.

RETHINKING LIFE GOALS
AS A RESULT OF DISEASE PROGRESSION

PWHIVs often despair that they do not have adequate time to achieve a meaningful life through valued and hoped-for accomplishments. These feelings may lead them to minimize their accomplishments, label their lives as unimportant, and resist making long-term goals (Allers & Katrin, 1988). Other clients respond with a deep desire to make a long-lasting contribution to society, to turn their despair into something positive, and to leave some legacy of their lives.

Overall, there is some support in the clinical literature for the idea that HIV disease can lead to disorganization in terms of life goals. It can also provide the client with an opportunity to refocus or redirect life goals in a manner that leads to creative and exciting new opportunities. What differentiates the person who uses this time in a creative, positive way from the person who cannot get beyond the despair? What types of strategies can assist clients in rethinking life goals and arriving at positive resolutions about what can be accomplished?

Solomon et al. (1987) suggest that persons who are long surviving have a commitment to life in terms of "unfinished business," unmet goals, or unfulfilled experiences. In other words, having things that you still want to do gives life a sense of purpose. For example, Alex, a 39-year-old white gay man became heavily involved in organizing a gay rights parade soon after he developed AIDS. He was able to devote energy, excitement, and his many talents to planning and implementing this goal over a period of two years. He became quite ill shortly after the parade and died within a few months. His goal seemed to keep him going and also served as the type of legacy he saw as defining himself. When the event was over, Alex was never really interested in getting invested in another commitment, nor was he able to.

Although changes in life goals and expected life roles have rarely been empirically examined in the HIV literature, my colleagues and I have specifically asked PWHIVs that we have interviewed about this issue. Based on responses to open-ended questions, several themes emerged. Prior to being diagnosed with HIV disease, these PWHIVs typically viewed life goals with a future orientation and viewed them as hoped-for events that would occur some years in the future. For example, Tom hoped to make enough money as an attorney to retire at age 50. Bill hoped to become one of the top financial analysts in the country. Many of these "pre-HIV" goals had to do with career achievement and material acquisition. In contrast, "post-HIV" goals seemed to shift to a wish to be connected with a significant other, to achieving something that would make one's life meaningful, or to simply finding ways to survive. For example, many PWHIVs expressed a wish to fall in love and to be loved in return. Others wanted to leave a legacy, such as having a child, or to do something meaningful so that they would be remembered. Others just wanted to have a job, health insurance, and housing. What this research suggests is that life goals shift as priorities and values are reexamined, but that goals remain important in organizing and motivating the PWHIV.

Interventions to Assist Clients in Rethinking Life Goals

HIV-infected clients may initially be resistant to setting new goals, especially long-term goals (Allers & Katrin, 1988). It is a challenging task for the counselor to assist the client in setting goals for what the client wants to achieve next in her or his life. One helpful strategy involves life review, which not only examines and evaluates where one has been, but also where one would like to go in terms of goals (Pickrel, 1989). By examining the past, the therapist is able to help the client identify past achievements and positive events, which may result in a sense of accomplishment or an increase in self-esteem. The client also examines negative past events and plans present and future changes to achieve some degree of resolution around these events. This review enables a client to decide on goals for the present and the future based on what is most rewarding and meaningful for him or her.

I have often been impressed by how frequently clients mobilize their resources and accomplish meaningful goals that had previously eluded them. For example, Jeffrey, an extremely bright and talented African American man who had dropped out of high school, become estranged from his family of origin because they were upset with him for being gay, and wandered aimlessly around the country for several years, stated that he had never finished anything, but had started "100 things and just quit." I was concerned that he would once again "quit" when he learned of his seropositive status. However, because of his antibody status, achieving life goals took on greater urgency. He decided that he needed to prepare to be financially independent and to be able to get health insurance. He decided to earn his GED, which he did, and he became employed. He also made a decision to let his family know of his HIV disease. To his surprise, he has able to reconnect with several family members in a positive, supportive way. Perhaps the possibility of a "time-limited" life served as an organizing and motivating force in Jeffrey's life. He became quite clear about what he wanted to do and what he wanted to change. His HIV also helped his family focus on the present and the future, rather than on past problems.

It is helpful if the counselor believes that some of the client's "best" may still lie ahead and if he or she believes strongly in the client's future. The instillation of hope in helping clients set goals may be a significant factor in the achievement of those goals. This often requires that counselors examine their own future orientation.

CHANGES IN EMPLOYMENT
AS A RESULT OF HIV DISEASE

Work and career are important and defining aspects of many persons' lives and represent one of the most important of life's goals and adult roles. Work supports feelings of worth, provides an important component of identity, is a source of social support, and provides financial independence. One of the first role losses that the PWHIV may experience is that of being a full-time worker. To illustrate, Phil, a 36-year-old white gay man, worked as a flight attendant for many years, eventually being assigned to the highly coveted international flights. As his disease progressed, he became less able to perform his share of cabin responsibilities, in large part because of the length of the flights. Rather than accommodating Phil by allowing him to try working short flights, he was placed on disability. Although Phil was able to live on his disability pay, it resulted in a significant drop in his income. Most important, Phil, who was used to traveling around the world, now had nothing to do all day but sit at home. He no longer had access to his long-time colleagues, who were frequently out of town on flights, and he no longer could work at a job that he had truly loved. Phil's situation illustrates many of the themes that emerge in counseling when PWHIVs either lose their jobs or anticipate this event.

Only recently has a handful of studies specifically examined the impact of HIV disease on employment. Some studies have tried to determine whether and at what points employment patterns change as HIV progresses. For example, using structured telephone interviews to examine the extent of work loss in men following onset of symptoms and the interval between symptom onset and cessation of work, researchers found that 86% of the men surveyed worked prior to onset of first symptoms (Yelin, Greenblatt, Hollander, & McMaster, 1991). Of these, 50% stopped working within 2 years of becoming symptomatic, and all had stopped within 10 years of symptom onset.

Other studies have tried to determine the factors that lead to a decrease in employment as HIV progresses. Impairment in health is one important factor that often leads to employment loss. For example, Kass (1990) found that persons with AIDS were significantly more likely to have been fired for health reasons than either seropositive or seronegative persons. Health factors were also examined in a study of employment status of men diagnosed with AIDS by gathering information on their employment situation and clinical status on a monthly basis (Metz, Fox, Odaka, & McArthur, 1990). Results showed that as early as 0 to 6 months post-AIDS diagnosis, a significant number of men ended full-time employment because of disease limitations. Several workplace characteristics facilitated longer employment, including flexible scheduling, work that could be done at home, such as computer work, and changing to less physically stressful work.

Other research has also shown that job or workplace characteristics are related to ongoing employment for PWHIVs. Although 76% of respondents in one study were working at the time they were diagnosed with AIDS, within 16 months this had dropped to 36%, with an additional 17% still employed, but out on disability or sick leave (Massagli et al., 1994). This study is informative because it also examined the

PWHIV characteristics as well as job characteristics that were associated with longer employment. Gay men were the most likely PWHIVs to have jobs at both diagnosis and at follow-up. Additionally, whites, college graduates, professional and clerical workers, and respondents who had no history of injecting drug use were also more likely to have jobs at follow up. In contrast, those without jobs were more likely to be nonwhite minority group members, women, or less educated, and to have previously held blue-collar jobs and have a history of injecting drug use. In terms of job characteristics, PWHIVs who had jobs requiring a lot of mental effort and little physical effort were employed much longer after being diagnosed with AIDS. However, even among those who continued to work, earnings postdiagnosis were only 62% of their previous earnings.

Other research suggests that neurobehavioral impairment contributes to unemployment (Heaton, Velin, McCutchan, & Gulevich, 1994). Using vocational difficulties as markers of clinically significant neuropsychological impairment, those with impairment had a significantly higher unemployment rate. For those who remained employed, neuropsychological impairment was strongly associated with subjective decreases in estimates of job-related abilities. These results could not be explained by depression or medical symptoms, which suggests that even mild neuropsychological impairment interferes with employment.

In addition to providing structure, social support, and a sense of accomplishment, work also provides necessary financial remuneration, in the form of salary and health insurance. In a study examining the financial impact of employment changes due to disease progression, PWHIVs were 2.7 times more likely than seronegative persons to lose full-time employment over a 6-month time period (Kass, Munoz, Chen, Zucconi, & Bing, 1994). Loss of employment was significantly associated with both loss of private health insurance and loss of income. The impact of this financial loss was reflected in both the difficulty PWHIVs reported in meeting their basic expenses when compared to seronegative persons (27% vs. 19%) and in not seeking medical care for financial reasons (15% vs. 9%).

Weissman et al. (1994) examined the impact of AIDS on changes in insurance status. The found that 36% of their respondents had a change in insurance coverage between the time of their AIDS diagnosis and a follow-up interview. For example, Medicaid coverage increased from 14 to 41%, signifying that an AIDS diagnosis corresponded with a significant drop in income. A sizable minority of their respondents also reported problems in obtaining medical and dental services. This group was primarily comprised of African Americans, the homeless, and PWHIVs with less than a high school education.

These studies are important for counselors because they show that employment changes are common and occur in most cases many years before the PWHIV dies. This has multiple implications for the PWHIV, ranging from feeling disconnected from others, losing opportunities to contribute one's energies and talents, and losing financial resources.

Interventions to Assist Clients in Maintaining Employment

Career interventions play an increasingly important role in counseling clients with HIV disease. Many people now learn of their positive antibody status years before they become symptomatic. It is likely that people will live longer with HIV because of early detection as well as progress in the treatment interventions. Those interventions aimed at assisting clients in finding and maintaining satisfying careers will be critical.

Several themes emerge from the research on employment patterns for PWHIVs and are important to consider when designing strategies to assist in maintaining or seeking employment. (1) Assessment and treatment of neurobehavioral symptoms as well as mood disorders may allow many PWHIVs to maintain employment for a longer period of time. (2) Careers and jobs that require mental work and rely very little on physical activity allow PWHIVs to work longer. (3) Work that can be done on a self-determined schedule, at home, or on a part-time or job-sharing basis can allow PWHIVs to work longer. What is apparent is that PWHIVs with little education, few job skills, a history of injecting drug use, and little or no employment history have greatly reduced chances of maintaining employment.

Multitasking Systems of New York, a specially created quick-print company, is one example of a response to the employment difficulties that people with HIV disease encounter (Laubenstein, Greene, Campbell, & Weisberg, 1989). This company employs people with AIDS and provides job counseling, placements, and vocational rehabilitation, including job training. This company also provides linkages between community-based agencies and government programs to provide needed support systems for PWHIVs.

Other PWHIVs contribute to their communities through volunteer work. This avenue, although it does not provide financial remuneration, provides many of the other benefits of work—a sense of mattering, a sense of structure, purpose in life, and social support. Volunteer work is often possible even when disease symptoms such as fatigue and cognitive impairment interfere with the demands and expectations of paid work. Volunteer work related to HIV is a way for many to create a purpose or a meaning that somehow helps to balance the negatives of being infected.

Work also needs to be defined more broadly to include homemaking. In most communities, about half of the women with young children are homemakers. This is an important role and clearly provides many of the same functions as employment outside the home. Therefore, interventions to help women (and men) continue their role as a homemaker and/or as a parent are important and contribute to self-worth and a sense of mattering for the PWHIV. Helping PWHIVs maintain these roles also contributes to the well-being of dependent children and other family members.

Given the centrality of work in the majority of persons' lives, it is striking that few studies have focused on employment changes. Few writings in the HIV literature specifically address employment changes from the perspective of the impact on the PWHIV. Work, however broadly defined, needs to be brought to the forefront in counseling interventions with PWHIVs. Interest in work roles on the part of the counselor conveys to clients that they do have a future—a future that is worth planning for in terms of education, job training, and commitment to a work role.

Therapists can also contribute to policy and program development regarding HIV disease. Policies and programs informed by knowledgeable and compassionate people might reduce stigma and lessen the likelihood of job discrimination. Job discrimination against PWHIVs should become less frequent with the passage of the Americans with Disabilities Act of 1990. Under this act, disability is defined as "A physical or mental impairment that substantially limits one or more of the major life activities of such individuals" (Public Law 101-336, 1990, pp. 933–934). This may include such medical conditions as epilepsy, cancer, AIDS, HIV disease, and emotional illness. This act, which became law on July 26, 1991, prohibits unfair and unnecessary discrimination in the workplace. However, protection under the law does not guarantee that a work environment will be supportive and free of stigma.

SUMMARY

Hoped-for life goals and expected life roles often change and need to be reframed when one gets a diagnosis of HIV disease or when the disease progresses. This is an important therapeutic task because goals motivate people and provide excitement, direction, and hope for both the present and the future. Moreover, many PWHIVs will live for a number of years, or indefinitely, following a diagnosis of HIV disease.

Becoming unable to work, or losing valued life roles, has the potential to destroy a sense of contribution and productivity. This process can also disconnect PWHIVs from both a sense of self-worth and the sense of something to work toward.

CHAPTER 11

Interventions to Explore Spiritual and Religious Adaptation to HIV Disease

> ... persons with AIDS often are challenged to engage the spiritual dimension of their lives on a deeper level than they previously have experienced. They face the spiritual issues of life's meaning, one's personal identity and value, love, one's image of God, and the need for forgiveness and reconciliation in a new and frightening context. They have a profound need for meaning and hope.
>
> —DUNPHY (1987, pp. 61–62)

A compelling and powerful aspect of most spiritual traditions is the focus on healing rather than curing. In this context, "healing" means simply "to restore to wholeness" (Bennett & Hendrickson, 1993). HIV disease leads many PWHIVs to define and redefine what it means to be whole. For some, the focus will remain on physical wholeness; for others, there will be a shift to a focus on spiritual wholeness. As seropositive persons face the prospect of death and dying, many find exploring spiritual and religious issues helpful in this process (Christ & Wiener, 1985; Gambe & Getzel, 1989; Nichols, 1986; Weiss, 1988). Clients may ask questions such as "What has my life meant?"; "Why me?"; Why am I dying now?" (Beckham, 1988). To explore the spiritual and religious issues of clients with HIV disease, it is helpful to understand the distinction between the two.

Spirituality is typically defined as a basic value around which one's life is focused and has been described as the dimension of life in which people find integration (Dunphy, 1987). Dunphy further describes the spiritual dimension of human experience as being concerned with issues of meaning, hope, self-identity and self-worth, one's image of God, forgiveness, and reconciliation. In other words, spirituality reflects the personal views and behaviors that express the individual's sense of relatedness to others and to something greater (e.g., God, nature) than him- or herself. In contrast, religions provide a more formal framework for an institutionalized system of beliefs, values, and codes of conduct.

There are few writings on the role of spirituality and religion in the lives of PWHIVs and even fewer empirical studies. Nevertheless, there is consistency in the view that HIV disease, like other serious illnesses, challenges people to explore the spiritual aspects of their lives (Belcher, Dettmore, & Holzemer, 1989; Dunphy, 1987; Fortunato, 1993; Yalom, 1980). Compared to other seriously ill persons, seropositive clients often have a greater spiritual struggle (and greater death anxiety) because of the stigma usually associated with this disease. Because of this stigma, PWHIVs are often faced with taking this spiritual quest alone, rather than as a part of a religious community. Moreover, they are often exploring spirituality and their views about what happens after death much sooner than their contemporaries. This means that counseling provides an important opportunity to explore spiritual concerns.

EMPIRICAL LITERATURE ON HIV DISEASE AND SPIRITUALITY

In a study examining the relationship between various coping strategies, stress, and high-risk sexual behavior (unprotected anal intercourse) in a sample of HIV-positive gay men, respondents who did not participate in high-risk sexual behavior participated in more spiritual activities than did those who participated in high-risk sexual behavior (Folkman, Chesney, Pollack, & Phillips, 1992). Over half of the spiritual activities (viewed as a type of coping response) involved social interactions such as attending religious or spiritual services, talking to others about spiritual concerns, and consulting a religious or spiritual leader. Although the exact relationship between spiritual activities and risky sexual behavior is not clear, this is an intriguing finding and suggests that spiritual activities may offer a sense of connection, support, and guidance for some PWHIVs. These findings are similar to previous research (on respondents with concerns other than HIV disease) that has found that reliance on spiritual beliefs is viewed by some as a way to get guidance and by others as a way to come to terms with painful life experiences.

Other research suggests that PWHIVs with existential well-being, defined as a sense of purpose in and satisfaction with life, express higher levels of hope and spiritual well-being than do those with religious well-being (defined as well-being related to God) (Carson, Soeken, & Shanty, 1993). These results are similar to findings of Reed (1987), who compared terminally ill adults with healthy adults and found a greater degree of spirituality in the terminal group. A relationship was also found between spirituality and well-being in this group. These studies suggest that spiritual well-being is different than religiosity and that spirituality is linked with positive emotions and behaviors in PWHIVs.

WRITINGS ON SPIRITUALITY AND RELIGION

Although there are few empirical studies that examine the role that religious and spiritual beliefs play in client's responses to HIV disease, the importance of these beliefs as a clinical theme has been noted by a number of writers (e.g., Bellemare, 1988; Gambe & Getzel, 1989; Saynor, 1988; Warner-Robbins & Christiana, 1989). A common theme found in these writings is the experience that many gay people express of feeling disavowed and condemned by formal religion because of their homosexuality. Kevin, an HIV-positive gay man raised as a Catholic, struggled to reconcile his view of God as loving and forgiving with his church's stance that as long as he continued to "sin" by having sex with other men, he could not participate in communion. His church's view is that God only loved people who behaved in certain ways. As Bellemare (1988) so aptly asks, "How do you reach out to gay patients who have consistently felt the brunt of a negative theology of sexuality in their regard?" (p. 58).

Another way that PWHIVs often express religious beliefs during counseling is through their concerns about the dying process and about what happens after death. Kelly (1985) speculated that the relationship between death anxiety and religious convictions depends on the specific religious beliefs of the individual rather than on the individual's degree of religiosity. This means that what a person believes, or has been taught, is influential even if the person is not presently practicing a specific religion. These religious beliefs are reflected in the individual's views of illness, disease, sin, and what happens, if anything, to the spirit after death.

Kelly (1985) suggests that the specific content of an individual's convictions about the afterlife may either decrease, or increase, death anxiety. He referred to those beliefs that decrease death anxiety as positive aspects, which include beliefs that death will unite one with God, that goodness will be rewarded, and that God has chosen one's time of death as part of a meaningful plan. Negative aspects include beliefs that one has disappointed God, that one will be punished for sins in hell, and that one is dying with unfinished business in terms of saving one's soul. Although Kelly was not specifically talking about PWHIVs, because of the stigma associated with most of the modes of transmission it is likely that many PWHIVs have beliefs that reflect negative aspects. To illustrate: Tawanna, an African American woman, believed that HIV had been sent as a plague by God to punish people who had sinned. The fact that she had acquired HIV meant to her that she was marked as a "sinner" who was going to go to hell. In contrast, Ginny, also an African American woman, felt that God had recognized how difficult her life on earth was and that by giving her AIDS had let her know that she would soon be joining her loved ones in heaven.

Another theme noted in the literature is that HIV disease increases the likelihood that clients will be willing to explore the spiritual side of themselves. According to Whitaker (1974), dying people have four major concerns: (1) to die with someone at their side who cares about them, (2) to suffer as little pain as possible, (3) to die with dignity and not grotesquely, and (4) to have some answer to the question, "What happens to me when I die?" This last question may actually contain many layers of questions: "Is there an afterlife?"; "Will I live on?"; "Will I be with those I love who have already died?"; "Will I be forgiven?" Often these questions reflect how distant and estranged the PWHIV feels from formal religion. Moreover, he or she may wonder how to reconcile spiritual and religious questions and concerns because of this estrangement.

Even when PWHIVs feel estranged from formal religion and its institutions, their spiritual needs are important to consider. Addressing these needs can help PWHIVs find meaning in what is happening to them, feel a sense of relatedness with both themselves and with their God, and find sustenance and support to help them through their physical and emotional pain.

INTERVENTIONS TO ADDRESS SPIRITUAL
AND RELIGIOUS NEEDS OF PWHIVs

Counselors can be most helpful if they are ready and willing to enter into what can be called "spiritual companionship" with their client (Attig, 1983). Through this companionship, the therapist and client can explore, identify, and articulate the client's various spiritual issues and beliefs. It is not necessary for the counselor and the client to share spiritual beliefs. Rather, entering into spiritual companionship means to simply listen with a posture of "curious openness"—to discover how your client's beliefs provide an understanding of what it means to have this disease in the context of his or her life. There is much about HIV disease that is inexplicable. Many PWHIVs struggle to find meaning in why this is happening to them. Spiritual and religious beliefs often provide understanding and meaning and bring order to that which seems inexplicable.

Another way of framing spiritual and religious discussions is to ask clients whether their thinking about their disease is shaped by their religious beliefs or traditions (Bennett & Hendrickson, 1993). It is helpful to avoid assumptions about clients' beliefs based on their denominational affiliations; for example, some Jews believe in Heaven (Fortunato, 1993). Some clients who feel abandoned or estranged from religious institutions would like to once again feel connected to organized religion. Encouraging these clients to seek institutions that openly embrace and support all who attend can be one way to find spiritual support. For example, some churches specifically welcome gay people which offers an opportunity for them to reconcile their sense of estrangement from traditional religious institutions.

Discussing spiritual beliefs also provides clients with the opportunity to discover views that offer them a sense of well-being, meaning, and hope as well as to come to terms with beliefs that might be "toxic" or negative. According to Fortunato (1993), these toxic beliefs can often be countered by antidotes from within the client's own religious or spiritual framework. He described an HIV-positive client who believed he should not take any pain medication because he was being punished by God for a sinful life. When this belief was explored and challenged, the client also noted that his God was a God of great mercy. Fortunato was ultimately able to get the client to view his God's mercifulness as extending to allowing the client to manage his pain through medication.

Another way a counselor can use an understanding of the client's view of spirituality is by normalizing that the client will have some degree of death anxiety (Kelly, 1985). Next, the counselor can explore the client's spiritual or religious convictions that are creating death anxiety. The client can then identify the positive and negative aspects of his or her beliefs and attempt to find a way to reduce these feelings of death anxiety. One way this might be achieved is by helping clients recognize and explore discrepancies between their spiritual or religious beliefs and their actions or behaviors and then find ways to resolve these discrepancies.

For example, Sharon, a 28-year-old married white woman, was raised as a devout Catholic who believed that adultery was sinful, yet she found herself having sex with numerous men to get drugs to feed her addiction to heroin. After learning that she was HIV-positive, Sharon decided that she had strayed far from the values she believed in. She began the process of recovery, in part to stop her sexual activities with men outside of her marriage so that she could once again go to church and accept communion. Clients can also achieve resolution between beliefs and actions by making amends to people they believe they have wronged, or they might reconcile with significant others from whom they have been estranged.

Spiritual issues may also be explored in HIV support groups (Beckham, 1988; Christ & Wiener, 1985; Gambe & Getzel, 1989) and in various 12-Step programs. Gambe and Getzel (1989) describe how they addressed spiritual issues in a group setting. Using Viktor Frankl's description of the tasks that must be undertaken to assist people in their struggles with human finitude, group members (1) addressed the meaning of their lives with regard to themselves, their sphere of relationships, and to society as a whole; (2) assumed responsibility for any aspects of their life over which they still have control; and (3) accepted the limits of their actions.

Other PWHIVs may express their spiritual and religious beliefs through attending religious services and through rituals such as confession and communion. They may have their needs met through programs for PWHIVs that are sponsored and administered by various religious groups. One such program is conducted by the AIDS Interfaith Council of Houston (Shelp, DuBose, & Sunderland, 1990). This group is an association of clergy and laity and provides educational and service programs as well as congregation-based supportive care to PWHIVs and their significant others. Respite care teams provided by this program offer social support, physical care, and emotional support, and respond to spiritual needs. Paired team members typically meet with the PWHIV once a week for several hours. As the disease progresses to AIDS, the team will often include 14 to 20 people who will take turns visiting the PWHIV daily. The intense and comprehensive focus of this program allows many people with AIDS to die at home. Impressively, this program has served about 16% of the people with HIV disease in the Houston area.

Despite the success of this program, several problems have occurred. For example, there has been some resistance from congregation leadership to being identified with AIDS because of its association with condom use, sexuality, and drug use. Related to this is the concern that discussing HIV issues is equivalent to promoting high-risk behaviors. These concerns mirror many aspects of the AIDS epidemic that contribute to stigma and that hamper effective and compassionate responses to those with HIV disease.

SUMMARY

HIV disease often creates anxiety-producing spiritual and religious concerns for some PWHIVs, whereas other PWHIVs find that spiritual or religious pursuits offer much-needed support and meaning. Entering into a spiritual companionship with clients, or being willing to truly explore spiritual and religious issues, can provide one of the most profoundly satisfying experiences in clinical work with PWHIVs. Perhaps this is because it is difficult for PWHIVs to feel restored to "wholeness" in so many other aspects of their lives, yet this is attainable when viewed in the context of spiritual wholeness. However, many PWHIVs feel estranged from and condemned by formal religious institutions because they are gay or because of behaviors such as injecting drug use. Helping clients find ways to explore and connect with their spiritual or religious beliefs is an important goal of clinical work with PWHIVs.

CHAPTER 12

Interventions to Prepare for Death and the Dying Process

Death is as much a reality as birth, growth, maturity, and old age—it is the only certainty of life.

—BEHNKE AND BOK (1975, p. 152)

HIV disease, especially when people become symptomatic, is associated with loss, the dying process, and death. The words of those with HIV reflect these themes. "It's a fact of life that everybody has to die, I just wish it wasn't so tragic." "Sometimes I just want to sit in a corner and cry. . . . It's like getting upset over something you can't do anything about." "It has put dampers on certain things I can no longer do. I mean I haven't worked any more, I'm on disability" (Werth, Duke, & Kunkel, 1994, p. 13).

In the words of some of the PWHIVs I have interviewed, "All I ever wanted was a job, a nice wife, and a family. . . . I guess I can have the job but I won't get the rest"; and "Somedays I have diarrhea so bad that I lay on the bathroom floor. It's so bad that I had to give up my little dog because I couldn't walk him." These words of PWHIVs reflect many themes of loss—physical changes, emotional changes, and losses of attained roles as well as hoped-for ones. As PWHIVs become symptomatic or develop AIDS, how do they manage these losses, focus on aspects of their lives that offer hope and sustenance, and prepare for dying?

Most persons with terminal conditions remain hopeful into the end stage of their disease (Levy, 1990). Levy, in describing responses to terminal illnesses, also described a shift in the object of hope that often occurs as death approaches. Initially, there is hope for recovery, but as disease progresses, there is often a shift in perspective to wanting to live for a certain event (seeing a child graduate, beginning a patch for the Names Project, living through Christmas, completing a book). Later, hope may shift to a focus on those significant others who will survive, such as children or a partner. This provides a sense of relatedness or connectedness to the future—although one will not be there physically, one lives on through significant others.

Finally, hope for oneself may shift to wishing for a peaceful or dignified death, often including a wish that it will be followed by eternal life. Levy's description of the shifting of perspectives that occurs as people go through the process of dying and death fits well with my observations of PWHIVs as well as the literature in this area.

EXPLORING DEATH ANXIETY

Although death anxiety has been explored fairly extensively in terms of other diseases such as cancer, there is little known about this area for PWHIVs. In the previous chapter, death anxiety was explored as a theme that often appears when PWHIVs explore religious or spiritual concerns. This chapter will examine other ways that PWHIVs often express death anxiety. In a study of death anxiety of both healthy and HIV-infected men, anxiety in the PWHIVs showed up in covert rather than overt ways (Hayslip, Luhr, & Beyerlein, 1991). It appeared that HIV resulted in redefinitions of one's life trajectory or course, which often created anxiety. If, for example, denial is used, death anxiety may be expressed in indirect rather than overt ways and counselors may need to listen closely. For many PWHIVs, death anxiety is expressed in both overt and covert ways—through words, through making plans, through dreams, through art, and sometimes through active avoidance of the subject. Death anxiety may also be expressed through impulsive or compulsive behaviors such as substance abuse that distract clients from concerns about death.

Death anxiety may be especially salient for PWHIVs who have seen others die from the disease. Often, HIV disease strikes multiple members of a social network. For example, both a mother and a child may be infected, or one's life partner, or one's injecting drug partners. Seeing others die from AIDS may lead to greater concerns about one's own health status and anxiety about the dying process. Losing a spouse or partner can lead to anxiety and to the question, "Who will be there for me when I die?"

One covert way that issues around loss and dying may be expressed is through dreams. Dream imagery can help therapists assist terminally ill patients by offering insights into unconscious processes related to the dying process. Using Jungian dream archetypes, Welman and Faber (1992) described a patient who continually denied his diagnosis (he had cancer, rather than AIDS). However, his dreams were laden with death imagery. Symbolically, his dreams shifted over time from confrontation, to realization, to acceptance, and enlightenment. The authors felt that this process, achieved through dream interpretation, allowed this man to face death with few signs of anger, denial, fear, or regret. How does this process occur? According to Jung, dreams anticipate and direct psychical changes that occur during critical developmental phases (or during life crises), including dealing with a serious or terminal illness, changes in health, and dying (Welman & Faber, 1992).

Hill (1996), in her research on dream interpretation, posits that dreams are important in enhancing awareness of thoughts and feelings, providing greater insight, resolving problems, and in leading to changes in behavior. Her three-stage model (exploration, insight, and action) for dream interpretation might be helpful in understanding death anxiety in PWHIVs as fears and issues of loss often emerge in dreams.

Dream interpretation can occur in individual therapy or in a group context. Bosnak (1994), in describing the dreamwork process in a group intervention for PWHIVs, concluded that the group experience facilitated dream exploration and provided a sense of belonging. He concluded that this approach is particularly helpful for people with HIV because it frees up energy that has previously been spent on repressing unconscious thoughts and feelings about HIV.

For many PWHIVs, dreams continue to provide a rich source of material at a time when other aspects of their lives may be narrowing. Dreams are valuable in suggesting important themes to be dealt with in therapy. This is especially true when dreams are particularly salient and troubling or when they are recurring. Issues such as death anxiety that are difficult for clients to explore in overt ways can often be explored through dreams.

Intervention: Exploring Death Anxiety through Dreams

According to Hill's (1996) model of dream interpretation, the clinical intervention process of exploring dream themes begins with a careful exploration of each image or aspect of the dream to help the client come to a cognitive awareness of the meaning of the dream. Central images that emerge connect the dream to both past and present issues in waking life. Insight is then achieved through exploration of thoughts, feelings, and images. Insight involves not only a deeper understanding of the dream but integrates this understanding into existing cognitive schemas, which often change to accommodate these new insights. Exploration and insight should lead directly to the final stage—action in which clients have an increased awareness of what they would like to change in their lives and how they might do this.

This process will be illustrated using a dream of Anthony, a 19-year-old African American gay man. Anthony came to counseling one day highly distressed by a dream he had had the previous night. He dreamt that he had wandered into a wake at a funeral parlor. Only nine young men were attending the wake, and his first reaction was surprise to see so few people. He walked up to the casket to see who was in it and saw a familiar-looking young African American man. He was shocked and upset that the young man's parents, siblings, and other relatives were not there. Suddenly, a minister strode into the room and angrily slammed the casket shut. Anthony awoke suddenly, feeling frightened and highly agitated.

Using Hill's (1996) dream interpretation model, we first focused on exploring the various images and associations Anthony had to those images. During this process, Anthony began to associate aspects of his dream to issues in his waking life. For example, he described how one of the members in his HIV support group had recently died and how he had been so upset that he stopped attending the group. Prior to that, Anthony had found the group to be highly supportive and helpful. In fact, the nine members of the group were the only people to whom Anthony had revealed his HIV status. He concluded that he was the young man in the casket and that the nine young men in his dream represented the men in his HIV support group. Nobody else could come to the funeral because nobody else knew he had HIV disease and that he had ultimately died.

Anthony also recalled the feelings he experienced when attending the recent funeral of his great-aunt. She had been sick for a number of years and had little contact with friends, so only a handful of people attended the funeral. This struck Anthony as profoundly sad. The sadness and anxiety he felt at her funeral were the same as the emotions he was experiencing when he awoke from his dream.

Anthony was raised in a conservative church that viewed homosexuality as a sin and gays as people who were too weak and sinful to control their behaviors. He associated the minister in his dream to his felt experience of his church "slamming" the door shut in his face.

Insight occurred as Anthony was able to incorporate his under-standing of his dream into his existing cognitive schemas. He became keenly aware of how estranged he felt from his family, friends, and church because he did not feel that they would accept his homosexuality. Because of this, he had told no one in his support network (friends and family) that he had HIV disease. He also became aware of how difficult it was for him to accept his sexual identity. Because of this, he had isolated himself from people he cared about and institutions that mat-tered to him. Now he was fearful of dying alone and unmourned and was afraid that no one would notice or miss him when he died.

Anthony used the insight gained from his dream to begin to decide on actions he wanted to take to change aspects of his life. He wanted to achieve a greater sense of self-acceptance as a gay man, reconnect with family members in a more honest and open way, and find a source of spiritual support. By exploring this dream over the course of a number of counseling sessions, Anthony was able to retain the intensity of the dream in a way that motivated him to use the dream to address several important themes in his life.

CREATING A LEGACY
AS A WAY OF PREPARING FOR DEATH

For many people, the awareness of death creates a "powerful yearning to make an enduring contribution, to turn one's personal tragedy into something valuable to others and in some way to be remembered after death" (Beckett & Rutan, 1990). A common counseling theme is the desire to leave a legacy that signifies the meaning of the client's life. Clients may not always express this wish in this way, but may instead express the wish that their life be viewed as meaningful and that they will be remembered by others. One way to prepare for death is to plan a legacy that allows one to live on in some personally meaningful way. A legacy can reflect the way one would like to be remembered, a way of reminding others of one's caring and love for them, a way of creating meaning out of one's disease, or a way of leaving an impact on the future.

There are many forms that a legacy can take. One of the best known is the Names Project AIDS Memorial Quilt, where a panel of a quilt is made to reflect important attributes or aspects of the life of a person who died from AIDS. In addition to the PWHIV's name, panels often contain photos, sayings, images that define the person, such as the sun or trees, poems, and birth and death dates. Some panels are planned and made by the PWHIV as a way of preparing for death.

Other PWHIVs use art as a way of expressing the progression of their disease or their feelings about loss or death. An analysis of artwork by more than 600 PWHIVs suggested themes and visual characteristics that identified emotional states (Edwards, 1993). Drawings made shortly after diagnosis reflected disorganization, fragmentation, and empty, dark places suggesting shock and helplessness. Sharp edges and opposing shapes expressed anxiety and rage, whereas abstract designs seemed to reflect anxiety and intense emotions. Dead trees and empty landscapes reflected depression and mourning. Tears, shrunken images, and drooping flowers were seen as representing sadness. As patients became more accepting of their disease, their artwork reflected more positive images, such as rainbows, the sun, home, and flowers (Edwards, 1993).

Themes related to HIV and the dying process were often present in works of art displayed at "Significant Losses: Artists Who Have Died from AIDS," an exhibit featuring works including paintings, sculptures, prints, photographs, and videos (Significant Losses Project, 1994). One artist, known for his still life portrayal of flowers, painted transparent vases through which an AZT capsule was visible. The capsule lay in the bottom of the vase, near the stems of slightly wilting cut flowers. Other displayed artwork included HIV-positive children's views of life with AIDS as told through narrative drawings. The purpose of this exhibit was to commemorate the artists rather than the disease. In this way, a powerful legacy was left that touched many.

PWHIVs may also reflect themes of loss and change through their writings. Noted author Harold Brodkey, using his writing to express his feelings and conflicts, described powerfully and poignantly his odyssey through a year of confronting AIDS by writing, "Dying too, has a certain rhythm to it. It slows and quickens. Very little matters, but that little is of commanding importance to me. . . . This something one must bear, beyond the claims of religion, not the idea of one's dying but the reality of one's death" (Brodkey, 1994, p. 84).

Many people want significant others to remember them and to know that they loved them and cared about them. A mother may make a videotape for her children as a way of letting them know about her, her life, her feelings for them, and as a way of saying good-bye. In their work with mothers who were HIV-infected, Taylor-Brown and Wiener (1993) used videotapes that the mothers made for their children. These videotapes served a number of purposes, including leaving behind developmental guidance, expressing love, letting children know their mother will always be with them spiritually, and reminding the child of the way their mother looked and talked.

Many women view their child or children as their most important legacy. Their child connects them to the future through the next generation. Some women believe that their child is the only one who will care about them and remember that they existed. This may be one reason why women with HIV disease decide to either become pregnant or to continue a pregnancy.

Others leave a legacy in their work. They may become advocates for others with HIV or bring awareness of significant issues related to HIV disease to the public at large. Others may bring about changes in their workplace that affect policy or awareness of HIV issues.

Underlying the issue of leaving a legacy is the theme of feeling connected to the future by living on in a meaningful way. One important aspect of death anxiety is the question "Will I have mattered—will my life have mattered?" Leaving a meaningful legacy is one way of feeling that one has mattered and that one will be remembered.

Intervention: Assisting Clients in Leaving a Legacy

There are numerous ways for a client to leave a legacy. Clients often begin this process indirectly by expressing a wish or a concern that may reflect underlying questions such as "Will my life have mattered?" "Will I be remembered?" For example, a client may express a desire to help others avoid the pain that he or she has experienced as a result of HIV, or a client may wonder if his or her child will remember them. These wishes and concerns often suggest meaningful ways in which clients might leave a legacy.

Sarah, a 22-year-old white woman, discovered that she was HIV-positive when she became pregnant with her daughter. Her health deteriorated rapidly throughout her pregnancy, and it soon became apparent that she would likely not live past the first few years of her daughter Lisa's life. Her greatest fear was that Lisa would not remember her and would not know of her great love for her. Sarah decided to make what she called a "life book" to tell her daughter about her life, to describe their time together, and to tell Lisa how much she loved her. She wrote about the songs she sang to Lisa, the stories she read to her, and about the things they did together. In a sense, she created a memory of herself and of a mother–daughter relationship for Lisa to have so that Lisa would always have the experience of having had a mother.

PLANNING FOR THE DYING PROCESS

Accepting the possibility of death and preparing for that phase of life is important not just for psychological and psychosocial reasons, but because it allows the PWHIV to make plans for his or her belongings, for those left behind, such as children and pets, and for how he or she would like the dying process to be. Clients might write a will, do financial planning, sign a power of attorney, or complete an advance directive. All of these can provide PWHIVs with a sense of control at a time when they may be experiencing less control over disease progression.

It is often helpful to begin making decisions about wills, advance directives, and life support before the PWHIV is diagnosed with AIDS. For some this may create anxiety and distress, but for many it allows the opportunity to make important decisions and to explore reactions to these decisions with significant others. Making these plans can assist in the processing of grief and in preparing for death (Lippmann, James, & Frierson, 1993).

One important way to make one's wishes known about medical interventions is through an advance directive, which combines both a durable power of attorney and a living will. With an advance directive, individuals can (1) indicate what medical treatments they do or do not want if in the future they are unable to make their wishes known, and (2) appoint someone to make medical decisions for them if in the future they are unable to make those decisions for themselves or to prevent others from making these decisions for them. Not only can the PWHIV have control over these important decisions, but the process of making these decisions often allows concerns about the dying process to be explored.

Making a will is especially important when a PWHIV wants money or belongings to go to someone, such as a partner, who might not automatically inherit under inheritance laws. Typically, the estates of persons who die without wills go to legally recognized next of kin. Wills are also important in providing for dependent children and for pets.

Financial planning is another way that PWHIVs can plan for the terminal stage of life. One organization that was founded specifically to offer financial strategies to persons coping with serious illnesses is Affording Care, founded by David Petersen, a financial planner living with HIV disease (*HIV Frontline*, November/December 1993c). In addition to running workshops in New York, this organization publishes a free bimonthly newsletter of financial advice addressing issues such as life insurance and medical insurance portability.

Other decisions that should be made include disposition of a home and personal belongings, establishing beneficiaries for pensions and insurance policies and guardianships for dependent children, and funeral and burial arrangements. *The AIDS Caregiver's Handbook* (Eidson, 1993) contains some useful forms in the appendices that can be helpful in getting one's affairs in order.

Intervention: Helping Clients
Complete an Advance Directive

Completing an advance directive serves the purpose of making one's wishes known about medical treatments in the event that one is not able to do so at a future time. The process of completing an advance directive is also invaluable in exploring and understanding anxieties, beliefs, values, and wishes about the dying process.

The first part of this document asks the PWHIV to appoint a person with durable power of attorney to make decisions about the PWHIV's medical care if a time comes when he or she cannot make those decisions. Appointing someone in this role encourages important discussions with that person regarding how the PWHIV feels about life-sustaining interventions, pain management, and other medical treatments. It also allows the PWHIV to appoint someone, such as a partner, who might not otherwise be legally recognized in terms of making decisions about the PWHIV's care.

Much can be learned about the values and beliefs of an individual from this process. For example, an individual who believes that the process of his or her dying should be in God's hands, or that dying is a natural part of the life process, may request that no medical interventions occur under the conditions detailed in the document. Persons in substance abuse recovery may need to explore how they feel about requesting drugs to keep them comfortable and free of pain. Others may be primarily concerned with how their choices affect their significant others.

EXPLORING THE POSSIBILITY
OF RATIONAL SUICIDE

As some persons with AIDS accept that the end is near and shift their focus to achieving death in the best possible way, they may want to initiate "end-of-life" discussions with their significant others, their therapist, or their health care professional. For example, they may be considering "rational suicide," which is an informed and well-planned decision to end one's life when one ascertains that quality of life has become intolerable and will remain intolerable. For years, rational suicide has created an ongoing debate in the health care field. For example, the president of the American Association of Suicidology stated recently that assistance with rational suicide is the single most important issue facing suicidology at this time (Motto, 1994).

In a study examining the attitudes of PWHIVs toward rational suicide, the AIDS Health Project distributed 92 anonymous question-naires to Positives Being Positive support group facilitators, who then distributed them to group members (Jones & Dilley, 1993). All individu-als who returned the survey described themselves as gay. Most had known their HIV status for a year or more. Slightly over half reported mild or moderate depression. Interestingly, over half of those who reported no depression in the past 6 months reported that they had considered suicide in the last month. In terms of their opinion about the concept of rational suicide, 64% were in agreement with it and only 1% (one person) objected to it. In fact, 18% knew someone who planned and completed a rational suicide, and 67% had considered this act as an option for themselves at some point since learning of their HIV status. This study suggests that many PWHIVs have thought about and con-sidered rational suicide. In many cases, considering rational suicide did not appear related to depression.

How can a clinician respond in a therapeutic way to a client who is considering rational suicide? In an excellent discussion of the issues involved in rational suicide, Motto (1994) discusses the evolution of this issue in terms of HIV disease. He noted that in a 1986 issue of *FOCUS*, Goldblum and Moulton (1986) recommended that for AIDS patients still contemplating suicide after examining the issues, "the clinician must consider taking more active measures, such as psycho-tropic medication or involuntary hospitalization" (p. 2). In contrast, Jones and Dilley (1993) state that "it is crucial for therapists to attempt to understand the patient's circumstances, and to consider a situation in which dying with dignity is more important than prolonged life" (p. 6).

Perhaps the shift represented by the attitudes in these two articles reflects an awareness that longevity and cure might not be the only or the most appropriate focus of interventions with PWHIVs. Rather, qual-ity of life and control over controllable aspects of one's life also represent important and significant issues. This shift may also reflect a greater understanding of the current limitations of medical interventions in altering the course of HIV disease.

Rational suicide within the context of HIV disease has also been addressed recently in the literature (e.g., Motto, 1994; Werth, 1992). The focus of Motto's (1994) article is on how clinicians might explore this issue with clients, and his suggested steps will be described later in this chapter in the strategies section. Werth (1992) considers a number of professional and ethical issues in his examination of rational suicide. In addition, he suggests steps to be considered when counseling PWHIVs who are considering rational suicide.

The importance and urgency of the issue of rational suicide has also resulted in professional organizations exploring their roles and responsibilities in assisting clients with end-of-life discussions. For example, members of the National Association of Social Workers (NASW) recently asked their organization to provide them with guidelines for discussing end-of-life options with terminally ill clients (*HIV Frontline*, November/December 1993d). The new policy of this group encourages social workers to openly discuss end-of-life options with clients, although it emphasizes that the professional should not promote or participate in assisted suicides. However, the policy does state that "If legally permissible, it is not inappropriate for a social worker to be present during an assisted suicide if the client requests that social worker's presence" (*HIV Frontline*, November/December 1993d, p. 4).

Other organizations have originated to assist people who are considering rational suicide. For example, Compassion in Dying is a Seattle organization founded in 1993 to support and respect the choices of people who want to make an end-of-life choice (Dunshee, 1994). This group validates the concept of rational suicide for those who are terminally ill and provides support in achieving this goal.

However, strict guidelines must be met, including that death is expected in a reasonable period of time—usually within 6 months. This information must be confirmed by a physician affiliated with the organization. In addition, the individual's medical condition must cause severe, unrelenting suffering that is unacceptable and intolerable for him or her. Persons must also have explored alternatives to suicide, including better pain management, hospice care, and in some cases, spiritual counseling. Requests for assistance must be made in writing or on videotape by the individuals themselves. These requests must be made on three separate occasions with at least 48 hours between the second and third request. Finally, the organization will not assist in a suicide if any close, involved family member, partner, or friend expresses disapproval of the choice.

Assistance involves informing the patient of medicines to be obtained from his or her own physician, including specific instructions about their effective use in ending one's life. The patient is expected to self-administer the medications, and it is up to him or her to decide when and where this will occur and who will be present. In summary, the process followed by Compassion in Dying involves a careful assessment of the patient's decision to commit suicide followed by providing the patient with the effective means to achieve this goal if the patient so desires. Recently, voters in Oregon voted in support of a law to allow physician-assisted suicide. The guidelines for assistance are very similar to those of Compassion in Dying.

Intervention: Exploring Rational Suicide

When clients are considering rational suicide, Motto (1994) describes steps a therapist can follow in exploring this issue. The first step is a thorough and realistic assessment of all relevant and available facts. This includes the client reviewing all aspects of his or her life to establish a clear perception as well as a realistic interpretation of the meaning of these facts. This might include how previous, seemingly unsolvable problems were approached in the PWHIV's life, the possible effects of suicide on the lives of significant others, how suicide fits the client's life philosophy including spiritual and/or religious beliefs, whether unfinished business needs to be completed, and the degree of ambivalence the PWHIV feels about the contemplated suicide.

The counselor, considering all of these factors, makes what Motto refers to as an "intuitive" judgment about the rationality of the client's proposed resolution. This part of the process is extremely hard to define, but is perhaps most similar to what therapists refer to as "clinical judgment." If the client at this point still opts for suicide, the clinician then makes certain that the client has thoroughly explored all reasonable alternatives (e.g., pain management) to suicide. Given that many suicidal persons shift their outlook due to time alone, it is helpful to ask the client to consider delaying the act, rather than relinquishing the option, to see if time changes the degree of certainty about this choice. It is wise for the therapist to refer the client for a consultation with another clinician to see if he or she might benefit from another perspective or approach. This also provides professional support for the clinician, who may be uncertain whether he or she has explored and understood the client's wishes adequately. It is also helpful, with the client's permission, to bring in significant others, including children, partners, or clergy. Leave taking, by any means, involves psychological preparation both within oneself and with one's network of significant others.

Motto (1994) believes that it is morally acceptable, if the clinician's own beliefs allow it, to assist with the lethal act. However, it is currently illegal and considered professionally unethical to do this. More commonly, a physician might assist indirectly and implicitly by providing a prescribed medication with information about what would constitute a lethal overdose. This allows the PWHIV to take the medicine within safely prescribed limits, or to know exactly what would be a lethal dose and to have the choice as to the timing and manner of his or her own death, if desired.

Werth (1992), in his review of rational suicide and AIDS, suggests three steps in the counseling process that are somewhat similar to those suggested by Motto (1994). First, he states that PWHIVs must have a realistic assessment of their situation, including their prognosis and an awareness of potential resources and alternatives. This step requires a passage of time to consider and reconsider suicide. Second, cognitive processes must be unimpaired by severe emotional distress or illness such as dementia that might rule out making a rational decision. Finally, the motivation for the decision should fit the conceptions of a "reasonable person."

Both Motto (1994) and Werth (1992) provide valuable suggestions for exploring rational suicide with clients. Because the exploratory process is thorough and often lengthy, significant issues may emerge that have been "masked" by the expressed wish to end one's life. For example, some clients may view suicide as the only way to manage physical pain as their disease progresses. Discussing this concern with one's therapist and then with one's physician may lead to better pain management and a desire to continue with one's life—at least for the time being. Because many issues can cause a PWHIV to consider suicide, and because suicide is a "final solution" that affects not only the PWHIV but his or her significant others, it is important to help the client explore and attempt to resolve these issues before reaching this decision.

My clinical experience has shown that many PWHIVs consider suicide at some point in time and seem to gain an important sense of control and dignity from feeling that options for their own management of their disease process exist. Through this process of exploration, PWHIVs clearly gain a sense of their beliefs, fears, and hopes about the dying process. They also learn about the fears and beliefs of their partners and family members, which can provide support and pave the way for the final aspect of the dying process—the concept of safe passage.

ASSURING SAFE PASSAGE

Nichols (1986), in describing the emotional stages that PWHIVs go through as their disease progresses, refers to the final stage as "preparation for death." Kübler-Ross (1969, 1987) refers to this final stage as "acceptance." Based on their interviews with PWHIVs, McCain and Gramling (1992) called the stage preceding death "getting worn out." Implicit in each of these descriptions is the PWHIV's emotional awareness of impending death as the physical aspects of the disease become overwhelming. An important aspect of this final stage is preparing for death in a way that is both meaningful and reassuring for the person with AIDS.

The focus of the clinical work may shift at this point from "seeking cure" to "assuring safe passage" (Clever, 1988; Lomax & Sandler, 1988), that is making the ending or passing of life as positive (from the perspective of the PWHIV) as possible. It is defined by each client in terms of his or her concerns and anxieties about the dying process and death. Safe passage is achieved through allowing the client to express these fears and by allaying these fears as much as possible.

Intervention: Assisting Clients in Seeking Safe Passage

Helping clients seek safe passage begins with the counselor exploring his or her own beliefs about "caring" versus "curing." It is difficult to accept that we cannot help clients "get better" in the traditional ways associated with psychotherapy. HIV disease often necessitates thinking about therapeutic outcomes in new ways. This is especially true when working with clients during the terminal stage of the disease.

Safe passage requires that both the client and the counselor value making the passing of life as positive as possible and view this as an important therapeutic goal. Clients will vary considerably in what they regard as most important in making this phase of life positive. For example, some clients will find connectedness to significant others to be most helpful in allowing them safe passage, whereas others will find their fears allayed through spiritual connectedness. Still others express the greatest concern over dying a painful or undignified death and will find reassurance when these concerns are addressed.

What is most important in interventions addressing the process of dying is the value of helping clients talk about what Bor and Miller (1988) refer to as "dreaded issues"—issues that both counselors and clients might avoid. These issues are defined by both the client's and the counselor's experiences and might include loss of physical control of bodily functions, notions of sin and redemption, and views of the afterlife. Existential concerns may also arise, such as whether one's life has had any meaning or whether one will be remembered once one is gone. These issues are rarely discussed in counseling with clients without terminal illnesses and are often ignored in counseling with terminally ill clients. Significant others often have great difficulty discussing these issues with PWHIVs. There is often a fear that talking about death implies a loss of hope. In actuality, the dying person may take this avoidance of the topic as a sign that discussions about death are too distressing to others and may then feel a need to reassure and comfort others. This diverts the PWHIV from the important task of leaving this life.

SUMMARY

The process of dying, when attended to, can help clients prepare for what they will leave behind and for what lies ahead, yet many counselors have great difficulty talking about the dying process. Poignantly describing this process, Levine (1982) writes, "The confrontation with death tunes us deeply to the life we imagine we will lose with the extinction of the body" (p. 3). Helping PWHIVs tune in to the losses they anticipate, helping them prepare for death in both concrete and emotional ways, will ultimately help them confront death in a more meaningful way.

CHAPTER 13

Case Examples: Applying the HIV Psychosocial Model

Case examples provide one of the best ways to illustrate the dynamic interplay between assessment and intervention that occurs throughout the course of psychotherapy with PWHIVs. The previous six chapters explored broad categories of adaptation to HIV disease and illustrated research and clinical concepts through brief case examples. In this chapter, detailed cases will be presented to illustrate how multiple aspects of the client's life are addressed. This will be done by showing how client resources are assessed using the HIV psychosocial model, how these resources affect adaptations to HIV disease, and how counseling interventions can then be used to enhance adjustment. Although these cases reflect typical concerns that PWHIVs bring to counseling, they are by no means exhaustive. Rather, an attempt was made to select cases that represented some of the most salient characteristics of PWHIVs as well as an array of concerns with which they often struggle.

KEN

Ken, a 34-year-old white gay man was diagnosed as HIV-positive around 1985. He has been in psychotherapy for 4 years; for 2 years with one therapist who then left the clinic where Ken was being seen and for the past 2 years with his second therapist. Ken has two master's degrees and is an accomplished singer. He has sung professionally in various symphonies and choruses for a number of years.

Both of Ken's parents were alcoholics. Another strong influence in his life was his traditional Catholic upbringing. In adulthood, Ken and all of his siblings became alcoholics. A theme that has permeated Ken's life is low self-esteem: "I've always felt that I could just never be enough—or good enough, to meet my family's expectations." For example, Ken's parents and siblings (as well as peers) suspected from a young age that Ken was gay or "different" and taunted and teased him. Ken's father battered him emotionally and physically when he was drunk. A second theme that has dominated Ken's life is guilt about his homosexuality in relation to the Catholic Church.

Applying the HIV Psychosocial Model

Defining Characteristics of HIV Disease

A recurring theme is Ken's internalized homophobia, which resulted from both his family's and his church's negative views about homosexuals. Therefore, Ken was fearful about telling his family when he learned he was HIV-positive and has since felt that their support has been erratic at best. Ken has become increasingly angry at the Catholic Church as his disease has progressed because of its intolerant views about homosexuality. Other than family members, Ken has not told any nongay people that he is HIV-positive because of his fear of being stigmatized. Ken also feels developmentally "off-time" with his contemporaries in two important ways. First, he is facing declining physical and neurocognitive health and retirement at a time when his seronegative peers are looking forward to many years of good health and career development. Second, Ken outlived every other member of his HIV support group, which made him feel out of sync with an important circle of friends. In terms of his support group, he feels that he has not died on time.

Social Support

Social support for Ken comes primarily from his HIV-positive lover of 4 years and his gay friends. Ken feels fairly satisfied with the social support he receives from these sources, although, as his disease progresses, he has sometimes been frustrated by perceived shortcomings in the sensitivity and support of his friends. Ken also receives some support from various family members but views his family as being ambivalent about being close to him because he is gay and has AIDS. Additionally, Ken has been successful in getting institutional support in terms of HIV-specific psychosocial and medical services. For example, he has received weekly individual psychotherapy, been a member of an HIV support group for gay men, and has received excellent medical care for his disease, including antiretroviral treatment. In the past year Ken's social interactions have decreased dramatically due to disease progression.

Unique Life Situation

Ken has been diagnosed with AIDS for over 2 years and has already experienced several AIDS-defining illnesses. He is suffering from HIV-associated dementia, which has led to cognitive confusion, rapid-paced, pressured speech, inappropriate social behavior, and motoric difficulties. Because of his dementia, Ken was fired from his job in a choir because he began singing or humming when he wasn't supposed to be singing. HIV-associated dementia has led to the loss of other roles in addition to that of employee. For example, Ken recently stopped interacting socially, he is often unable to satisfactorily communicate with his partner, and he recently ended therapy (and then returned after 2 days) because he believed his therapist was telling everyone in the waiting room that he had AIDS. Ken has found the dementia-related neurocognitive changes the most difficult and frightening aspects of HIV disease.

Personality and Demographic Characteristics

Much of Ken's psychotherapy has focused on the personality and demographic characteristics component of the HIV psychosocial model. Low self-esteem leading to emotional distress and poor coping skills has dominated Ken's life and had its origins primarily in his alcoholic, dysfunctional family life and in his early difficulties finding any validation or support for being gay. In part because of his internalized homophobia and resultant adjustment difficulties, and in part because of his strong familial history of alcoholism, Ken has been an alcoholic since his teens. He attributes his many years of unsafe, casual sex in large part to his heavy drinking. Ken has also been diagnosed with major depression, and it is likely that prior to learning he was HIV-positive, he suffered for many years with a dysthymic disorder.

Adaptation to HIV, Goals, Interventions, and Other Counseling Issues

During the first year of Ken's therapy, an important goal was to manage his emotional distress, which was caused in part by loneliness, low self-esteem, and worry about having HIV disease. This response was addressed in several ways, including helping him form a committed relationship with his partner, Ted. Ken and Ted met soon after both were diagnosed with HIV disease. Ken attributes his increasing motivation to make things work in his relationship with Ted to HIV disease. This is the only committed relationship he has been in. HIV disease made him realize how important such a relationship is to him and how difficult it might be to find another HIV-positive partner with Ted's qualities. An important goal of therapy was helping Ken redefine ways that he could view his sexuality and sexual activities and to learn to communicate with his partner about these issues.

Increasing self-esteem and understanding its link to Ken's internalized homophobia and his depression has been an ongoing goal of the therapeutic work. Interventions have included building a positive gay identity and creating an open and involved relationship with some members of Ken's family of origin.

As Ken's HIV disease has progressed and he has experienced major depression as well as HIV-associated dementia, much of the focus of the counseling has been on monitoring and managing these conditions. Strategies have included assessing, monitoring, and medicating. Ken's depression was helped significantly through antidepressant medication. However, when he became increasingly demented he was put on other medications to manage his agitation and insomnia.

Ken has primarily coped with HIV disease by making a number of positive changes reflective of an active behavioral coping style. For example, he joined AA 4 years ago and has been in recovery since that time. Additionally, he began psychotherapy and joined an HIV support group at about the same time. Ken has also taken antiretroviral medications as well as antidepressants and other medications to manage his depression and HIV-associated dementia. Finally, Ken uses humor and wit as ways to cope and bring emotional balance to his life.

Counseling issues and interventions shifted dramatically as Ken's health and neurocognitive skills declined. Ken began to have difficulty coming to sessions. For example, one day when he was walking his dog in his neighborhood he became disoriented and got lost for several hours. He insisted on driving himself to sessions in his car despite experiencing difficulties remembering directions. In addition, Ken had increasing difficulty expressing and focusing on issues because of his neurocognitive problems. He often became upset with his therapist because she was in good health. As his speech and thinking became increasingly fast-paced and pressured, he began to view his therapist as "too relaxed" and "indifferent" to his distress. Ultimately, the sessions became more difficult and stressful because of his HIV-associated dementia.

ANTHONY

Anthony, a 19-year-old African American gay man, discovered he was HIV infected while being treated for an unrelated illness. Overwhelmed by his HIV status as well as by interpersonal and job concerns, he attempted suicide. Anthony describes experiencing emotional ups and downs since being diagnosed, concerns about his future, and feelings of isolation from his peers.

Anthony also describes his interpersonal discomfort and shyness as having increased as he anticipates rejection from anyone who is not gay. He has had difficulty separating being gay from being HIV infected and expects that others will also associate the two. Additionally, he avoids close friendships with gay men as he fears becoming physically intimate and running the risk of infecting them or of being rejected because of his seropositive status.

Applying the HIV Psychosocial Model

Defining Characteristics of HIV Disease

A recurring clinical theme is Anthony's fear of being stigmatized for being both HIV infected and gay. He views his religion, as well as his small-town community, as being intolerant of homosexuality and PWHIVs. He tries to anticipate situations where he might experience discrimination or exposure of his HIV status and, as a result, avoids many social interactions. He wanted to enter a nurse training program but did not do so out of concern that he might have to take an HIV test and might be barred from practicing. He also feels that he is going through significant life events at a different time and rate than his contemporaries. For example, he views his peers as "having no pressures" and "partying all the time." In contrast, he worries constantly about his health and his future, and fears that others will discover that he has HIV disease.

Social Support

Anthony has little social support because he is avoiding close friendships to hide being gay from heterosexuals and to avoid revealing his seropositive status to other gay men. Anthony has not told any family members or friends that he is HIV-positive for fear of rejection. He does not personally know anyone else with HIV disease. He has also had difficulty finding institutional supports with which he is comfortable. For example, he wanted to join an HIV support group but felt very uncomfortable at the first one he attended because most of the men were older, white, and highly educated. Later, he joined a group for young HIV-infected men. Although he is the only African American among them, the group provided him with his first opportunity to identify with other young men who were also coping with HIV. Even though Anthony grew up in a predominantly African American community, his developmental stage (late adolescence/young adulthood) was the most salient issue for him in terms of his seropositive status. He longed for a connection with other young men to see how they were managing relationships, thinking about careers and jobs, and relating to their families.

However, after one group member died and another became too ill to attend, Anthony abruptly left the group because he found it too distressing (see Chapter 12 for an interpretation of a dream Anthony reported around the time of leaving the support group).

Unique Life Situation

Anthony is still emotionally adjusting to his HIV diagnosis, as he is experiencing intense, labile emotions such as depression, guilt, shame, and anxiety. His shame focuses around how he acquired HIV disease— through sex with men. He feels guilty because he has let down his parents by being both gay and HIV-positive. He also worries that his hometown friends will reject him. Although the individual counseling has been helpful to him in managing these emotions, his isolation from other young, HIV-infected gay men (especially African American men) affects his adjustment as he has had no peer group with which to share his emotional ups and downs.

Although his CD4+ cell count is dropping rapidly, Anthony is asymptomatic. He is medically qualified to begin AZT, but because of his socioeconomic status he has no health insurance and cannot afford to pay for the medication. He is waiting to receive Medicaid.

Personality and Demographic Characteristics

Anthony is experiencing an adjustment disorder with mixed emotional features. For example, he is highly anxious at times and depressed at other times. He is having the most difficulty coping with his sense of shame and resultant loneliness. He is also having difficulty accepting his sexual orientation because he has internalized the messages about being gay that were common in his African American community and in his church.

Anthony also worries about how he will support himself and afford medical treatment, as he has no personal or familial financial resources upon which to depend. His family lives in poverty and is unable to help him financially. Anthony is in a GED program and has no viable job prospects until he completes the program. Additionally, he has no marketable skills such as carpentry, retail experience, or computer training.

Adaptation to HIV, Goals, Interventions, and Other Counseling Issues

Anthony had two issues that he wanted to address in counseling: managing his emotional reactions (e.g., shame, internalized homophobia, depression, increased interpersonal anxiety) and learning more effective coping methods, including health-promoting behaviors. To address some of his emotional reactions to having HIV disease, Anthony wanted to increase his social support. Several interventions addressed this issue: (1) Anthony first explored his internalized homophobia in counseling because his fears of being rejected for being gay and HIV-positive interfered with seeking any type of social support. (2) To reduce social anxiety, his counselor assisted Anthony with a stress management intervention involving progressive muscle relaxation as well as an imagery component. Additionally, Anthony role played social interactions. (3) To increase social support by seeking family support, Anthony decided which family members he felt safest approaching first. He decided to disclose his HIV status to his mother and one of his brothers. (4) Finally, Anthony decided to return to his HIV support group and to use this group as an adjunct to individual therapy.

Anthony responded well to trying new ways of coping, such as active cognitive-behavioral approaches. For example, he entered a job skills training program so that he could complete his GED and get job training. These would offer him some degree of financial security and would also give him the satisfaction of feeling successful and productive. Because his health was good, Anthony preferred focusing on building a "safety net" for his disease rather than focusing exclusively on HIV. His counselor assisted him by helping him locate community resources, including a live-in job training program to allow him to continue his education and training.

In addition, Anthony adopted several health-promoting behaviors. For example, he no longer drinks or uses recreational drugs and is very interested in nutrition. He is motivated to make active behavioral changes (such as exercise) to foster good health.

Several other counseling issues have emerged in working with Anthony. Although Anthony feels very comfortable in the one-to-one counseling relationship, he easily gives up in interpersonal situations outside of counseling. Therefore, it has been difficult for him to keep his momentum in his attempts to increase his social support network. Returning to the support group has been helpful in addressing this issue. At times he resents the boundaries of the counseling relationship in terms of length and frequency of sessions because it was initially his only source of support. When he felt frustrated by these limits, he sometimes felt ashamed for "needing" the sessions. His shame would at times get projected onto his therapist, whom he would then view as being "disgusted" and "fed up" with him because he was so needy and demanding.

MARIA

Maria, a 28-year-old Latina woman, sought counseling because of worry about her HIV status and because her injecting drug use was interfering with taking care of her 3-year-old son, Eddie, who is HIV-negative. She began counseling by expressing two major fears. She worried that the Department of Social Services would take away her son, and she was concerned that her partner, Ed, would die from HIV before she did.

Maria has injected drugs (heroin and cocaine) daily for many years. Although she has never entered substance abuse treatment, both she and Ed stopped shortly after she began therapy about a year ago. However, she continued to use alcohol. When Ed died from AIDS several months ago, she felt depressed and overwhelmed and quickly relapsed and began injecting drugs again on what would have been his birthday.

Maria left school in the 10th grade when she was pregnant with her oldest son, who is now 13 years old. This son lives with her mother. She feels that she has failed in her attempts to be a good mother for her older son and is determined not to fail with her younger son. After Ed died, Maria felt that the only thing she had left in the world that mattered to her was her little boy.

Applying the HIV Psychosocial Model

Defining Characteristics of HIV Disease

Maria has a strong concern that she will experience stigmatization if others find out about her HIV status. Other than her mother (and Ed), she has told no one. She worries that her friends and neighbors would not even say "hello" if they were to find out.

Social Support

Maria's social support is nearly nonexistent. Ed was basically her only source of support, other than her little boy. Now that Ed has died, she feels alone and helpless. He provided the apartment for them to live in, financial assistance, and emotional support. Her mother gives lip service to wanting to help her out, but almost always turns down her requests to babysit. Many of Maria's friends are injecting drug users with whom she has virtually no contact other than within the context of shooting up.

Unique Life Situation

Maria's CD4+ cell count is just above 500, and she is asymptomatic. However, her emotional adjustment to HIV disease is very poor. She witnessed Ed's excruciatingly painful dying process and is terrified of what she will go through. She also worries that she will die alone. Because of Maria's lack of education, lack of job skills, and her injecting drug use, she has never had a job. The roles by which she has defined herself are being a mother and being Ed's common-law wife. She has lost this latter role because of HIV and now fears losing her role as a mother.

Personality and Demographic Characteristics

Maria has very low self-esteem because she feels that she has "messed up her life" by getting pregnant, leaving school, using drugs, and getting HIV disease. Further, she has very low self-efficacy in managing sexual and drug situations, she almost always goes along with what others want. In part, this might be attributable to gender-role expectations in Maria's Latino culture.

Maria has a dual diagnosis, HIV disease and substance-related disorder, and she has also been very depressed since Ed's death. There is the possibility that she had an affective disorder prior to becoming HIV infected. Additionally, Maria lives in poverty, as she is unemployed and lives on a small check from public assistance and on food stamps. Because she has never worked, has no job skills, and is an injecting drug user, there are no current prospects for bettering her economic situation.

Maria has many life-style issues that contribute to her difficulties in managing her HIV disease and in improving her overall life situation. She has never learned health-protective behaviors such as safer sex and drug practices, good nutrition, or regular exercise. Moreover, in the context of her addiction these types of behaviors have not seemed important or relevant.

Adaptations to HIV, Goals, Interventions, and Other Counseling Issues

Maria's response to HIV that concerns her the most is her return to using alcohol and heroin. Her goal for therapy is to begin the process of recovery and in the process adopt health-protective behaviors. Because she has been unsuccessful doing this on her own, her therapist recently told her that she needs to enter a treatment program and attend Narcotics Anonymous if they are to continue to work together. Maria's therapist worked hard to form a strong therapeutic alliance so that Maria would not leave therapy when she was given this ultimatum. Maria recognized that if she could not begin the process of recovery, she would lose her little boy.

A second adaptation to HIV that Maria wants to address in counseling is managing her anxiety about being HIV-positive as well as her grief over losing Ed to this disease. She has also expressed much anxiety about the dying process and concerns about what will happen to her after death. She feels that she has been a "bad" person and fears that she may go to hell.

Maria would also like to develop better coping skills so she can become a better parent. She often neglects Eddie when she is using drugs. Moreover, she has difficulty managing her anger and disciplining him effectively. She feels that she was a terrible mother to her older son and fears making the same mistakes again. This goal has been addressed many times in her therapy sessions. Additionally, Maria's therapist is attempting to enroll her in parenting classes but has been unsuccessful in finding this resource in her community. Maria's parenting skills will also likely improve if she is successful in her substance abuse treatment.

Finally, Maria would like to get a part-time job. She has never worked and feels that she has missed out on having a sense of accomplishment. Additionally, a job would provide structure and might alleviate some of her boredom, which she believes has often led to drug use. Maria is investigating several job training programs for people who lack adequate education and training.

Counseling has also focused on building a strong therapeutic bond to increase the likelihood that Maria will enter and complete a substance abuse treatment. Therapy has often progressed inconsistently, as Maria has missed sessions when she was high. Additionally, her counselor has at times felt overwhelmed by Maria's high level of need in nearly every area of her life and the very few resources available to Maria to address these needs.

MARCUS

Marcus, a 23-year-old African American man who became HIV-positive through heterosexual contact, has not told anyone of his HIV status. He associates HIV disease with gay men and injecting drug users. He is convinced that others also make this association and that they will not

believe how he acquired HIV. Therefore, he now avoids close relationships with both women and men. He is afraid to date because he doesn't
think anyone will want to get close to him "once they know" and because
he is terrified that he will "put someone else through what I'm dealing
with." Marcus is also isolated because he knows no other HIV-infected
persons.

Marcus struggles financially as he has only been able to find part-
time work. He won't seek medical treatment as he fears being labeled
"gay" at the clinic. He also views life with a stoic acceptance and believes
that he "got himself into this" and now must "deal with it." Marcus
states that all he ever wanted was "a good job, a nice wife, and a family."
He despairs that, at most, he will be lucky if he gets the job.

Applying the HIV Psychosocial Model

Defining Characteristics of HIV Disease

Marcus has not told anyone that he is HIV-positive because he expects
that he will be rejected. His small rural community views HIV disease
as contagious and considers that those afflicted are a danger to others in
terms of any type of contact. For example, a family that enrolled an
HIV-positive child in the local school system experienced so much
ostracism that they moved out of the area. Marcus also feels that he no
longer has anything in common with his contemporaries. Young men
his age are spending their time with girlfriends and beginning careers.
He feels excluded from these activities because of having HIV disease,
with its uncertain future.

Social Support

It is apparent that Marcus is lacking in social supports. Because he fears
telling his family about his serostatus, he avoids going home for visits.
He is concerned that his mother will be able to tell that something is
seriously wrong. Marcus will not date, and he ignores and discourages
women who show an interest in him. He is afraid of "doing this to
someone else."

Unique Life Situation

Marcus's CD4+ cell count is just below 500. However, he is not interested
in beginning antiretroviral therapy. He is experiencing recurrent genital
herpes and generalized lymphadenopathy. Emotionally, he seems stoic
and resigned at times and worried at other times. His usual response

when he ponders what he should do about his disease is to conclude that he should "just let what happens happen—a man's gotta do what he's gotta do."

Marcus experiences the most sadness and anger over feeling that life roles that were important to him will not be achieved. He wanted to be a husband and a father and believes that will not be possible. He also wanted to be a "productive member of society" and now wonders if that will happen. Marcus often wonders who gave him HIV, and believes it was a former girlfriend whom he loved. He wonders if she was deceitful about being monogamous or about her past, and he feels betrayed. This has translated into a distrust of women.

Personality and Demographic Characteristics

Gender identity and racial identity, along with socioeconomic status, have been the most defining personality and demographic characteristics in Marcus's psychotherapy. For example, he feels that the essence of what it means to him to be a man—being with a woman, having children, being proud of his body—has been taken away by HIV disease. He also believes that his African American community can never accept him as a man with HIV disease. Moreover, he lacks material resources such as adequate income and health insurance, that would help to buffer his present life situation.

Marcus alternates between blaming himself for acquiring HIV disease and blaming his former girlfriend. In both cases, he is making negative attributions that cause him distress. His coping style has isolated him from others and has interfered with him taking an active role in coping with his disease. For example, his avoidant style has led him to believe that there is little that he or anyone else can do since he cannot be "cured." Because of this, his plan is to not tell any family members or friends that he has HIV until he is near death.

Adaptation to HIV, Goals, Interventions, and Other Counseling Issues

Emotional distress, caused by self-blame, fear of rejection, and social isolation, and poor coping skills were common responses to HIV disease that defined Marcus's earlier counseling sessions. After working with his therapist for several months, Marcus became more optimistic about setting goals that might be helpful in managing these reactions to HIV disease. He agreed that he would like to increase his social support to help with his loneliness and depression. Specifically, he would like to have a girlfriend again, make contact with old friends, and let several of his family members know about his HIV status. Strategies included helping Marcus focus on emotional intimacy as a precursor to physical intimacy in relationships with women. He also learned health-promoting behaviors such as safer sex practices that made him more confident to begin trying to date again.

Marcus has yet to disclose his HIV status to any family members, but he is exploring his fears of disclosure and practicing ways that he might effectively disclose. One option is to use his counselor as a resource to provide information to family members to alleviate their fears about casual contact and HIV transmission. Alternatively, he could bring his family members to a counseling session so he can have professional assistance in disclosing his HIV status.

Another issue that Marcus would like to address is his difficulties finding a vocation. He decided to begin by acquiring more job skills. To address this goal, Marcus recently enrolled in a city-run job training program. This program arranged for him to work as a junior apprentice to a plumber to further develop the basic plumbing skills he had learned in a previous training program.

Finally, Marcus's counselor is helping him to develop a more effective repertoire of coping responses. To do this, Marcus is being taught cognitive-behavioral techniques that fit the characteristics of a particular stressful situation (e.g., learning to manage emotional intimacy before initiating a sexual relationship based on safer sex).

The most challenging counseling issue that Marcus's counselor has experienced is motivating him to believe that what he does, or does not do, can make a difference in his quality of life "post-HIV." Initially, Marcus was not committed to pursuing counseling, but this has changed as he has become more hopeful and more allied with his therapist. Marcus had little previous experience with self-disclosure and emotional intimacy, and his therapist has often felt as if she were "pulling teeth" to get Marcus to talk about any aspect of his life or his feelings. Additionally, Marcus has no reliable means of transportation and was often late for sessions. As he became more involved in the therapeutic work, these issues were resolved.

SUMMARY: THEMES AND COUNSELING ISSUES THAT DEFINE THE CASES

Several themes are present in all of these cases and suggest that HIV may contribute to the emergence of these themes in counseling. Each of these clients is struggling to forge a positive identity in terms of gender, sexual orientation, or race. This struggle has been exacerbated by HIV disease.

For example, Anthony and Ken both struggle with internalized homophobia as well as the reactions of others to their gay identity. Marcus struggles with what it means to be an African American man with HIV disease. Maria's primary identity has been to be someone's mother or girlfriend.

Other common themes are low or diminished self-esteem, the feared loss of valued or hoped-for life roles, disrupted or aborted life goals, and varied and multiple losses. It is interesting that most of the themes these clients present in counseling are about the desire for interpersonal relatedness, rather than specifically about health or disease progression. In many ways HIV disease seems to bring these issues more sharply into focus.

These cases of clients living with HIV disease also lead to several important points for therapists to consider:

1. The importance of a thorough assessment of client concerns before intervening.
2. The necessity of keeping an open mind by considering multiple hypotheses. Clients present with multiple issues, and it is important to collaboratively identify and prioritize what is most important and salient to address first. This may or may not directly relate to HIV disease.
3. The importance of helping clients learn about HIV disease so they may understand the ways in which it affects their life, their goals, and their emotions, so they may play an active role in managing their disease.
4. The importance of maximizing the clients' interpersonal effectiveness both within the context of HIV disease and in the larger context of their lives.
5. The value of considering other resources (in addition to individual counseling) to enhance and support client change. These resources might include medications for mood disorders, substance abuse treatment, group counseling or other modes of therapy, systems support such as families and friends, and community resources and support such as churches, community recreation services, and other agencies in the PWHIV's community.

PART III

THE PSYCHOTHERAPEUTIC CONTEXT

> ... all psychotherapies involve ... a relationship
> between healer and patient. Within this
> relationship, the task of the therapist—whatever
> his or her technique—is to clarify symptoms and
> problems, inspire hope, facilitate experiences of
> success or mastery, and stir the patient's emotions.
> —FRANK AND FRANK (1991, pp. xiii–xiv)

Therapeutic relationships flourish when the counselor and client develop a strong therapeutic alliance, understand the boundaries of the counseling relationship, work through transferential and countertransferential themes, and together facilitate client change. Although these aspects are at the heart of all counseling, at times the psychotherapeutic context may differ with PWHIVs. Counseling boundaries, such as session length and location, may shift as the PWHIV experiences the physical, emotional, and neurocognitive effects of HIV disease. Transference and countertransference themes often reflect reactions to stigma, the dying process, and death. The psychotherapeutic context will also be shaped by multicultural variables. This is because multicultural variables, defined broadly to include gender, sexual orientation, race/ethnicity, age, socioeconomic status, and affiliations, have in large part defined this disease. Ethical dilemmas may also intrude in the clinical work and cause the therapist to struggle with how the rights of the PWHIV should be weighed against the rights of society to curb the epidemic. The counseling relationship, multicultural considerations, and ethical issues are discussed in Chapters 14, 15, and 16.

Many aspects of HIV disease, including stigma, modes of transmission, and its fatality rate, create challenges for those who offer care to PWHIVs, including counselors. Yet the enormity of what is happening to the client with HIV disease often diverts attention from the impact of the disease on significant others, including caregivers. Chapter 17 examines the impact of caring for PWHIVs on informal (e.g., partners, spouses, family members) and formal (e.g., counselors, nurses) caregivers. Moreover, as will be seen in Chapter 18, few counselors have received the type of HIV-specific, or even HIV-related, training that could help them more effectively offer services to PWHIVs.

Frank and Frank (1991) note that the goals of all therapies are to clarify issues, instill hope, and facilitate experiences of mastery within the connectedness of the counseling relationship. These goals are certainly important and necessary components of therapeutic work with PWHIVs. But as will be seen in the following chapters on the psychotherapeutic context, the ways in which the counselor and PWHIV redefine what it means to care, heal, and to make whole is perhaps at the heart of the psychotherapeutic journey.

CHAPTER 14

The Counseling Relationship: Boundaries, Transference, and Countertransference

Counseling is an interpersonal and intrapsychic process in which the development of the counselor–client relationship is central to the therapeutic impact. Interpersonal aspects of the relationship focus on the interplay between the counselor and client. For example, as the PWHIV becomes symptomatic, both the client and the counselor may react in a number of ways, such as becoming more anxious, that might affect the boundaries or structure of the relationship. Intrapsychic processes, which often reflect core personality dynamics, may be expressed through transference and countertransference reactions. Several broad themes will be explored in this chapter to illustrate the counseling relationship: the changing boundaries of the relationship, transference reactions, and countertransference reactions.

To illustrate these counseling issues and themes, case examples will be used and will be referred to throughout the chapter. These cases portray issues that often define the counseling relationship with clients with HIV disease, provide insight into the complexity and challenge of the work of the counselor, and provide a view of the therapeutic alliance.

QUINN

Quinn, a 21-year-old white gay man, sought counseling when he entered a job/educational training program. He had learned of his HIV-positive status about a year prior to entering the program but had received no follow-up counseling. Quinn described a long history of emotional abuse from his mother and sexual abuse from his father. From the age of 12 he spent 4 years at a boys' ranch for emotionally disturbed boys. Shortly after arriving at the boys' home he was raped by an older boy. In Quinn's eyes, this replicated the sexual abuse he had experienced at the hands of his father and began a long-standing pattern of being emotionally and sexually victimized by older, more powerful boys and men.

Quinn was motivated to work on family of origin issues as well as self-esteem. He worked very hard in his counseling sessions to make changes in his life. He was extremely bright and well read about HIV disease and understood safer sex practices. However, about once a month he described finding himself almost irresistibly drawn to go to a neighborhood where there were a number of gay-oriented bookstores and clubs. Once inside a club, he enjoyed the attention and sense of closeness. Quinn was very good looking and looked much younger than his years. Older men were drawn to him and often commented that he must be healthy as he was too young to be infected.

He usually ended up going home with an older man, often not knowing the man's name or where they were going. On two occasions, he ended up fearing for his life once he went to the man's home. These evenings typically ended with Quinn agreeing to have unprotected anal intercourse. When he described these experiences in his next counseling session, he presented ambivalent feelings about the encounter. He described how wonderful it felt to be taken care of and desired. He also expressed disgust with himself and disappointment that he could not seem to change his life patterns. On another level, he felt powerful because this man might now get HIV.

GEORGE

George, a white bisexual man in his 30s, had been in psychotherapy for over 2 years prior to learning of his seropositive status. George had a master's degree and had always been successful in his career, but felt that his problems revolved around interpersonal issues and had therefore focused in his therapy on intimacy and relationship concerns. After learning of his seropositive status, issues that had been examined by George early in the therapeutic work, such as feelings about his bisexuality, entered into the therapeutic work again. George had worked hard to move from a series of casual, short-term relationships and was finally feeling successful and happy in a long-term, committed relationship with his lover. Instead of being able to enjoy his achievements in his interpersonal relationships and his promising career, George felt that

HIV symbolized a "payback." It was as if a "long arm from the past" had snatched him back to "account for his behavior."

Over the next few years George's physical health deteriorated to the point where he frequently missed work and eventually could no longer work full-time. He did not reveal his seropositive status to anyone at his work place, although he believed that some colleagues suspected the reasons for his many health-related absences. Because George eventually had to shift to part-time work, he lost his health insurance, had a significantly reduced income, had mounting medical bills because he did not qualify for Medicaid, and had to be seen in counseling for a reduced fee. George increasingly could not come to office appointments because of his health. Most of his time and energies were directed to the development of an AIDS task force at his place of work.

Eventually he was hospitalized a second time for *Pneumocystis carinii* pneumonia (PCP). When George realized he might be dying, he decided to tell his family of origin that he had AIDS and that he was bisexual. While in the hospital he asked his therapist to come to the hospital to offer supportive counseling while he "came out" to his family. Shortly before his death, George was nearly blind, was emaciated due to chronic diarrhea, and often showed marked disturbances in his cognitive processes due to AIDS-related dementia. In one of the last sessions that he was able to make at the therapist's office, he got diarrhea during the session and his therapist needed to assist him in cleaning himself and the chair. Shortly before George died, both he and his family asked his therapist to attend and to participate in his funeral.

STACY

Stacy, a 19-year-old African American woman, became HIV-positive from heterosexual transmission. She learned of her antibody status when she became pregnant and was tested as a part of routine prenatal care. She miscarried soon after that and was referred to the counseling unit of her clinic to assist her to cope with her seropositive status and her miscarriage. Stacy enjoyed being in counseling for a variety of reasons. She valued close interpersonal social support and felt that counseling provided this.

During the turmoil of her pregnancy loss, her positive antibody test, and her mother's death, her counselor provided a source of safe, supportive, and steady contact in a world that felt chaotic and unsafe. In many ways, Stacy was able to use her therapy to make changes in her life and to cope on a day-to-day basis more effectively than she had in the past.

Soon after beginning counseling, Stacy began dating a new man and soon fell in love. Initially, she planned to tell him that she had HIV disease as soon as they got to know each better and before initiating a sexual relationship. However, around this time Stacy's mother died from cancer and Stacy's boyfriend became her "lifeline" in terms of offering daily love and social support. She gave every indication of consistently practicing safer sex, despite desperately wishing to have a baby at some point in time. At the same time, she became increasingly guilty about not telling her boyfriend that she had HIV, yet was extremely fearful that he would leave her for a variety of reasons including fear of contagion, a desire to find someone else to marry who could safely have children, and anger and distrust toward her due to her deceit. This issue escalated as Stacy became symptomatic and her worried boyfriend implored her to let him know what was wrong with her.

The cases of George, Stacy, and Quinn illustrate some of the complex therapeutic issues of clinical work with clients with HIV disease. These issues include (1) rethinking typical therapeutic goals, including setting new goals and identifying psychotherapy themes; (2) changing the boundaries of the psychotherapeutic relationship, including issues of working with clients for the duration and working in nonoffice settings, time and money concerns, and decisions about self-disclosures; (3) understanding and working through transference and countertransference reactions; and (4) counselor helplessness, stress, and burnout. Interpreting moral, ethical, and legal guidelines, and consulting with other professionals are issues that arise in the context of the preceding topics. In illustrating all of these issues, I will refer back to the three cases presented above.

RETHINKING TYPICAL THERAPEUTIC GOALS

Counseling is typically conducted as if the client has a number of years ahead and many dreams, hopes, and aspirations may be realized. The client might move, change careers, fall in love, get married, or become a parent. Goals are made as if there is not only a present but also a future waiting to be created in which the client has the major role. It is as if the client has a canvas and a palette of paints and can select colors, shadings, and themes, and can decide what will be the figure and what will be the ground.

Counseling goals for clients with HIV disease may at times stand in sharp contrast. The therapist may be balancing belief in the client's potential to paint a meaningful and moving canvas while wondering if the day-to-day issues of HIV, the unrelenting progression of the disease, or the reactions of others will intrude on the canvas that he or she is encouraging the client to create. How can a therapist help a client manage these issues so that they do not solely determine what appears on the canvas?

Interventions to assist the PWHIV in rethinking life goals have been discussed previously. In addition to these interventions, several therapeutic perspectives are helpful for counselors in reframing counseling goals for clients with a progressive disease such as HIV:

1. A commitment to maintain (or assist the client in obtaining) a counseling relationship throughout the duration of the client's disease, if desired by the client (Lomax & Sandler, 1988); many clients continue to value and benefit from a counseling relationship as they cope with ongoing adjustment to the ever-present shifts brought about by disease progression.
2. A recognition that depending on when the client began counseling, he or she may have many years of functional and productive living ahead.
3. A recognition of the importance of hope and a positive attitude (Frank & Frank, 1991; Lomax & Sandler, 1988); both the client and the counselor need to believe in the power of realistic hope in coping and achieving a meaningful quality of life.
4. The value of a directive approach around issues of safer sex and drug practices for the client and others, as opposed to a nondirective approach (Cochran, in Landers, 1988).
5. Changing the therapeutic goal from "seeking cure" to "assuring safe passage" (Clever, 1988; Lomax & Sandler, 1988), or from "seeking to cure" to "seeking to care" (Ramsey, 1971). Safe passage refers to making the passing or ending of life as positive as possible. To assure safe passage is to explore these fears about death and the dying process and to support hopeful expectations as much as possible by allowing the client to express these concerns in the counseling relationship (Lomax & Sandler, 1988).

George's case illustrates his therapist's commitment to be with George for the duration of his illness. This meant drastically reducing his fee, changing the site of counseling from the formal structure of the office to the client's home, the telephone, and the hospital, as needed, adjusting to physical changes along with the client, changing the focus of the therapy to cope with here-and-now issues of loss as well as fears around impending death, and participating in a significant rite of passage with his client—George's funeral. George's case illustrates a reframing of the therapeutic goals from the more typical view of the future to a different view of the future achieved through "safe passage."

In this case, the therapist also suffered a loss—the loss of George as he was when they began their therapeutic journey together and the loss of seeing the complete fruition of their therapeutic work as they had once envisioned it. Because they had begun their therapeutic work long before George learned he was seropositive, the therapist also had to reframe the goals of their work together. Once he was able to do this, George's therapist viewed this as one of the most meaningful and poignant therapeutic journeys he had taken. Some of the goals that had seemed impossible in the "pre-HIV" stages of their work became possible: George forming a loving and committed bond with his partner, and coming out to his family, reconnecting with them, and working through past rifts. He also felt moved and awed by George's powerful wish to live after years of depression and his strength, courage, and dignity as he died. Hope is an essential feeling that allows one to go through adversity, to make plans, and to believe in a future. The opposite of hope is demoralization. In working with clients with HIV disease, the focus of hope might shift from a goal of living to be very old to leaving a legacy, finishing loose ends, making reconnections, raising a child, or achieving a "good" death. In Stacy's case, she reframed her "hoped-for" goal of "marriage sometime in the future" to being in love and being loved in a relationship in the present. She was less focused on goals she had previously had, such as having a long marriage, living to be old, having a great career, and so on. Thus, her reluctance to tell her boyfriend of her seropositive status reflects her fear that her dearest hope would be destroyed. Because having goals is a marker for hope, helping clients hold on to goals through reframing, modifying, or coming up with new ones is an essential aspect of the therapeutic work. To not do so might be to collude with the client's sense of giving up.

Quinn, because of his difficulties practicing safer sex, illustrates the value of a directive approach around safety issues for the client and others. Since Quinn was not involved in an ongoing relationship and was essentially engaging in anonymous unsafe sex, it was not possible to use the support of the other person to alter his behavior or even to warn or protect the other persons if that had been required by law. Instead, the counselor had to work very hard within the therapeutic relationship, and with some degree of urgency given the seriousness of the situation for both Quinn and others, to help Quinn understand and alter these behaviors. Quinn often felt overwhelmed with trying to cope with his disease, so it was helpful for him to focus on one aspect of this process: how he took risks in order to feel close, intimate, and in control.

CHANGING THE BOUNDARIES
OF THE COUNSELING RELATIONSHIP

"For therapists whose patients have HIV or AIDS, setting boundaries might seem oxymoronic, especially when the nature of the work requires continuous flexibility. The changing health status of patients alone demands that boundaries change with their needs" (*HIV Frontline*, March/April 1994b, p. 4). In contrast to this view, during graduate school we are taught about the importance of maintaining therapy boundaries. Counseling sessions are typically held in an office, at a designated time, and for a specified amount of time (typically 50 minutes). The client is expected to attend regularly, to be on time, to work actively on his or her issues between sessions, and to keep up on the payments for his or her sessions. Counseling center policies, insurance policies, theoretical frameworks, and mutually agreed-upon psychotherapeutic goals typically limit the number of sessions to what amounts to a relatively small portion of the remainder of the client's life. These parameters often change when counseling clients with HIV disease. Decisions need to be made based on the specific situation of the individual client—balancing the importance of the client finding the therapy accessible and responsive to his or her ever-shifting needs, yet not overburdening the therapist's resources.

Working with Clients for the Duration

I have already briefly discussed the importance of counselors being prepared to work with their clients with HIV disease until the client's death (Lomax & Sandler, 1988; Nichols, 1986) or until the client is ready to terminate the counseling relationship. There are times when that may not be possible or may be unlikely for a variety of reasons, and it is important to make these limits clear to the client. When a client who already has HIV disease seeks counseling services, the therapist needs to have a clear sense of what the commitment will mean, including questions such as "Am I willing to reduce my fees to what my patient can pay?"; "Am I willing to make myself accessible, at a minimum for phone messages and calls, during weekends and late evenings?"; "Am I willing, or able, to make home or hospital visits?"; "How do I feel about family members or significant others coming to sessions or calling me?"; "How do I feel about letting my client know more about me? Such as my sexual orientation, my health status, or any other issues that might come up with shifting boundaries?"

Namir and Sherman (1989) described this process as that of therapists struggling with the "rules" they have assumed in the way they practice psychotherapy. These rules or issues are important to explore before committing to work with a client with HIV disease. However, if a client who has been seen in an ongoing counseling relationship learns that he or she is infected, the counselor may also need to explore his or her competence as well as willingness to make the commitment to the clinical work that will be required.

At the beginning of the therapeutic work, if the client is fairly healthy or asymptomatic, sessions will typically be structured, in terms of time, place, and so on, much as any counseling sessions are. This begins to change as the client becomes symptomatic. If the client is hospitalized, counseling sessions might be conducted in the hospital or in the client's home. If the client recovers from the medical crisis, he or she may resume structured counseling sessions at the counselor's office. Nevertheless, a change may have occurred in the dynamics of the relationship due to the shift away from typical boundaries during the medical crisis. The impact of this shift should be examined within the therapeutic relationship. Shifting boundaries, as well as sharing a deeper intimacy around the issues stimulated by death anxiety or other aspects of the dying process, may change the counseling relationship. At this point, significant others may become an informal or adjunctive part of the therapy. Partners may call the counselor to let him or her know that the client is quite depressed or suicidal or to ask for help in managing a situation. In other words, significant others may become "informal" clients.

George's case illustrates the transformations in the counseling relationship as George learned he was HIV positive and then gradually died after developing AIDS. George began therapy unaware of his HIV status. His health had already begun to decline by the time the antibody tests were developed, and at that point he had devoted significant time and energy in his therapy to issues other than HIV. His diagnosis represented not only a major life crisis, but a major shift in the focus of the therapy. As George's health deteriorated, the changes this brought about in the therapeutic relationship were notable.

Working with Clients in Other Settings

Although the literature on HIV disease describes the counselor–client relationship as an ongoing commitment, this may not always be possible given the setting where the client is seen. That is, some settings may impose time limits on the counseling relationships (e.g., university counseling centers or a community mental health center). For example, university counseling centers will likely offer services to increasing numbers of students who have just learned of their HIV positive antibody status and are in a state of crisis. These clients may seek counseling to cope with the initial diagnosis of seropositivity. Interventions might include working through emotions, understanding what it means to have HIV disease, learning about health-promoting behaviors, deciding whom to tell, and learning about ongoing sources of psychological assistance. Other clients may prefer to see a counselor "as needed." For example, they might seek counseling to assist with the initial stages of the crisis and later when symptoms affect relationships or work. Time-limited therapy, with its emphasis on selecting a specific focus or theme, is a helpful approach when warranted by clients or settings.

What is most important is that the counselor clearly convey to the client any limits that the setting might place on their continuing work. The counselor, before deciding to work with a client with HIV disease, needs to commit to work with the client as long as his or her setting allows and to assist the client in seeking other psychological services if necessary. It is also important that the counselor have the necessary skills to work with clients with HIV disease and an awareness when consultations with or referrals to other professionals are warranted in order to provide the best care for the client.

Time and Money

Time and money are often central issues in clinical work. Behaviors such as missed sessions, being late for sessions, running over allotted time, and problems with payment are interpretable issues. These boundary issues often take on additional, and at times different, meanings with clients with HIV disease. That is, boundary issues may sometimes have less to do with the inner dynamics of the seropositive client and more to do with the realities of the PWHIV's current life situation. Crises for PWHIVs often occur at unexpected and unpredictable times. For example, counselors may need to be available in the middle of the night and on weekends (Landers, 1988). To illustrate, the day before George died, a Saturday, he had his father call his therapist to ask him to come to the hospital as quickly as possible to say good-bye.

Clients may arrive late for sessions because of the physical efforts required to get ready to leave their home and to get to the session. They may need to rely on others or public transportation if they have lost the means (e.g., income, vision) that would allow them to own and operate an automobile. They may not have the energy to participate in a full-length session. Likewise, they may have cognitive deficits that make this difficult.

The majority of persons with full-blown AIDS are unemployed and often uninsured. They may not be able to pay the usual fee, if any fee, for their sessions. Even for clients who have some ability to pay for sessions, therapists may feel uncomfortable "taking money" from dying clients (Maloney, 1988). Although fees can be adjusted or therapy can be pro bono, for many PWHIVs this represents a loss of independence or pride. These issues represent real, in-the-here-and-now events as well as possible manifestations of the transference relationship.

Although I am an advocate of sliding scales so that therapy is accessible to many individuals, this value is not shared by everyone, nor is it possible to do this if many of one's clients have this need. It is common for both physicians and therapists who are successful in establishing rapport with PWHIVs to find that through word-of-mouth many other PWHIVs seek their services. To avoid feeling overburdened either financially or emotionally, some mental health providers maintain boundaries by limiting the number of PWHIVs they will see at any given time. Another option may be to run therapy groups to provide psychotherapy and support in a way that is not only beneficial to clients, but that allows more people to receive help at a more affordable cost.

Self-Disclosure

Self-disclosure is another important and significant boundary issue and may be especially salient with PWHIVs. Many gay therapists believe that because of internalized homophobia, it is important for clients to know that the therapist is gay and is comfortable with some degree of public acknowledgment. Another issue arises when the therapist has HIV disease: Will knowing this be helpful to the PWHIV? There are a multitude of other issues where self-disclosure might be considered as an important way to connect in the therapeutic work.

Self-disclosure can be one of the most powerfully healing therapeutic tools available to us or it can serve our own anxiety or needs. Perhaps the best guideline is to ask yourself why you are considering sharing personal information (about any aspect of your life) and whether it is "in the service of the client." In terms of timing, you may consider how it might be interpreted by the client, how it might benefit the client, and how it will foster the therapeutic bond. Poorly timed self-disclosure often has the impact of moving the focus of the therapeutic work away from the client, closing off or redirecting the focus of further exploration, causing the client to want to protect or take care of the therapist or to worry that the therapist will not be there for him or her.

TRANSFERENCE

Transference can be viewed as expectations based on past experiences, such as conflicts with significant others, that color current experiences.

For example, a gay man who has typically experienced homophobia from heterosexuals might expect to experience that reaction from his heterosexual therapist. Clients may also experience reactions in the context of the counseling relationship that do not fit the definition of transference. Yet all of these emotional reactions, whether transferential or not, are important and meaningful to examine as an integral part of the therapeutic work. These reactions may help or hinder the counseling depending on whether they are explored as an integral part of the relationship and worked through, or ignored and avoided.

Transferential reactions from any client often contain underlying themes: those reactions pertaining to sexuality and intimacy, loss, and caretaking and dependency. These same themes, as well as themes of death and dying, become intensified when working with clients with HIV and AIDS (Nichols, 1986).

Reactions to Sexuality and Intimacy

Intimacy issues for clients with HIV disease may be merged with the client's view of his or her sexuality as well as with having acquired HIV. For example, Quinn had never experienced a sense of intimacy without being involved with someone sexually. He initially responded to his male therapist in a highly seductive and sexualized manner as he attempted to form a therapeutic alliance. He did not know how to be intimate without being sexual. However, because he associated his gay identity so closely with becoming HIV-positive, he initially saw his therapist's behavior as a rejection of him because he was gay and was HIV-positive. Clients may have projections about their counselor's sexual history as well as projections about what the counselor thinks about the client's sexual history (Bartnof, 1988). During another session, Quinn described a weekend where he went home with a man he did not know and had unprotected sex. His counselor had to unexpectedly cancel their next session due to illness. Quinn became convinced that because he was such a terrible and disgusting person he had made his therapist sick.

Reactions to Loss and Therapist's Health

Clients may express rage at the counselor's apparent good health as their own health deteriorates (Lopez & Getzel, 1984), or they may be concerned that the counselor may also become ill and abandon them. They may also feel that their counselor cannot understand what they are going through because he or she has good health. Clients may bring up feelings of envy or hostility for what the counselor has, such as the child the client may never have. Stacy, mourning both the loss of her failed pregnancy as well as the possibility that she might never become a mother, became focused on wondering about her therapist's own children. She alternated between feeling that the therapist's children took her therapist's attention away from her, and envying her therapist for having children.

The client may vacillate from seeing the therapist as the rescuer (perhaps the only one who can help) or as one of the enemy (a part of healthy society or a part of the health care profession that cannot save the client). As such, the therapist may be viewed as an idealized object or a disappointing object, with shifts in these views occurring frequently (Nichols, 1986).

Reactions to Caretaking and Dependency

Illness and impending death may also stimulate many unresolved fears and issues around dependency. After George had missed several sessions by canceling at the last minute, his therapist discovered that George was so ashamed of his lack of control over bodily functions and fear of what his handsome and healthy therapist would think that he chose to remain in his house alone, despite wanting desperately to come to the sessions.

Dependency issues for the client with HIV may also take the form of making additional demands on the counselor in terms of extra sessions, phone calls, nonoffice visits, and problems with payments. This may further stimulate client conflicts about dependence and helplessness.

Reactions to Disease and Death

Clients may also express anxieties about disease progression and death in the form of transference. For example, they may fear that the counselor fears contagion from them or that the counselor will not be able to tolerate their appearance (Bartnof, 1988). After George learned that he had HIV disease, he began to anxiously scan the sofa where he sat during sessions to make sure he had not left a coffee cup or tissues that his therapist would have to touch. He also canceled an appointment at the last minute because he had developed a visible Kaposi's sarcoma lesion that he did not want his therapist to see. When his therapist later explored these situations, George was able to talk about how ashamed he was of his disease and his feeling that he was "contagious." He feared making his therapist uncomfortable by having to get too close to his disease (i.e., touching a tissue or seeing a lesion).

Exploring transference is a major part of many therapies. However, it may play an even greater role with seropositive clients given the intensity, realities, and disequilibrium of their situation. Research suggests that clients often do not share with their therapists what they are thinking and feeling (Hill, Thompson, Cogar, & Denman, 1993). This issue may be especially salient for clients with HIV disease who are struggling with concerns and reactions around issues such as sexuality, dependency, and shame that may be extremely difficult to raise. Counselors need to be exquisitely tuned in to transference reactions clients may be experiencing.

COUNTERTRANSFERENCE

Countertransference can be viewed as counselor expectations based on past experiences, such as conflicts with significant others, that color current experiences. Counselors may also experience reactions in the context of the counseling relationship that do not fit the definition of countertransference. Yet all of these emotional reactions, whether countertransferential or not, are important and meaningful for the therapist to examine to optimize his or her clinical work. Understanding and managing reactions and countertransference is best done through supervision, by talking to colleagues, or in the therapist's own therapy.

Countertransference reactions can usefully be placed into several broad categories: those reactions pertaining to (1) disease and death, (2) sexuality and intimacy, and (3) the notion of caretaking or being taken care of (McKusick, 1988), and (4) life-styles that differ from the therapist's (e.g., injecting drug users). At the root of these countertransference reactions are deeply embedded values about sexuality, life-styles, disease, and death (Meisenhelder & La Charite, 1989).

Reactions to Sexuality and Intimacy

HIV disease has been associated with sexuality, gay men, and injecting drug users. "Indeed, to get AIDS is precisely to be revealed, in the majority of cases so far, as a member of a certain 'risk group,' a community of pariahs" (Sontag, 1989, pp. 24–25). Countertransference reactions may revolve around negative feelings about homosexuals as well as about behaviors clients may have engaged in to become infected, such as same-sex intercourse, sex with hundreds or thousands of partners, anonymous sex, prostitution, and injecting drug use. Unresolved reactions about sexuality and sexual practices may make it difficult for counselors even to explore specific sexual practices, which is highly relevant and necessary in working with clients with HIV disease (Macks, 1988).

Homophobia is another reaction that counselors may experience. Homophobia has been defined as negative attitudes toward gays and lesbians that are based on prejudice and arise from fear or dislike of homosexuality (Martin, 1982; Morrison, 1989). Because everyone has been exposed to homophobic beliefs, it is likely that these have been internalized to some extent. This may be true for both gay and straight therapists, as demonstrated in Cadwell's (1994) study of gay therapists, who reported concerns about homophobia as a factor in identifying with gay clients with HIV.

Unexamined and unresolved emotional and attitudinal issues, such as discomfort and conflicts about men having sex with men, might compromise the counseling relationship. For example, in a study of health care workers currently caring for AIDS patients, homophobia was highly correlated with fear of contagion (O'Donnell et al., 1987). In a study of male counselors' discomfort with gay and HIV-infected clients, homophobia predicted their discomfort with gay male clients, regardless of whether they were HIV infected or not (Hayes & Gelso, 1993). However, counselors experienced greater discomfort with seropositive clients than with uninfected clients, suggesting that these reactions might be rooted in counselors' anxieties about death.

To illustrate counselor reactions to issues of sexuality from one of the cases described earlier in this chapter, Quinn's therapist sometimes felt it was all he could do not to shout at Quinn after hearing of a weekend of anonymous, unsafe sex, "What do you think you're doing? That's the sleaziest thing I've ever heard!" His therapist worked hard to get past feeling shocked about Quinn's behavior and to work with Quinn on changing that behavior and understanding how his client was seeking closeness and intimacy through sex.

Lack of knowledge about or comfort with men being intimate with men or the culture of injecting drug users can also give rise to countertransference reactions (Morrison, 1989; Sheridan & Sheridan, 1988). This can make exploring issues around intimacy, sexuality, or drug practices difficult for both the client and the counselor. Gay or lesbian counselors (although usually familiar with many of the issues that confront gays and lesbians) may struggle with whether or not to disclose their own sexual orientation to their client. They may need to examine the meaning of disclosing or not disclosing that information (Nichols, 1986). This may be particularly salient for the counselor who is HIV-positive. Hearing about how seropositive clients became infected or how they struggle to find and maintain relationships while at times avoiding disclosure and/or putting others at risk may also elicit countertransference reactions from counselors. Hearing the story of a client whose sexual history is highly similar to the counselor's can create anxiety or overidentification.

Human sexuality is taught as part of the curriculum in fewer than half of counseling and clinical psychology programs (Campos, Brasfield, & Kelly, 1989). Because HIV is in large part a sexually transmitted disease, lack of training in sexuality, as well as the counselor's unresolved conflicts around sexuality, might stimulate fears in counselors about their own sexual behaviors and antibody status. Yet exploring patterns of intimacy and sexuality, as well as frank discussions about sexual practices (e.g., condom use) that are often initiated by the therapist, are integral and essential aspects of the clinical work with clients with HIV disease.

Reactions to Other Ways of Living

As discussed in the previous section, counselors often have reactions to ways of living that they are unfamiliar with or that seem dangerous or negative. This is often the case in counselors' reactions to injecting drug users. In a survey of social workers, the majority reported that they would have difficulty working with clients who continued to engage in risky behaviors (Gillman, 1991). Of those who were working with PWHIVs, only 10% felt that working with gay clients was difficult, whereas 41% viewed working with injecting drug users this way. This suggests that injecting drug users, who not only use illicit drugs but who may also engage in prostitution or trades of drugs for sex, may be viewed with strong reactions by therapists.

Reactions to Caretaking and Dependency

Clinicians enjoy the rewarding, collaborative role they experience with their clients. Their clients' gains and movement toward autonomy, individuation, intimacy, and important life roles are sources of pleasure and are intrinsically rewarding. In contrast, the client with advanced HIV disease may become increasingly dependent both psychologically and physically, thus stimulating reactions from the counselor as his or her role moves from a collaborative role to more of a caretaking role. When George suffered diarrhea in his therapist's office and the therapist had to assist him, this not only felt shameful to George but stimulated his therapist's fears of becoming dependent on others to manage everyday tasks and bodily functions.

When I teach my graduate-level seminar on psychosocial issues of HIV disease, the most prevalent "dying process" fear that my students express is the fear of becoming dependent on others to do everyday things. Their own discomfort with dependency and helplessness may cause feelings of frustration and anxiety when their clients become increasingly dependent.

Therapists may also feel helpless to intervene successfully in the psychological and physical impact of this disease (Macks, 1988). This may result in a powerful sense of professional inadequacy in their work with clients with HIV disease (Land & Harangody, 1990; Macks, 1988). The debilitating and serious nature of HIV disease may also stimulate a wish on the therapist's part to "rescue" the client (Land & Harangody, 1990).

Reactions to Disease and Death

Therapists, despite understanding how HIV is transmitted, may still have fears of contagion. This theme emerged as an issue reported by gay therapists working with gay PWHIVs in Cadwell's (1994) study of overidentification with HIV clients as well as in other clinical writings on HIV (Macks, 1988; Maloney, 1988). Why is fear of contagion such a powerful aspect of HIV disease? According to Sontag (1989), three elements add to the perception of an illness as being contagious: mystery (e.g., where did it come from?), death, and punishment (e.g., what did they do to get it?). Thus, fear of contagion represents the fear of the unknown, the unpredictable, and the uncontrollable aspects of existence (Meisenhelder & La Charite, 1989). In talking to other clinicians, many say that they intellectually do not fear contagion but that emotionally they find themselves worrying. Fear of contagion may cause counselors to avoid shaking hands with their client, to worry about touching tissues the client has used, and to wonder what to do with coffee cups the client has used. These fears, if unresolved, can create a distance between the counselor and the client (Adler & Beckett, 1989).

A dying client may stimulate feelings of helplessness because training emphasizes "cure" as the only acceptable outcome of counseling (Dunkel & Hatfield, 1986; McKusick, 1988). In fact, "forming relationships with young people who are dying" and "dealing with death and dying issues" were the items most often mentioned as being difficult for social workers working with PWHIVs (Gillman, 1991). Witnessing physical and mental debilitation is also often cited as a reaction that is difficult for therapists (Gillman, 1991; Maloney, 1988). Seeing this happen to a client may also cause the counselor to feel guilty about his or her own good health (Land & Harangody, 1990; Maloney, 1988).

Therapists may also experience anxiety about the dying process and what happens, if anything, after death. Whether therapists have confronted issues about death and dying in their own lives is a common focus of the literature on countertransferential reactions to clients with life-threatening illnesses (e.g., Clarke, 1981). Explicit in these writings is the belief that therapists are better prepared to help others who are dying if they have successfully examined these issues.

A dying client may also stimulate the therapist's unresolved issues with loss as well as anticipatory grief for the loss of the relationship with the client. In a study of the relationship of therapist history of personal loss to therapist reactions to termination (in a symbolic sense, a loss of the counseling relationship), Boyer and Hoffman (1993) found that therapists with significant loss histories were more depressed at termination than were those who reported less loss in their lives. Although this study did not focus on therapist terminations with HIV-positive clients, it suggests the powerful role of the therapist's own life history in responding to clients, especially in terms of their own unresolved issues.

Stacy began counseling expressing the theme of "loss" due to her recent HIV diagnosis and her recent pregnancy loss. Her therapist, who had also suffered recent pregnancy loss and also longed for a child as did Stacy, felt very pulled by the issues of loss that were explored in their work. When Stacy's mother unexpectedly died, her therapist had a fantasy that she would adopt Stacy to protect her from further loss. Stacy had truly experienced an unusual number of losses in her young life, so the theme of loss was unusually salient and poignant in the clinical work. Yet her therapist, who was very experienced in working with PWHIVs, felt unusually pulled by the loss themes in her work with Stacy. As Stacy's health declined and it was apparent that she had developed full-blown AIDS, her therapist found counseling Stacy through the dying process more difficult than she had previously experienced with other PWHIVs.

The dying process and death also stimulate our own fears about dying. For example, a counselor might have anxiety about premature death or fears about the dying process, about having to depend on others, about loss of attractiveness and disfigurement, and about diminished life quality (e.g., loss of mental capacity, loss of body control, loss of job, and social isolation; see Bartnof, 1988; Hoelter, 1979). This might be especially salient for therapists who identify with their client along some important dimension (e.g., being gay) or who have experienced the loss of multiple clients to AIDS.

Therapists working with PWHIVs also need to examine their own beliefs about spirituality, such as God, death, and the afterlife, because these beliefs may have a powerful effect on the course of counseling (Kelly, 1985). Beliefs about God as forgiving or punishing (or that there might not be a God) may become stimulated by our clients. For example, by blaming the PWHIV for "unacceptable" behavior in the eyes of God, the therapist can continue to view God as rewarding "good" behavior. Therapists' views about God and the afterlife will also influence their ability to explore end-of-life issues and to consider rational suicide when raised by a client.

It is helpful to recall that countertransference reactions are based on deeply held values, beliefs, and conflicts about life-style, sexuality, disease, loss, and death. The stigma attached to HIV as a disease is layered on preexisting stigma and reactions that may exist toward marginalized groups (Herek & Glunt, 1988). Despite our training as therapists, we are also human beings who are shaped by social and cultural values and who are immersed in clinical issues with our seropositive clients that are complex, challenging, changeable, and poignant. Our internal reactions as therapists need to be attended to, understood, and managed so that they serve, rather than impede, our therapeutic work (Gelso & Carter, 1985).

COUNSELOR HELPLESSNESS, STRESS, AND BURNOUT

There is no other counseling issue that I can think of other than HIV disease that requires so much from therapists in so many ways. Enormous demands may be placed on one's energies as well as on one's professional skills and resources, possibly resulting in feelings of helplessness, stress, and burnout, as well as unexplored and unmanaged countertransference. AIDS-related burnout is one of the main causes of turnover and absenteeism among caregivers in AIDS/HIV agencies (*HIV Frontline*, November/December 1993b). There are few studies of counselors exploring these issues, but a study examining burnout in physicians treating PWHIVs is relevant.

In this study, Horstman and McKusick (1986) concluded that practitioner burnout was less a function of years spent working with these patients than of concentrated (percentage of time per week) exposure. Amount of time per week spent with AIDS patients also correlated with depression and overwork. This suggests that an important contributor to burnout is experiencing difficulties in emotionally or physically separating from an intense situation.

A related phenomenon is called "helper helplessness syndrome" (Horstman & McKusick, 1986) and is caused by feelings of helplessness, depression, and anxiety as a result of working with dying patients. Physicians who worked with HIV patients and identified themselves as gay were more likely to report increased anxiety, overwork, and fear of death than were heterosexual physicians who worked with HIV patients. The researchers concluded that this was due to the gay physicians' perceptions of being at risk for HIV as well as overidentification with their gay patients. It is possible that some of the physicians were sero-positive and may have reacted strongly to seeing the progression of the disease in others. The women physicians reported being less personally threatened by AIDS and felt less stress than did the men. One could speculate that most of these women believed that they were seronegative and perceived their future risk of infection to be low.

This study is important because it highlights an aspect of HIV disease that differentiates it from other diseases—the high fatality rate and the impact of that on the caregiver. Within years of treating his first patient with HIV, an empathic and skilled internist I know found nearly his entire practice consisting of patients dying from this disease. He had entered medical school excited about the possibilities of medicine to "cure" in the traditional sense of the word. Entering his waiting room day after day and seeing dying young men became so difficult for him to handle emotionally that he abruptly moved his practice to an area with a very low incidence of HIV.

I do not think that this example reflects an indifference to or devaluing of working with patients with HIV. Rather, it reflects the struggle many health care providers face when what they envisioned to be their work with patients is threatened too often or when they find that they cannot emotionally cope with or escape the demands of the situation. After only 8 months of counseling with PWHIVs, Fritz described feeling "an overwhelming sense of numbness, isolation and separation because death had become a constant companion" (in *HIV Frontline*, November/December 1993b, p. 4). For some practitioners, HIV is not only the focus of their professional life, but is present in their personal life. Experiencing HIV as an unremitting thrust of one's professional or personal life can lead to feeling overburdened and to experiencing burnout.

There are several ways that counselors might avoid burnout. As a first step, acknowledging the emotional and physical demands and stresses created by work with PWHIVs is important. Colleagues and other professionals are an essential part of this process. Nichols (1986) suggests being involved in some type of support therapy (formal or informal). It is especially helpful to talk to other professionals about coping with loss and death and to explore how our own issues are contributing to stress in our work. Individual therapy and supervision are also helpful in this process. Horstman and McKusick (1986) found that many of the physicians in their sample (65%) coped by teaching others about AIDS. By reshifting some of the focus of how one works with HIV, such as, from working only with clients to including training or research, one can contribute in a way that feels emotionally more balanced.

SUMMARY

HIV disease leads to some complex therapeutic issues that can impact the counseling relationship. These include (1) rethinking typical therapeutic goals; (2) changing the boundaries of the therapeutic relationship; (3) understanding and working through transference and countertransference issues that are stimulated by HIV; and (4) counselor helplessness, stress, and burnout. Successful management of these issues makes the counseling relationship a powerful vehicle for helping clients with HIV disease.

Although events in our clients' lives are often painful and difficult, we can use the counseling relationship to help them understand and manage their reactions to what is occurring. The support, hope, and opportunities for exploration and mastery provided by the counseling relationship help clients ask questions such as "How am I going to deal with this?" and "What can I learn from this?" rather than simply "Why is this happening?"

CHAPTER 15

Multicultural Considerations in Counseling Persons with HIV Disease

> Being black and being a woman, I been on the outside looking in my whole life. Now that I got to deal with this AIDS thing, I'm even way beyond the outside. I went and tried one of those groups to talk about my situation, but that was no good cause I'm not gay, I don't use needles, I'm not white. . . . I just couldn't relate.
>
> —SELMA, *a 29-year-old, HIV-positive, African American woman*

Broadly defined, multiculturalism acknowledges the importance of cultural variables such as demographics (e.g., race, gender, age), status (e.g., social, economic), ethnography (e.g., ethnicity, religion), and affiliations (formal and informal) in working with all clients (Pedersen, 1991). Specifically, race and ethnicity, gender and sexual orientation, age, socioeconomic status, and subculture affiliations have emerged as important multicultural variables to consider when counseling HIV-infected clients.

A multicultural perspective is essential in working with HIV-infected clients because this epidemic has been defined by cultural variables that are linked to private, intimate behaviors (Hoffman, 1993). This is true both in terms of the transmission of the virus and in the psychosocial issues that have emerged. Consequently, multicultural issues often define the types of concerns that clients bring to counseling. Selma, quoted above, felt isolated because she knew no other African American women with HIV disease. She worried about her rapidly declining health, who would take care of her young daughter if she got sicker or died, and how she would pay for food, housing, and medical bills when she was no longer able to work at her low-paying job. Her initial attempts to get counseling and other HIV-related services left her feeling even more alone and alienated from the mainstream. Selma was eventually successful in finding counseling services that reflected the multicultural variables that in part defined her experience of living with HIV disease. Considering multicultural issues strengthens the therapeutic relationship and enhances the effectiveness of counseling interventions.

Complex cultural issues that have long existed in our country and that been intensified by this epidemic are reflected in the demographics of AIDS cases to date in the United States. Understanding what these demographics reflect about the lives of PWHIVs is important for counselors. Figure 3 shows that of all AIDS cases to date, 53% have resulted from men who have sex with men, 25% from injecting drug use (including both female and male heterosexual), 6% from men who have sex with men and inject drugs, and 7% from heterosexual contact (Centers for Disease Control and Prevention, 1995). Race has also defined this epidemic, as African Americans (29%) and Latinos (17%) have comprised 46% of cases in males and 75% of cases in females (54% and 21%, respectively) as well as 79% of pediatric cases (Centers for Disease Control and Prevention, 1995). Many of these persons are also economically disadvantaged (Fullilove, 1989) and are likely to find their financial situation even more precarious as their health deteriorates.

Whereas the first "wave" of HIV infection in the United States primarily affected gay men, the second wave, which has included many injecting drug users (both men and women), has disproportionately affected African Americans as well as Latinos. More recently, an increasing proportion of heterosexual men and women who are partners of injecting drug users has become infected, with the overwhelming majority being African American and Latino (Centers for Disease Control and Prevention, 1995).

These statistics underscore the importance and necessity of considering multicultural variables in clinical work with HIV-infected clients. Although there is some universality in terms of the impact of HIV disease on the individual (e.g., a chronic, progressive disease that carries stigma), and often some universality when HIV-positive persons share specific cultural variables (e.g., being a gay man, being African American), there is also great diversity that reflects the unique experiences of each person. The challenge for therapists is recognizing and addressing cultural variables in a way that acknowledges the individual's unique experiences within his or her social and cultural context.

OVERVIEW OF HIV LITERATURE FROM A MULTICULTURAL PERSPECTIVE

The HIV literature on gender, sexual orientation, race, age, affiliations (e.g., injecting drug use), and socioeconomic status highlights the effects these variables have on psychosocial responses to HIV disease and points to the need to consider multicultural issues in clinical work. For

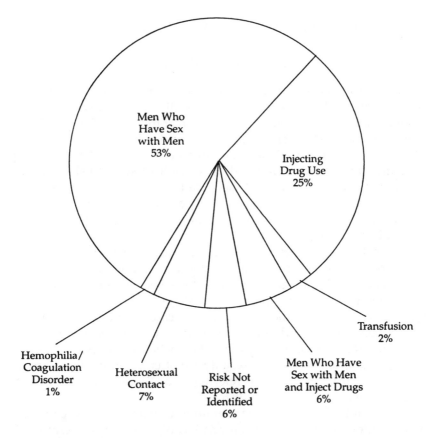

FIGURE 3. Cumulative AIDS cases for adolescents and adults (males and females) in the United States by mode of transmission through 1994.

example, variables such as sexual orientation and ethnicity affect multiple aspects of the client's life, including interpersonal support, access to HIV-related support services, and discrimination and stigma.

This review of the literature on multicultural aspects of HIV disease is not exhaustive. Rather, transmission variables and psychosocial responses that are especially influenced by a social and cultural context will be emphasized. Just as ignoring multicultural variables can be problematic in clinical work with PWHIVs, so too can attending to these issues in a way that is stereotypical and that misses the unique perspective of each client's life situation and meaning-system. What is most helpful is being aware of the importance of cultural variables in shaping the lives of all people and exploring the cultural variables that are most important and centrally defining for the client.

GENDER AND SEXUAL ORIENTATION

Gay/Bisexual Men

Gender and sexual orientation have been major defining variables for this epidemic in the United States. Nearly all of the early cases of AIDS involved homosexual/bisexual men. Even at this time, Figure 4 shows that the majority of current cases (68%) and deaths from AIDS involve this group (Centers for Disease Control and Prevention, 1995). Most of these men have become infected as a result of sexual behaviors (as opposed to injecting drug use). Because the majority of the literature presented in this book has been primarily based on the responses of gay men to HIV disease, only a few of the more salient cultural issues for gay men will be discussed.

From the beginning, HIV disease in the United States has been associated with the sexual behaviors of gay men. Consequently, homophobia and a backlash against gay men have been defining reactions to this epidemic. As a result, many gay men have contended with homophobic reactions from others, and, in some cases, with their own internalized homophobia and oppression that may resurface as a result of acquiring HIV disease. Feelings that they believed had been resolved about sexual orientation and sexuality are often recapitulated. Resolution of these feelings has been referred to as "coming out as a PWA [person with AIDS]" (Nichols, 1986, p. 212).

This epidemic has also had profound effects on how gay men manage interpersonal and sexual relationships. The HIV literature is replete with studies on changes in sexual behaviors (e.g., condom use, fewer partners, closing of bathhouses) in response to the high rate of infection in many parts of the country. Although many studies present encouraging results about changes in attitudes and behaviors that have led to significant decreases in unsafe sexual practices in this population, a small but significant percentage of gay men continue to engage in highly risky sexual activities (Ekstrand & Coates, 1990). This high-risk group is comprised mostly of younger gay men, and a disturbing trend has been reported in recent literature suggesting that the rate of infection in young gay men is once again on the rise.

This trend among gay men portends the difficulties that challenge efforts to contain the epidemic. It is extremely difficult for many individuals, as well as communities, to make and maintain behavioral and attitudinal changes that involve social, cultural, and interpersonal aspects, as does HIV transmission. However, as Leigh and Stall (1993) note,

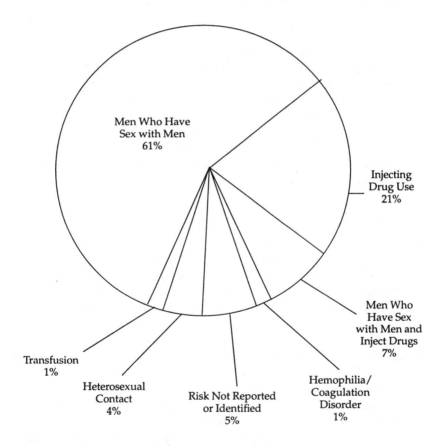

FIGURE 4. Cumulative AIDS cases for males (adolescents and adults) in the United States by mode of transmission through 1994.

most of this research is based on convenience samples in HIV epicenters such as San Francisco. Much less is known about the impact of HIV on gay men in smaller cities and rural areas, and about the impact of HIV on patterns of intimacy such as monogamy and the importance of sex within the context of the overall relationship. This is an important area for future research.

Finally, many HIV-infected gay men (and gay men in general) have experienced what has been referred to as AIDS-related bereavement. Multiple bereavements often occur at the same time that HIV-positive gay men are contending with their own sense of loss due to their disease. As discussed in an earlier chapter, this bereavement has had a major impact on the social support systems and community structures of many gay men. The large numbers of deaths in communities such as San Francisco has also caused some gay men to feel fatalistic about this epidemic and their own ability to make and maintain the necessary changes.

Compared with other groups, the gay community has committed considerable resources to providing educational, medical, and psychosocial services to address this epidemic. In some cases, these efforts have unified both gay men and lesbian women across racial, gender, and class lines. At the same time, many gay men of color experience racism in white organizations and homophobia in their communities of color (Ostrow et al., 1989). Although they may have a primary identity with one community over the other, they may often feel that they do not truly fit in this community.

Common Themes in Counseling Gay Men

Gay men with HIV disease often present the following themes in counseling: (1) experiencing stigmatization or discrimination from others because of homophobia as well as reactions to HIV; (2) finding that nonrecognition (legal or from friends or family) of their partner leads to discrimination in terms of hospital privileges, insurance, burial decisions, and the like; (3) experiencing their own internalized homophobia, in many cases intensified by becoming seropositive; (4) coping with the death of a partner or lover; (5) rejection by a partner or lover because of their HIV disease; (6) difficulties making changes in initiating and maintaining intimate relationships post-HIV diagnosis; (7) loss of support network due to deaths of friends and acquaintances; (8) isolation and loneliness; (9) estrangement from potential sources of support, such as family of origin; (10) loss of material support, such as job and health insurance; (11) loss of physical health or attractiveness; (12) the need to leave a legacy or feel that their life matters; (13) wanting to reconcile aspects of their lives with religion or spirituality; and (14) not wanting the remainder of life to be defined by HIV-related activism simply because they are gay.

Common Resources and Barriers to Resources

Typically, gay men (particularly white gay men) (1) have greater access to HIV-specific psychosocial and medical resources including clinical trials than do other populations affected by HIV; (2) are better understood in terms of their responses to HIV because of the extensive body of research on this population covering all aspects of HIV; (3) have greater support and acceptance of their HIV disease in their community (if they have a primary or strong identification with the gay community); (4) have greater awareness than other groups of legal rights and legal documents (e.g., living wills, advance directives); and (5) have more "rituals" to achieve a sense of meaning and legacy regarding their disease (e.g., Names Project, AIDS benefit walks, planning one's funeral).

In terms of barriers, many gay men experience (1) legal and interpersonal barriers to having their relationship with a partner or life partner recognized; (2) discrimination from medical/professional caregivers because of stigma due to both homophobia and HIV disease; (3) a lack of access to resources outside the gay community because of homophobia; (4) estrangement from family of origin, and fear of discrimination; (5) little access to HIV-specific services in smaller towns and rural areas; (6) and, for many gay men of color, the experience of racism from services that seem designed for white men.

Women

Women, as a group, represent the fastest growing category of new HIV cases in this country. As a group, lesbians have the lowest rate of infection via sexual transmission, but are represented among injecting drug users. At present, women comprise about 13% of persons with AIDS and over 30% of new cases. Until recently, the majority of women with HIV became infected through injecting drug use. However, Figure 5 shows that the proportion infected through heterosexual contact has recently increased to about 36% (Centers for Disease Control and Prevention, 1995). In contrast, the proportion of women infected through injecting drug use is 48% and the mode of transmission is unknown or unreported for 11% (many of these women are assumed to be infected through heterosexual contact) of women. The Centers for Disease Control and Prevention lists only one risk category per person, so it is difficult to accurately assess the mode of transmission in women since injecting drug users are often sexually active, leaving open the possibility of an even greater rate of heterosexual transmission.

It is difficult to understand the issues that most HIV-infected women face without also examining the impact of race, sex, social class, and poverty (Bell, 1989). The majority of HIV-infected women in the United States are African American or Latina (Centers for Disease Control and Prevention, 1995). Research suggests that nearly 90% of these women have dependent children (Levine & Dubler, 1990). In most cases, these women are single parents, and many have also lost their husband or partner to AIDS. Because of the difficulties coping with debilitating health and single parenthood, most of these women are also struggling with poverty.

Interestingly, little of the literature on HIV-infected women has

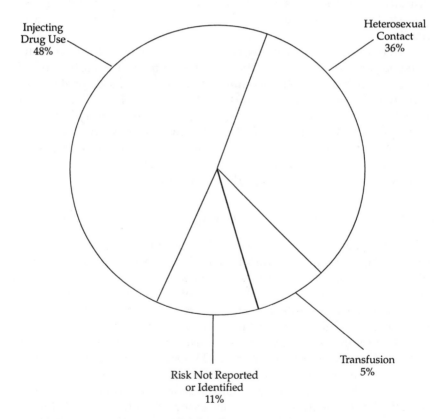

FIGURE 5. Cumulative AIDS cases for females (adolescents and adults) in the United States through 1994.

focused on the impact of the disease on the woman herself (i.e., as the literature on gay men has), but rather on her role as a disease vector or transmitter of the disease to others as well as on the related issue of whether she should bear children (Levine & Dubler, 1990).

In responding to this issue, Dr. James Curran of the Centers for Disease Control AIDS program commented: "Someone who understands the disease and is logical will not want to be pregnant and will consider the test results when making family planning decisions" (*CDC AIDS Weekly*, 1988, p. 2). A philosopher, responding to this issue, asked, "What kind of moral universe do these women live in, anyway?" (in Levine & Dubler, 1990, p. 322). These quotes imply that the decision-making process women with HIV engage in regarding pregnancy or continuing a pregnancy is logically and clearly defined. What the comments ignore are the values and norms that direct women's sexual and reproductive lives as well as the social, economic, and cultural forces that contribute to these norms (Levine & Dubler, 1990).

To understand these forces, a more complex understanding of the role of childbearing in women's lives is important. Childbearing is valued across cultures and can be viewed as a theme that unifies women of diverse backgrounds. For many women, motherhood may provide one of the most important, or one of the few, avenues for self-definition, esteem, and a link to the future. Social class and ethnicity also play an important role in understanding this issue, as these cultural issues in part define attitudes about childbearing (Levine & Dubler, 1990). Finally, having a child is often viewed by HIV-infected women as a powerful incentive to make a commitment to the future in such ways as giving up drug use or leaving a legacy.

What are the risks that women with HIV face in transmitting the virus to their unborn children? Until recently, the risk of maternal transmission was about 25–30%. A recent study administering AZT to HIV-infected women and then to their infants found that this resulted in a transmission rate of just 8%, as compared with a rate of 26% among the placebo group (Centers for Disease Control, 1994). It is important to note that at this time, most pregnant women with HIV disease do not receive AZT during their pregnancy, so their rate of transmission is much higher. Babies born to women with HIV are born with the mother's antibodies, and the baby's own serostatus cannot be known with certainty until he or she is about 15 months old. This creates stress and uncertainty about the baby's serostatus for a lengthy period of time.

There is a paucity of psychosocial research on the impact of HIV on the woman herself. What is known is that women with HIV are more likely than men with HIV to be unemployed, to have sole responsibility for children, to be a member of an ethnic minority group, and to have few HIV-specific supports available (Gentry, 1993). Women have also been underrepresented in clinical trials for a variety of reasons, such as their potential to become pregnant during the experimental protocol. P. J. Kelly (1993) also described a number of other social and cultural factors that often lead to the underrepresentation of women in HIV clinical trials: social barriers (e.g., sexism, socioeconomic problems), institutional barriers (lack of meaningful incentives, child care, convenient scheduling), and personal barriers (being primary caregiver, transportation, cultural beliefs). Further, until the Centers for Disease Control and Prevention's recent change in the definition of AIDS, many women did not meet the criteria for AIDS, which were based on earlier cases that primarily included men.

It is apparent that women with HIV disease face an array of issues that most seropositive men do not, such as coping with dependent children, concern and guilt about bearing an HIV-infected child as well as physically caring for that child, and concern about leaving their children when they become sick and die. Concerns for the welfare of dependents often occur at the same time that these women are struggling with the physical and emotional effects of their own illness.

Common Themes in Counseling Women

Women with HIV disease often present with the following concerns: (1) experiencing sadness about the possibility of not becoming a mother; (2) feeling guilty and worried about having transmitted HIV to their children, or worrying that they will do so; (3) experiencing concern about what will happen to their children if they die; (4) dealing with stress due to caretaking of others when their own health is declining; (5) feeling isolated from others with HIV; (6) lacking material resources, such as money and housing; (7) lacking access (due to personal, institutional, or social barriers) to HIV-specific psychosocial and medical resources; (8) lacking adequate social support; (9) losing a husband or partner to AIDS; (10) wanting to make or remake a religious or spiritual connection; (11) experiencing multiple sources of powerlessness or oppression due to gender, ethnicity, and/or poverty; and (12) needing substance abuse treatment.

Common Resources and Barriers to Resources

Women routinely report few resources to assist in coping with HIV. Some women report the following resources: (1) spiritual beliefs reflected through activities such as prayer, (2) religious institutions, such as churches, and (3) family support (including children).

In contrast, women experience a number of barriers to HIV resources, including (1) difficulties in obtaining and maintaining HIV-specific psychosocial and medical services due to institutional, personal, and social barriers (lack of child care, perception that services are for gay men); (2) lack of financial resources, including adequate income and health insurance; (3) not having a primary care physician, as economically impoverished women often rely on services such as emergency rooms; (4) day-to-day issues, such as inadequate housing and child care that interfere with HIV care being a top priority; (5) fears of stigma and discrimination if their HIV status becomes known in their community; and (6) little awareness of the issues that HIV-positive lesbian women face and very few services specifically for this group.

Heterosexual Men

Gender issues also play a significant role for HIV-infected heterosexual men. However, there is a dearth of research on these seropositive males, other than those who are injecting drug users and hemophiliacs. The focus of the research on men who inject drugs is on their substance use and transmission risk to others rather than on the impact of HIV on the man himself. Most noteworthy is the lack of literature examining how HIV impacts the sexual identity and gender roles of this group of men. Men who became HIV-positive through having sex with women comprise 4% of AIDS cases, and heterosexual men who acquired this disease through injecting drug use represent 21% of cases (Centers for Disease Control and Prevention, 1995). It is not known what proportion of this latter group became infected through their drug use or through sexual activities.

Based on my clinical work with heterosexual men who do not inject drugs, most report feeling isolated because they do not know any other HIV-infected persons. They frequently express concerns that they will be labeled as "gay" or as "IV drug users" if others discover their HIV status. For these reasons, they may be reluctant to seek support services, such as groups, and in many cases are unwilling or uncomfortable seeking services offered at clinics that serve a primarily gay clientele. Additionally, 71% of men infected through heterosexual contact are African American, which suggests that research and interventions are needed that address the needs of these men.

Based on interviews with a small sample (10) of HIV-positive heterosexual men, a surprising consistency was noted when they were asked to describe their present and future goals in terms of how HIV had affected these goals (Hoffman & Driscoll, 1993). Almost every man (8 of 10) used nearly the same phrase, "One goal that has been shattered is getting married, having the house, the white picket fence, the kids" (a 39-year-old African American man). Interestingly, the phrase "white picket fence" was used by most of these men and seemed to be a metaphor for "traditional family life." Often what seems to emerge when people struggle with HIV is their sense of loss over the life role or roles that were most defining of who they are or had hoped to be, and that now seem to be most threatened.

Common Themes in Counseling Heterosexual Men

Heterosexual men with HIV disease often present with the following concerns: (1) feeling isolated because they know few or no men who became infected this way (this is especially true for those who are not injecting drug users); (2) worrying that others will think that they are gay because they have HIV; (3) worrying that people will think they got HIV from injecting drug use; (4) worrying that they will not be able to find a girlfriend or wife because of HIV; (5) needing to learn how to initiate and maintain relationships with women, given their HIV status; (6) feeling sad because they will likely never have their own children; (7) telling few people, if anyone, of their status out of fear of stigmatization; (8) lacking access to HIV-specific resources directed toward heterosexual men; and (9) worrying that they will not be able to achieve the career and financial goals for which they had hoped; and (10) in some cases needing substance abuse treatment before they can address managing HIV disease.

Common Resources and Barriers to Resources

In contrast to heterosexual women with HIV, heterosexual HIV-positive men typically report (1) greater access to material resources (e.g., jobs, health insurance) and (2) fewer responsibilities (than women) as a primary caretaker to dependents, which allows them more time and energy to devote to managing their disease.

However, this group of men encounters a number of barriers to obtaining HIV-related resources, including (1) difficulties obtaining HIV-specific psychosocial and medical services due to institutional, social, and personal barriers (e.g., viewing services as being designed for gay men, fear of stigmatization and discrimination) and (2) fears of stigmatization and discrimination if their HIV disease becomes known to others in their community.

RACE/ETHNICITY

African Americans and Latinos are overrepresented in AIDS cases in the United States in all categories: among homosexual/bisexual men, among injecting drug users, among women, and among children (Centers for Disease Control and Prevention, 1995). Figures 6 and 7 show how African American and Latino men and women are disproportionately represented by AIDS cases in the United States. This translates to an estimated cumulative incidence of AIDS cases reported in 1991 per 100,000 persons of 31.4 for African Americans and 41.5 for Latinos as compared with 11.7 for whites (both Asians/Pacific Islanders and Native Americans/Alaskan Natives at present have relatively low rates of infection and will not be included in this discussion). Although these

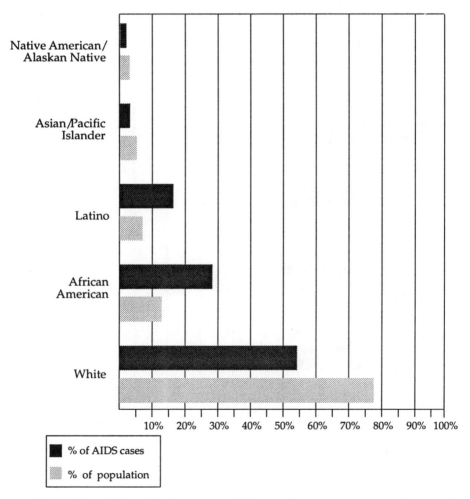

FIGURE 6. Male AIDS cases and United States population by race/ethnicity.

statistics point to a high rate of infection for African Americans and
Latinos, it is unclear what factors are responsible for this disproportionate rate (Wyatt, 1991).

Some have speculated that factors such as poverty, alienation, and
boredom may be related to the initiation and maintenance of drug use
(Friedman, Des Jarlais, & Sterk, 1990). These factors might account in
part for the high rate of HIV infection in injecting drug users of color.
Others have suggested that African American and Latino communities
differ from gay communities, which have provided the model for re-

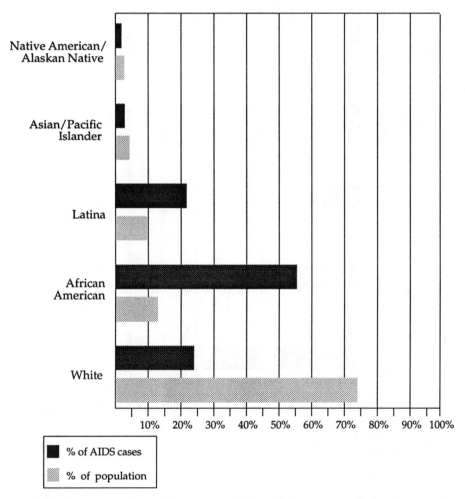

FIGURE 7. Female AIDS cases and United States population by race/
ethnicity.

sponsiveness to HIV, in terms of social class and access to resources relevant to both prevention and treatment (Freudenberg, Lee, & Silver, 1989).

Less access to health care and other HIV-related services also differentiates African Americans from whites. In a review of studies comparing survival time between African Americans and whites, conflicting results were found, although most studies found that whites survived longer (Curtis & Patrick, 1993). These results are suggestive of differences in socioeconomic status and access to health care, as African Americans were not consistently shown to have lower survival time (which would have suggested biological differences).

Several HIV-related issues specific to African American and Latina women were previously discussed. Two additional issues often arise when counseling HIV-positive African American or Latino clients: what it is like to be an HIV-positive gay or bisexual man in a community of color, and the experience of some clients of color that HIV disease is not the most pressing issue they are dealing with in the context of their overall life situation.

There is a large body of literature on the psychosocial issues of HIV-infected gay men. In actuality, the majority of this literature examines the experiences of white gay men. Because gay and bisexual men frequently divide into subgroups along racial lines (Williams, 1986), much of the research on HIV-infected gay men may not reflect the experience of minority gay men. These men may have a stronger tie to their ethnic community than to what they view as the primarily white gay community (Ostrow et al., 1989).

Researchers have speculated that this lack of identification with the gay community is due to a variety of factors. For example, this division may result from differences in the acceptance of being gay in an individual's subculture (Dalton, 1989; Williams, 1986), from the ethnic minority gay man's own level of self-awareness in the coming-out process (Morales, 1990), and from racism. Some Latinos define homosexuality by the role the man plays in the sexual encounter rather than by same-sex partner choice alone. For example, the partner who is penetrated is viewed as feminine and therefore homosexual (Gonzalez, 1995).

Socioeconomic differences may also be a factor (De La Cancela, 1989; Freudenberg et al., 1989). From a counseling perspective, often an important difference between ethnic minority and white gay men is the primary community with which they identify. For example, gay Latino men may have a primary identification with their ethnic community and may view a gay identity as representing a white political movement rather than a sexual preference (Morales, 1990).

Race may also play a role in determining the relative importance of

HIV disease in the context of the individual's life situation. For many African American and Latina women, the place that HIV occupies in their hierarchy of daily needs and demands is especially important to consider. Many of these women also struggle with other serious problems such as poverty, additional health problems, lack of health insurance, unemployment, and housing (Cohen, Hauer, & Wofsy, 1989). A disease that may claim their lives in the distant future of 5 to 10 years may not seem as pressing or urgent as these other issues, which intrude sharply on the present. This is especially true for HIV-infected persons who are addicted to substances, the majority of whom are African Americans or Latinos. The urgency of an addiction is likely to dominate one's life on a day-to-day basis to a greater extent than concern about one's HIV status. What this literature suggests is that race is often confounded with substance use and socioeconomic impoverishment for many African Americans and Latinos who are HIV-positive.

Finally, members of groups other than gay men are often unaware of their HIV status until they become symptomatic or have to take an antibody test for reasons such as pregnancy or entering the military. This is illustrated by the results of a study of seroprevalence in an urban African American cohort in the New York City area (Brunswick et al., 1993). This group was not selected because of high-risk behaviors. An alarming 8.4% of the sample were found to be seropositive, with men having 1.8 times the infection rate of women.

Several things are important and striking about this study. The majority of both men and women were unaware and unsuspecting of their seropositive status, and the male–female ratio was much closer than the ratio reported for actual AIDS cases in African Americans in the same city. One can conclude that current AIDS case reports seriously underestimate HIV infection among some African Americans, especially women, and that widespread ignorance about one's infection status and level of risk can contribute greatly to transmission rates in this population. The results of this study also show the need for prevention interventions for groups who do not perceive themselves as being at risk for HIV disease.

Common Themes in Counseling
Racial Minority PWHIVs

Minority PWHIVs often bring the following concerns to counseling: (1) feeling oppression, stigmatization, or discrimination because of their race as well as their HIV status; (2) experiencing a lack of acceptance and understanding of their disease in their community; (3) for gay men, experiencing a sense of racism from the white gay community and a lack of acceptance of homosexuality from one's minority community; (4)

lacking access to material resources (e.g., jobs, health care, housing); (5) viewing family as the most important source of social support; (6) worrying that HIV has affected the support structure of their family of origin because of multiple HIV-related deaths or rejection due to HIV; (7) distrusting the medical establishment; (8) worrying that HIV may be a government-based attempt at genocide against certain groups of people; and (9) viewing religion as a source of support.

Common Resources and Barriers to Resources

African American and Latino PWHIVs are more likely to perceive barriers to HIV resources rather than access. However, in HIV epicenters, there are an increasing number of HIV-related services that meet the medical, social, and cultural needs of these groups.

Barriers to HIV-related services often include (1) difficulties receiving HIV-specific medical and psychosocial services due to institutional, personal, and social barriers; (2) barriers to HIV-specific resources, including logistical barriers, psychosocial barriers, and cultural barriers (e.g., distrust of traditional medical establishment; not having a primary care physician); (3) not self-identifying as a gay or bisexual man and therefore not getting appropriate services; (4) lack of material resources, such as adequate income, housing, and health insurance; (5) lack of adequate access to addiction treatment services; (6) relatively low participation in research studies and clinical trials, resulting in less being known about this group of PWHIVs; and (7) experiencing multiple sources of stigmatization due to HIV, ethnicity, injecting drug use, and/or poverty.

INJECTING DRUG USERS

In some HIV epicenters such as New York City, over half of the injecting drug users are estimated to be HIV-positive. Injecting drug users often come to counseling with multiple psychosocial concerns because they are contending with both an addiction and with HIV disease. For example, their risk of transmission to others can be either through unsafe drug practices or unsafe sexual practices, so interventions need to address both areas. Addictions may cause difficulties in many other aspects of these PWHIVs' lives, including transmission to spouses/partners and children, inability to maintain a stable job, poverty, estrangement from significant others, and inability to focus constructively on making health-promoting changes.

Contrasting injecting drug users to other groups of PWHIVs, Newmeyer (1990) concluded that this group had a shorter life expectancy, fewer self-help programs, widespread infection of partners and children, a disproportionate representation of African Americans and Latinos, and marginalization due to the combination of HIV, drug use, ethnicity, and poverty.

Injecting drug users are probably underestimated among those with both HIV disease and full-blown AIDS. For example, it is likely that many of them die from other causes such as drug overdose and other illnesses before HIV runs its course (Newmeyer, 1990). Because many injecting drug users who are HIV-positive appear to be unaware of their serostatus, the risk of their transmitting the virus to others is greater. This is illustrated by a study of male and female injecting drug users entering treatment at two methadone clinics in California (Reardon et al., 1993). Thirteen percent of the sample was HIV-positive, of which 45% were unaware of their status. There were no significant differences in the percentages of men and women infected. However, 37% of African Americans and 8% of Latinos were infected, as compared with 3% of whites. Although African Americans had the highest infection rate, they were 3 times less likely to know they were infected. Interestingly, all homosexual/bisexual injecting drug users in this sample who were HIV-positive were aware of their antibody status. This suggests that many groups of persons, other than gay men, are unaware and often unsuspecting of their positive antibody status.

Common Themes in Counseling Injecting Drug Users

Injecting drug users often present for counseling with the following themes: (1) wanting treatment first for their addiction, rather than for HIV; (2) needing counseling services directed at dual or multiple diagnoses (e.g., addiction, affective, or personality disorders, HIV); (3) lacking compliance and commitment to counseling if addiction is untreated; (4) lacking material resources such as adequate income, housing, health insurance; (5) feeling that HIV services often fail to adequately address their addiction and that addiction services often fail to address their HIV adequately; (6) estrangement from family, including family of origin; (7) losing custody of children due to addiction; and (8) losing social support due to HIV-related deaths of partner/spouse, children, and friends.

Common Resources and Barriers to Resources

Although many injecting drug users have access to addiction treatment services, a common barrier is that these services are often inadequate to serve all people seeking services. Other barriers to HIV-related resources include the following: (1) addiction services often do not adequately address HIV-related needs; (2) community agencies are often conflicted about how HIV-positive injecting drug users are best served (drug treatment clinics or HIV-focused clinics); (3) HIV-positive injecting drug users may perceive a lack of access to medical and psychosocial HIV-related services due to institutional, personal, and cultural variables (e.g., not being motivated to address addiction); and (4) addiction may dominate life so that HIV concerns are often not addressed until addiction is managed.

ADOLESCENTS/YOUNG ADULTS

Most people with HIV contract the disease when they are young—in their teens, 20s, and 30s. This means that they may miss out on many aspects of the developmental tasks of adolescence and young adulthood. This is especially salient for people who acquire the disease and learn that they are HIV-positive during their teens and early 20s. Adolescence is typically a time for developing one's own identity through the process of exploring various vocational, sexual, moral, and political paths (Elliott, 1993). Peers and peer acceptance become the primary source of identification and approval. Adolescents may have less impulse control at the same time that they perceive themselves to be immortal, resulting in greater risk taking (Elliott, 1993). Learning one is seropositive can disrupt this important and necessary exploration.

Cases of AIDS in adolescents and young adults (13 to 24 years of age) represent 4% of cases in adolescents/men and 7% in adolescents/women (Centers for Disease Control and Prevention, 1995). Because PWHIVs usually develop AIDS 7 to 10 years after initial infection, many persons with AIDS in the 25- to 29-year-old age group likely acquired HIV during their teens and early 20s. This means that about 18% of men with HIV and 24% of women became seropositive in their teens or early 20s.

It is also helpful to look at gender, modes of transmission, and race/ethnicity in adolescents and young adults with AIDS. For example, 76% of cases in this age group are males (Centers for Disease Control and Prevention, 1995). For this group, 64% became infected from having sex with men; 13% from injecting drug use, and 11% from both. Only 3% report heterosexual contact as their only risk variable. In contrast, 49% of females became HIV-positive from heterosexual contact and 34% from injecting drug use. In terms of race/ethnicity, African Americans and Latinos are disproportionately represented. For males with AIDS in this age group, 53% are African American or Latino (Centers for Disease Control and Prevention, 1995). For females, 75% are African American or Latina. These statistics suggest that the cultural variables of gender, race/ethnicity, and mode of transmission are important to consider when counseling adolescents and young adults.

Data from Job Corps, which has screened all residential students entering the program since 1987, provides one important picture of seropositive rates (as opposed to actual AIDS cases) in adolescents (in this population, ages 16 to 21; St. Louis et al., 1991). Overall, the seroprevalence rate in both males and females entering the Job Corps was about 10 times higher than that of same-age applicants for the military. Rates were slightly higher for males versus females and more than twice as high in African American students as in white students. Rates were also more than double in urban versus rural areas. These rates are striking for several reasons: They are quite high; rates in males and females show a very different pattern than Centers for Disease Control and Prevention statistics for AIDS cases; and African American students show much higher rates than do white students. Although the Job Corps is a federal training program for economically disadvantaged, out-of-school youth, it is the only program that routinely screens a national sample of youth for HIV and therefore provides valuable data on infection rates. Rates are higher in this group of adolescents and young adults than in military recruits and college students. However, other groups of adolescents, such as runaways and crack addicts, likely have even higher rates.

What are the variables that put adolescents at risk for acquiring HIV disease? This question was examined in a study of high school students in urban and suburban New York City, an AIDS epicenter (Walter, Vaughan, & Cohall, 1991). Although the HIV status of the respondents was not known, 28% engaged in risky behaviors such as inconsistent or no condom use and multiple sexual partners. Additionally, 79% reported using alcohol, cigarettes, and/or marijuana, which can affect immune functioning. Additionally, alcohol and marijuana were often paired with sex, reducing the likelihood of safer sex practices.

This study of adolescent risk factors supports the findings of a study examining the characteristics of HIV-infected adolescents participating in a New York City program addressing AIDS (Futterman, Hein, Reuben, Dell, & Shaffer, 1993). Respondents in this study were predominantly African American and Latino. Both infected and uninfected adolescents engaged in many HIV-risky behaviors, such as substance use and unsafe sex. The vast majority of HIV-positive males reported having sex with other males, although many did not see themselves as gay. Some of this behavior was in exchange for drugs or for money to get drugs.

In contrast, most of the girls identified heterosexual intercourse as their only known exposure, but were very unaware of the specific risk behaviors of their partners. Consistent condom use among this group of adolescents with HIV was rare. Nearly half of the females reported more than 50 lifetime partners, and nearly half of the males reported 10 to 50 partners. Most striking, only 12% of the females and 30% of the males informed sexual partners of their HIV status.

Although this study was based on an urban sample of primarily ethnic minority at-risk teenagers, many of the themes have relevance for teens across the United States—inconsistent or nonexistent use of condoms, pairing alcohol and drugs with sex, multiple sexual partners, little communication with sexual partners, and reluctance to discuss HIV-positive status with partners.

Common Themes in Counseling Adolescents

Adolescents with HIV disease often present for counseling with these concerns: (1) feeling out of sync with their peers because they are dealing with HIV-related issues that are developmentally "off-time"; (2) disclosing their HIV status to peers (maintaining peer acceptance); (3) initiating intimate relationships given their HIV status; (4) feeling isolated because they know few or no peers with HIV; (5) fearing or experiencing family estrangement due to their HIV-positive status; (6) wondering how to set life goals in the context of HIV; (7) denying the significance of their HIV status; and (8) having difficulty making and maintaining changes in risky behaviors.

Common Resources and Barriers to Resources

There are few HIV-specific resources for adolescents/young adults in most towns and cities. Other barriers for this age group include (1) lacking psychological and emotional resources (including maturity) to cope with HIV; (2) finding few available HIV-related medical and psychosocial resources that are developmentally appropriate; (3) lacking material resources such as adequate income and health insurance; and (4) needing resources that address issues (in addition to HIV) such as substance abuse.

SOCIOECONOMIC STATUS

Socioeconomic status is the final multicultural variable that will be considered. AIDS cases are beginning to shift from gay, primarily middle class white men to inner-city populations, and some cultural observers have predicted that, "understanding and patience are going to dwindle across the political spectrum, to be replaced by animosity and/or indifference" (Murray, 1988, p. 22). Many inner-city persons live at or near the poverty line and are already experiencing the alienation and neglect that often accompany poverty. This underscores the importance of socioeconomic status, and specifically poverty, in understanding responses to HIV.

One in five AIDS patients has no health insurance, and of those with insurance, 40 percent are covered by Medicaid (Fineberg, 1988). The percentage of uninsured seropositive individuals is growing as the demographics of this epidemic continue to change. Increasingly, treatment of HIV is being covered by Medicaid (Jonson & Stryker, 1993). However, few studies have looked specifically at the impact of socioeconomic status on HIV antibody status or on responses to HIV. A growing body of research has linked other sexually transmitted diseases (STDs) with an enhanced likelihood of HIV transmission, most likely through lesions caused by these STDs (Anderson & May, 1992). This is especially true when sexually transmitted diseases go untreated. Socioeconomic status and access to health care likely play a role in the early treatment of STDs.

One study, which found an association between low income and HIV infection in men, explained this in terms of the link between poverty and poor health (Krueger, Wood, Diehr, & Maxwell, 1990). The study on seroprevalence in Job Corps students, discussed earlier in this chapter, also suggested a link between low socioeconomic status and HIV (St. Louis et al., 1991). Low socioeconomic status, which is often paired with less access to health and support resources, also appears to be linked to HIV survival time (Curtis & Patrick, 1993).

What is known is that quality of health care in general is linked to socioeconomic status (Ginzberg, 1991). Higher income typically correlates with having adequate health insurance as well as access to health care. Estimated lifetime cost of medical care for a seropositive person is about $40,000 to $80,000 (Bloom & Carliner, 1988; Joneson & Stryker, 1993). Thus, HIV-infected persons who do not have adequate health insurance but do not qualify for Medicaid, may have difficulty getting the medical care they need. Poverty may also lead to people feeling disenfranchised from the health care system. At the least, poverty amplifies the problems of coping with HIV disease. For a variety of reasons, socioeconomic status, and specifically poverty, will play a major defining role in both the future of the AIDS epidemic and in responses to this epidemic.

Common Themes in Counseling Economically Impoverished PWHIVs

Impoverished PWHIVs often express the following themes in counseling: (1) feeling overwhelmed by other demands of their life, which are exacerbated by lack of resources, including housing, food, child care, and transportation; (2) experiencing HIV disease as relatively low on the hierarchy of day-to-day concerns and struggles; (3) feeling abandoned by "the system," including the medical establishment; and (4) having other psychological concerns, such as addictions.

Common Barriers to Resources Experienced by Economically Disadvantaged PWHIVs

Many inner-city clinics, especially those providing STD services, offer HIV-related services for economically impoverished persons. However, this group of PWHIVs often experience many other barriers to HIV services, including: (1) lack of material resources such as adequate income and health insurance; (2) lack of resources such as transportation and child care to allow physical access to HIV services; (3) not having a relationship with a primary care physician; (4) feeling that psychosocial services such as counseling and support groups do not address their needs; and (5) viewing management of HIV as less urgent than other day-to-day demands related to survival.

SUMMARY: MULTICULTURAL FACTORS AS AN OVERARCHING FOCUS

Considering multicultural variables can inform and enhance assessment and counseling interventions with HIV-infected clients. Because HIV disease has been defined in the United States by cultural variables, the role of these variables in shaping every aspect of this epidemic should be considered when counseling clients with HIV disease. Broadly defined, multicultural variables include race/ethnicity, gender, sexual orientation, socioeconomic status, and membership in subgroups such as injecting drug users. These variables often define what it means to have HIV disease, they affect the types of concerns that PWHIVs bring to counseling, and they have implications for access to HIV-specific services.

CHAPTER 16

Ethical and Professional Issues in Counseling Persons with HIV Disease

> A therapist should not be encouraged routinely to reveal such threats . . . unless such disclosures are necessary to avert danger to others.
>
> —*Tarasoff v. Regents of the University of California* (1976, p. 347)

HIV disease has led to a myriad of ethical, moral, and professional dilemmas that often enter the therapeutic context. Some of these ethical issues, such as the PWHIV's right to treatment and the issue of confidentiality, often directly affect the therapeutic relationship. Other issues, such as the PWHIV's experience of discrimination, may become concerns that he or she wants to explore during counseling. Perhaps the issue that has received the most attention is whether or not the *Tarasoff* decision, quoted in part above, requires a therapist to warn others about an HIV-positive client. It is helpful to view these ethical issues related to HIV disease as fitting two broad themes: measures intended to protect society and measures intended to protect the individual (Manuel et al., 1990). Basically, ethical dilemmas that have occurred in response to HIV typically balance the rights of the individual versus the rights of others (or society) to protect against the spread of the disease.

OVERVIEW OF MEASURES TO PROTECT
THE INDIVIDUAL VERSUS OTHERS

According to Manuel et al. (1990), the following categories, beginning with the most coercive, fit under the theme of "measures intended to protect society":

1. Quarantine and isolation of HIV patients (to prevent spread of the disease).
2. Discriminatory measures concerning specific population groups (e.g., excluding PWHIVs from jobs, schools, or insurance coverage, or from entering borders of a country).
3. Nonrespect of the confidential nature of medical information (e.g., advising spouse or partner of patient's HIV-positive status).
4. Application of the penal code (e.g., viewing transmission of HIV as a criminal offense).
5. Screening, compulsory notification, and registration (e.g., requiring that all AIDS cases be reported, or that all instances of positive antibody tests be reported).
6. Protection of blood given for transfusion (e.g., refusal of donors with certain risk behaviors; notification of donors when they test HIV-positive).
7. Research on drugs and vaccines (e.g., therapy vs. placebo).
8. Information and education.

Measures intended to protect the individual include:

1. Right to confidentiality.
2. Right to information (e.g., about screening, aspects of the disease, and therapeutic options).
3. Right to treatment (e.g., refusal to treat).

These categories are helpful to clinicians in understanding the array of ethical issues that are posed by HIV. However, some of these issues are more likely than others to affect the work of the counselor, and these will be briefly discussed.

ETHICAL ISSUES OFTEN RAISED IN COUNSELING

Early in the epidemic it was not uncommon for PWHIVs to experience job discrimination, such as by being fired, or to be excluded from schools or training programs. This type of discrimination is less common now for several reasons. For example, more is now known about the transmission of HIV and the lack of risk from casual contact. In addition, passage of the Americans with Disabilities Act of 1990 (which became law on July 26, 1991) has limited job discrimination based on HIV status.

However, other types of discrimination are often reported by PWHIVs, such as being rejected for health and life insurance, discrimination against gays by closing bathhouses and bars, and legal nonrecognition of relationships such as life partners. This last issue is often a focus in counseling. To illustrate: Tim and Alex were life partners, had bought a house together, and had each named the other as their sole heir in their wills. When Tim, who was HIV-positive, became too ill to work, he lost his health insurance. Because his relationship with Alex was not legally recognized, he was unable to get health insurance through Alex's policy. When Tim had to be hospitalized unexpectedly, Alex was not allowed to visit him in intensive care. As soon as Tim was out of intensive care, his parents were given legal rights as his guardian and moved him to a nursing home in their hometown.

Another pervasive ethical issue that many PWHIVs contend with is being refused treatment because they have HIV disease. There are a number of studies, some of which were discussed in Chapter 3, reporting the experience of PWHIVs being refused medical and dental services. Health care providers have an ethical duty to treat people with HIV disease (Gostin, 1990). Some providers argue that their refusal to treat is based on lack of clinical competence to treat HIV disease rather than on discrimination. However, most professionals are governed by laws or guidelines that expect them to have a level of competence that is "commensurate with the standard that prevails in their specialty" (Gostin, 1990, p. 2089). Because of the prevalence and duration of this epidemic, increasingly professionals are expected to have some minimal level of competence to treat people with HIV disease. In contrast to health care providers, there are few guidelines for mental health professionals in terms of "duty to treat." As will be seen in Chapter 18, many lack the training and competence to provide counseling for this population.

A somewhat related issue is the PWHIV's right to access to services. This might mean that a community with a number of PWHIVs would be required to provide HIV-specific services such as antibody testing, counseling when test results are given, and HIV-specific medical services. This could also be interpreted to mean that an adequate level of treatment would be made available.

CONFIDENTIALITY AND DUTY TO WARN

The ethical issues that have been presented are important and are often raised in counseling, yet the ethical dilemma that has received the most attention by therapists is that of patient rights in terms of confidentiality. A review of the literature for various mental health providers finds this issue discussed almost to the exclusion of other issues. As will be seen in the following discussion, it is likely that therapists rarely violate confidentiality. Yet I believe that this issue worries and concerns counselors because it threatens that which is at the very core of the counseling relationship—trust. Counselors may also fear being placed in an adversarial role if they should come to view a particular client as an irresponsible and dangerous person from whom others must be protected.

It is helpful to first examine the psychosocial aspects of HIV disease that create dilemmas in terms of safety of others. Dishonesty to sexual partners regarding one's sexual history and infectious state appears to be common. For example, Kegeles, Catania, and Coates (1988) found that 12% of gay or bisexual men obtaining HIV testing did not plan to tell their primary sexual partners if they received positive test results, and 27% said they would not tell nonprimary partners. In another study, Elias (1988) found that 20% of heterosexual men stated that they would lie about being HIV-positive. Additionally, 35% of the respondents said that they had lied to female partners about their past sexual behavior.

Although both of these studies posed the hypothetical situation "If you are positive, would you. . . ?" to the participants, it is likely that a number of PWHIVs continue to engage, at least part of the time and with some partners, in sexual practices that carry a degree of risk without informing their partner of their status.

Several studies have addressed this issue by asking respondents who already know that they have HIV disease whether they have disclosed their status to significant others. In a sample of seropositive men (most of whom were gay or bisexual) being treated at a public HIV clinic located in a predominantly Latino section of Los Angeles, 76% had disclosed their status to an intimate lover and 83% had told their spouse (Marks et al., 1992). In a similar sample of men, the greater the number of sexual partners, the less likelihood of status disclosure (Marks et al., 1991). Of the men with only one sexual partner since diagnosis, 69% had disclosed their serostatus, whereas only 18% of the men with five or more partners had disclosed to at least one of these partners. Nearly half of the sexually active men had participated in unprotected anal intercourse without disclosing their status to their partner. These rates of disclosure to partners are considerably lower than those found in other studies. For example, a sample of gay, non-Latino white men in San Francisco reported a disclosure rate of 98% to lovers (Hays, McKusick, Pollack, & Hilliard, 1993).

These studies on disclosure of seropositive status suggest that many factors may influence this process. Having one partner or spouse seems related to a relatively high level of disclosure, whereas having multiple partners does not. Some people in this latter group may be engaging in anonymous sex where there may be no emotional investment in their partner. Cultural and social class variables may also be important. For whatever reasons, many PWHIVs have difficulty disclosing their status to some or many of their partners. What is not known is whether PWHIVs in counseling are similar to the men in these studies. It is not known how often clients honestly and accurately tell their counselors about the safety of their sexual behaviors. These situations create a dilemma for therapists who suspect or know that their HIV-infected client may be posing a threat to uninformed partners.

The *Tarasoff* Decision

An understanding of the *Tarasoff* decision and how it might be interpreted in the case of clients with HIV disease is helpful. A number of persons have written about this issue (E. D. Cohen, 1990; Ginzburg & Gostin, 1986; Gray & Harding, 1988; Harding, Gray, & Neal, 1993; Kain, 1988; Kermani & Weiss, 1989; Knapp & VandeCreek, 1990; Melton, 1988). The *Tarasoff* decision states that three criteria must be met before breaching confidentiality (*Tarasoff v. the Regents of the University of California*, 1976). I will discuss these criteria in the context of the client with HIV disease.

1. A fiduciary (or special) relationship must exist. The relationship of special trust between the counselor and the client meets this criteria (Knapp & VandeCreek, 1990).
2. There must be an identifiable potential victim. The duty to protect extends only to identifiable victims rather than to all persons the client could conceivably infect. Spouses and partners who live under an assumption of monogamy or exclusivity would most likely meet this criteria (Knapp & VandeCreek, 1990). The duty to protect would not be extended to anonymous partners as well as casual partners who are unknown to the counselor.
3. An assessment of dangerousness must be made. The issue of foreseeable danger is the most difficult of the criteria to assess. Three factors need to be considered: (1) the certainty that the

client has HIV disease (Kain, 1988), (2) the extent to which the client engages in behaviors that carry a high risk of transmission, and (3) the use (or nonuse) of safer sex practices to reduce the possibility of transmission (Kain, 1988; Knapp & VandeCreek, 1990; Lamb, Clark, Drumheller, Frizzell, & Surrey, 1989).

Several problems make the determination of danger difficult. I have heard some therapists worry about their client presenting a risk to others, without even knowing if their client is infected, simply because their client belongs to a group (e.g., gay men) with a high rate of HIV. Further, not all sexual behavior is high risk with regard to transmission. Consequently, not all sexual practices require informing one's partner of one's positive antibody status (Kain, 1988). Except in the case of rape, sexual partners can avoid practices that carry a degree of known risk (Kain, 1988). In theory this may be true, but in practice it may be more complicated. Persons who believe that a spouse or partner is monogamous may not perceive a need for practicing safer sex. For example, if a female partner of a seropositive man is using some form of birth control other than condoms, or is trying to become pregnant, she would not be focusing on safer sex. Practicing safe and safer sex requires the cooperation of both persons.

Another distinction between the *Tarasoff* decision and the potential danger from a client with HIV is that in the case of *Tarasoff*, a direct verbal threat against a specific person's life was made (Kermani & Weiss, 1989). This is rarely the case with seropositive clients, where the threat can be defined in most cases as passive. Very few PWHIVs expressly tell their therapist that they plan to infect others. When this intention is expressed, it may reflect a phase of dealing with the disease and may represent an expression of rage or an attempt to shock rather than a willful plan to harm others. If an HIV-infected client engages in high-risk sexual practices with an identifiable and uninformed partner, the three criteria for breaching confidentiality under the *Tarasoff* decision may have been met (Kain, 1988).

Guidelines of Mental Health
Professional Organizations

What guidelines do professional organizations such as the American Psychological Association use to address this issue? I will only provide an overview of the policies of several professional organizations because these policies are continuing to evolve.

The policy of the American Medical Association is the most specific and offers less leeway for the discretion of the physician than others (Daniolos, 1993). This policy states: "Where there is no statute that mandates or prohibits the reporting of seropositive individuals to public health authorities . . . the physician should 1) attempt to persuade the infected patient to cease endangering the third party; 2) if persuasion fails, notify authorities; and 3) if the authorities take no action, notify the endangered third party" (Council on Ethical & Judicial Affairs, 1988, p. 1360). It is important to note that the statements "attempt to persuade" and "if persuasion fails" leave a great deal of room for interpretation. For example, one physician may allow five visits to persuade a patient whereas another physician may think that one should be sufficient.

The American Psychiatric Association AIDS Policy on Confidentiality and Disclosure directs the psychiatrist to notify the patient of the specific limits of confidentiality if a patient refuses to change his or her behavior or to inform his or her partner. At that point, if the psychiatrist's interventions have not been successful, "it is ethically permissible for the physician to notify an identifiable person who the physician believes is in danger of contracting the virus" (APA Ad Hoc Committee on AIDS Policy, 1988, p. 541).

The policy of the American Psychological Association states the following:

1. A legal duty to protect third parties from HIV infection should not be imposed.
2. If, however, specific legislation is considered, then it should permit disclosure only when (a) the provider knows of an identifiable third party who the provider has compelling reason to believe is at significant risk for infection; (b) the provider has a reasonable belief that the third party has no reason to suspect that he or she is at risk; and (c) the client/patient has been urged to inform the third party and has either refused or is considered unreliable in his/her willingness to notify the third party.
3. If such legislation is adopted, it should include immunity from civil and criminal liability for providers who, in good faith, make decisions to disclose or not to disclose information about HIV infection to third parties. (American Psychological Association, 1991, p. 1)

As with the policy of the American Medical Association, different psychologists might interpret aspects of this policy quite differently, such as "the client/patient has been urged to inform the third party" and "is considered unreliable in his/her willingness."

The guidelines of the National Association of Social Workers state:

>In the absence of standard statutory or regulatory guidelines, practitioners and agencies may perceive a responsibility to warn third parties of their potential for infection if their spouses, other sexual partners, or partners in intravenous drug use are HIV infected and the partners refuse to warn them. . . . Social workers should first use the strength of the client-worker relationship to encourage clients with HIV infection to inform their sexual or needle-sharing partners of their antibody status. (National Association of Social Workers Delegate Assembly, 1990, p. 5)

Finally, the guidelines of the American Association for Counseling are the least specific of these policies, as the organization directs its members to "understand the ethical and legal issues raised by the AIDS epidemic and develop a framework for ethical decision-making, especially as it relates to issues of client confidentiality" (American Association for Counseling and Development Governing Council, 1988, p. 3).

Each of these organizations' guidelines emphasize the importance of confidentiality for the counseling relationship. Each requires that practitioners first attempt to change the behavior of the client or patient both in terms of his or her unsafe practices and in informing his or her partner(s). Implicit in these guidelines is the value of the counseling relationship to influence the behavior of the client and ultimately to provide for the protection of others. Therapists need to be aware of what their state laws mandate, how their ethics board views their responsibility, and whether the laws and ethics are in agreement. Because this type of situation is often so difficult to judge, ideally, statutory protection should be provided when therapists feel compelled to warn others of risk (Knapp & Vandecreek, 1990).

Utilizing the Counseling Relationship to Protect Others

In a complex examination of this issue, Driscoll (1992) suggests that there are two basic considerations regarding breach of confidence: "What purpose will breaching therapeutic confidence serve? Whose needs will be met in breaching therapeutic confidence?" (p. 704). Other researchers have tried to examine how potential clients might react to therapist breach of confidentiality. In a study of gay men and lesbians, respondents were asked whether a psychotherapist should breach confidentiality to protect a third party from HIV exposure (Georgianna & Johnston, 1993). Results showed that 80% of the respondents, when placed in the role of a psychotherapist, would not inform a third party, and 76% said that an actual psychotherapist in a similar situation should not disclose the serostatus of a client. In fact, 60% said that they would sue counselors who disclosed their HIV disease to a third party.

Although this study posed a hypothetical, albeit realistic, situation to what was most likely a well-informed group of respondents, these findings are noteworthy in the message this sample conveyed about the importance and value of confidentiality in the counseling relationship. Although guidelines such as the *Tarasoff* decision are designed to protect the public, a number of clinicians, such as Driscoll (1992) and Kain (1988), believe that the counseling relationship offers the best means to alter risky client behavior. Both raised concerns that a focus on whether to breach confidentiality might overshadow more critical counseling issues, such as *why* a client is not telling sexual partners about his or her HIV positive status.

Using the concept of ethics of covenant, Driscoll (1992) believes that the counseling relationship can be compared to a covenant—a special, sacred, and intimate relationship between people, with the basic relational dynamic of the covenant being trust. When this dynamic is upheld within the counseling relationship, the client is often able to move toward insight and behavioral change. Driscoll suggests that in this process of exploration, the counselor and client can become aware of how the client's outward behaviors (e.g., engaging in unsafe practices; dishonesty with partner) may reflect an internal process of struggle or conflict. She believes that understanding and resolving this conflict, within the context of a covenantal relationship, will ultimately provide the greatest good for others as well as for the client.

According to a study by Totten, Lamb, and Reeder (1990), many therapists who have experience in working with clients with HIV disease apparently share this view about the value of resolving these issues in the context of the counseling relationship rather than breaching confidentiality. In this study, clinicians assessed the likelihood of their breaching confidentiality in hypothetical scenarios involving gays, bisexuals, prostitutes, and injecting drug users. Therapists with no experience working with clients with HIV were significantly more likely to breach confidentiality than were those with experience with this population. HIV-experienced psychotherapists considered degree of dangerousness to be the most important factor (more so than identifiability of the victim) when making decisions to warn a third party. The researchers concluded that therapists with experience with seropositive clients have developed ways other than warning third parties to handle the potential risk to partners.

Helping clients become educated about what it means to have HIV disease, teaching them the specific steps to take to protect self and others, helping them understand inner conflicts and barriers to change, and helping them to overcome barriers to making these changes will likely protect the greatest number of people. Clients may also need assistance in how to tell partners that they are HIV-positive. Many therapists, especially those with less experience with seropositive clients, may feel great anxiety and a sense of urgency about the safety of third parties as well as their own ethical and legal responsibilities and liabilities.

Driscoll (1992) suggests some extremely useful guidelines to follow in this case: (1) It is essential to get an explicit understanding of what the client means by continued sexual activities or substance-using activities. Do these activities actually pose a risk to others? (2) A client with HIV who continues high-risk behaviors does not present as imminent a danger as the situation presented in the *Tarasoff* decision. For example, not every unsafe act results in infection, and it is often not possible to pinpoint the specific incident of exposure that led to infection. (3) One cannot rule out the possibilities that any potential partners of the client are exposing themselves to multiple sources of HIV, or that they themselves are infected. (4) In the case where a client has one committed partner, it is highly likely that the couple has been engaging in various insertive sexual behaviors and exposure and possible infection has already occurred. In these cases, the counselor cannot negate previous exposures. The gist of Driscoll's argument is that there is a window of time when the most beneficial intervention is the therapeutic alliance within the context of the counseling relationship.

Once counselors determine that there is a risk to others, they need to explore the barriers their client faces in informing partners of his or her HIV status. Is the client afraid of losing a relationship with a significant other? Is the client exchanging sex for money, drugs, or shelter and does the client risk losing these if he or she negotiates for safer sex? Does the client feel powerless because of sex-role dynamics or intimidation from a partner? The studies on whether or not seropositive persons inform sexual partners suggest that disclosure is uncommon in less significant relationships (e.g., anonymous sex or sex with many partners). There are a number of possible reasons for this. For example, people who have more difficulty with intimacy (and communication) may be more likely to engage in anonymous sex; there may be less concern for the person involved; or the seropositive person may be acting out anger and hostility.

In situations where the client is engaging in anonymous sex, it is not possible to identify (and warn) a victim. Therefore, the counseling relationship provides the best avenue of intervention, as illustrated in this clinical example. Bob, a 50-year-old white gay man with HIV disease, sought counseling because of concerns about his sexual behaviors. For over 25 years, Bob had been engaging in anonymous, often unprotected, sex—frequenting parks, bathhouses, and bars. During this time he had never been involved in a committed relationship. At the beginning of therapy, he continued to engage in these sexual activities. He would eagerly seek out such encounters, find momentary pleasure, and return home beset with extreme guilt and self-deprecation. As Bob began to identify how his depression—fueled by his own sense of internalized homophobia and anxiety—contributed to his high-risk sexual behaviors, the frequency of these behaviors decreased. Moreover, he realized that when he was most lonely he would engage in these encounters for "contact" with another person. For him, wanting contact and having sex were synonymous. As counseling progressed, he began to examine his negative self-attitudes and develop other ways of inter-acting and having contact with men.

This example illustrates how the best avenue to protecting others is often through the counseling relationship. Several aspects of this case are important to note. First, there was no identifiable victim; next, men with whom Bob had sex could likely insist on using condoms or refuse sex; and, most important, understanding the reasons for Bob's behavior not only protected others but allowed Bob to find more positive and rewarding ways of connecting with others.

Finally, some clinicians believe that many of the problems related to breach of confidentiality could be circumvented if clients were in-formed of the limits of confidentiality in the initial counseling session (Erickson, 1990; Gray & Harding, 1988; Lamb et al., 1989). For example, written formats might facilitate the informed consent process (Han-delsman & Galvin, 1988). However, others have raised concerns about the legalistic nature of some written documents delineating the ground rules of counseling that clients must sign before counseling begins. Specifically, these documents may not reflect the mutual trust and the counselor's integrity that are essential for successful counseling (Jordan & Meara, 1990). Others have expressed concerns that informing the client of the limits of confidentiality before asking questions related to sexual behavior may discourage clients from disclosing their HIV posi-tive status or from sharing important information about their practices relevant to HIV transmission. They may then leave counseling, sub-sequently contributing to the greater spread of HIV (Driscoll, 1992; Kain, 1988; Kermani & Weiss, 1989).

SUMMARY

Professional mental health organizations view the counseling relation-ship as offering one of the best means of helping clients with HIV disease to prevent the spread of the virus to others. Counseling interventions offer an invaluable window of opportunity to help clients explore the contexts in which risky behaviors occur and to work through barriers to making difficult and lasting changes in these areas so that others are protected. The client's trust and confidence in the therapist is what allows the therapist to fully support the client in practicing self- and other-protective behaviors. Counseling also provides opportunities for clients to explore other concerns that affect their adjustment to HIV disease, including discrimination in the workplace, lack of access to HIV-specific services, and lack of legal acknowledgment of partners.

CHAPTER 17

Counseling the Caregivers: Significant Others and Health Care Providers

> Loss of a loved one has been acknowledged
> throughout history as one of the most profound
> life experiences . . . during protracted,
> life-threatening illness family members
> accompany loved ones on a journey through
> deterioration, multiple losses, and dying.
> —BROWN AND POWELL-COPE (1993, p. 179)

Caregivers are often forgotten when the psychosocial impact of HIV disease is considered. Yet many aspects of this disease have a powerful effect on both formal and informal caregivers to PWHIVs. Informal caregivers are partners/spouses, friends, parents, siblings, and other family members, whereas formal caregivers are professionals, such as mental health providers and medical and nursing personnel. It is important to understand how HIV disease differs from other serious illnesses and the implications these differences have for both informal and formal caregivers. Traditionally, the informal caregivers cited in the literature have been parents, spouses, and adult daughters of widowed mothers (Brown & Powell-Cope, 1993; Folkman, Chesney, & Christopher-Richards, 1994). The focus of these studies typically described caregivers for diseases such as Alzheimer's and for elderly dying family members. Caregiving for HIV disease is unique both because of the characteristics of the disease as well as the psychosocial issues that accompany the disease process.

According to Folkman et al. (1994), certain disease characteristics create stress for caregivers, including the unpredictability of the disease, uncontrollability of symptoms, and debilitating or disfiguring effects. By these criteria, HIV is one of the most stressful diseases. Similar to other serious illnesses and diseases, caregivers of PWHIVs assist with daily living activities such as shopping, running errands, and transportation to appointments and so on. However, several psychosocial aspects of this disease create a unique situation for many caregivers.

These psychosocial aspects include the stigma associated with this disease, fear of contagion or becoming infected, the young age of most who are receiving care and of those providing care, and the fact that many caregivers themselves are infected with the same disease. The stigma associated with HIV disease may lead to isolation for both the HIV-positive individual and the caregiver (Lippmann et al., 1993). For some parents who are caregivers, learning of their son's or daughter's disease may occur at the same time that they learn of major issues such as sexual orientation or injecting drug use.

CHARACTERISTICS OF INFORMAL CAREGIVERS FOR PWHIVs

Traditionally, informal caregivers have been family members—most often a wife or adult daughter caring for a husband or a widowed mother (Turner, Catania, & Gagnon, 1994). This sharply contrasts with the characteristics of HIV caregivers described by Turner et al. (1994) in their study examining the prevalence and characteristics of HIV caregivers in the United States. The results are briefly summarized below:

1. Fifteen percent of all respondents (including those who were not HIV caregivers) know or have known someone with HIV disease (this increases to 24% of respondents in central cities).
2. Of those respondents who know or knew someone with HIV, 20% of the national sample (24% of central cities sample) have provided care or assisted someone with HIV. This translates to 3% of the national sample and 6% of the central cities sample having assisted someone with HIV disease.
3. Respondents in the 18- to 39-year-old age group were more likely to have provided care to a PWHIV, as were those respondents with higher incomes.
4. A similar proportion of men and women have provided assistance, but more men do so in the central cities.

5. In terms of the sexual orientation of central cities caregivers, 3.4% of heterosexual men and 5% of heterosexual women had provided care, in contrast to 54% of gay men and 33% of lesbian women.

6. For men who know or have known someone with HIV, 64% of all gay or bisexual men and 19% of heterosexual men have provided some type of care.

7. Approximately one-third to one-half of gay men with HIV disease are cared for by gay partners or friends.

The results of this study are noteworthy in several ways: It is based on a national sample; a significant proportion of persons who know someone with HIV have provided some type of care; men are as likely as women to be caregivers, unlike the caregivers for other diseases; most HIV caregivers are young; and gay men and lesbian women have provided a disproportionate amount of the care to those with HIV. It is important to note that caregiver characteristics in large part reflect the demographic characteristics of those with HIV. This may change as the demographics of the epidemic shift.

In a study interviewing caregivers in the Seattle area (Brown & Powell-Cope, 1993), the majority were found to be partners or spouses (38%) or friends (43%). The remainder of the caregivers were members of the HIV-positive person's family of origin (13% were parents, 4% were siblings, and 4% were other family members). As in the Turner et al. (1994) study, a disproportionate number of the caregivers were young (mean age was 36) and gay or lesbian (66%).

These two studies lend support to Folkman et al.'s (1994) conclusion that four key dimensions differentiate caregivers of men with HIV: (1) Caregiving partners are likely to be young or middle-aged; (2) the family support available to caregiving adult children, spouses, and parents is often not available for HIV caregivers, due to physical and emotional distance; (3) there are few models of male caregiving to guide caregivers of those with HIV because caregiving is typically a female role in the United States; and (4) a significant number of HIV caregivers are themselves HIV-positive. Although Folkman et al. (1994) were describing the literature on caregiving for men with HIV, at least some of their conclusions are salient for most caregivers of PWHIVs.

ISSUES AND THEMES ASSOCIATED
WITH INFORMAL CAREGIVING

A number of issues and themes are associated with caregiving provided by significant others. First, significant others are also experiencing both loss and the anticipation of loss as they provide care for a loved one with HIV disease. In addition, they often experience many of the same issues that PWHIVs do, such as stigmatization and contending with multiple HIV-related losses.

Anticipatory Grief

Anticipatory grief is particularly salient for caregivers of PWHIVs. Defined by Rando (1984) as "the phenomenon encompassing the processes of mourning, coping, interaction, planning and psychosocial reorganization that are stimulated by the awareness of impending loss of a loved one (death) and the recognition of associated losses in the past, present, and future" (p. 24), the process of anticipatory grief allows the reality of loss to be absorbed gradually over a period of time. During this time there is the opportunity for caregivers to express feelings and resolve past conflicts with the dying person. Other aspects of anticipatory grief include depression, mentally rehearsing the loved one's death, planning a funeral, and anticipating and adjusting to the consequences of the death.

In their interviews with AIDS caregivers, Brown and Powell-Cope (1993) found that anticipatory grief was an integral part of facing loss or the anticipated void in their life.

Anticipatory grief is common to many illnesses—especially those that are not sudden and where there is an opportunity to think about and experience the losses that lie ahead. There are many aspects of HIV that sharpen the intensity of anticipatory grief when compared to many other illnesses: for example, the multitude of losses that occur, the associated stigma and isolation, and the off-time nature of HIV. Tim, a 35-year-old white gay man, has been mourning the impending death of his partner, Jack, for nearly a year. Jack has experienced multiple AIDS-defining illnesses, but has continued to cling to life. Because of Jack's physical fragility, Tim rarely leaves the house for longer than an hour. Jack is also contending with HIV-associated dementia and can no longer converse with Tim in the manner that they both valued. Additionally, Tim is also HIV-positive and has recently become symptomatic. Tim is grieving the loss of Jack as he once knew him, the anticipated loss of Jack through death, and of his own life as he once knew it.

Multiple Losses for HIV Caregivers

HIV disease is often described as affecting all aspects of one's life. This is often true for caregivers, too. Loss was a central theme of interviews with informal caregivers, with most reporting multiple losses—dreams for the future, personal freedom, previous life-style, and interpersonal relationships (Brown & Powell-Cope, 1993). These losses also affected

other relationships, work, and recreational activities. The most pervasive and painful loss was the anticipated loss of the loved one. As the
disease progressed, caregivers acutely felt the loss of the relationship
with the loved one as it was known prior to HIV. They also lost most of
their personal freedom, as their time was consumed by the disease and
its demands. To illustrate: Russ and David became life partners 6 years
ago, founded a business together, and then learned shortly thereafter
that Russ was HIV-positive. They had dreamed not only of a long life
together as partners, but of a long future together as business partners
who would see their venture grow. As Russ became ill, he virtually lost
all interest in their business. David spent more and more time taking
care of Russ, and the business began to founder. By the time that Russ
died, David felt that he had truly suffered multiple losses: the loss of his
relationship with Russ, the loss of the lifelong relationship with Russ
that he had hoped to have, and the loss of a successful business that
symbolized something they had created together.

Brown and Powell-Cope (1993) note that the literature often describes these losses (e.g., employment, time, finances, and social activities) as "changes," which does not capture the psychological and emotional meaning of these events.

The Impact of Stigmatization on Caregivers

Societal stigmatization may also add to the burden of grief that
caregivers experience. Most PWHIVs have become infected through
stigmatized routes of transmission (i.e., men having sex with men, and
injecting drug use). Consequently, some caregivers experience stigmatization or fear that they will be stigmatized if others know. Murphy
and Perry (1988) have referred to these people as "hidden grievers"
who fear stigmatization if their secret is known. The wish that the
person with AIDS will die is especially common when the caregiver
feels stigmatized or secretive about the cause of the illness (Lippmann
et al., 1993).

Other caregivers may not experience a sense of shame or secretive-
ness around their loved one's disease, but may find that stigmatization
from others (e.g., bosses, coworkers, clergy, friends, family members)
leaves them feeling that they do not have adequate interpersonal supports for coping with their caregiver role.

The Impact of Caregiving as an Off-Time Event

One of the most pervasive and significant aspects of HIV disease is that
it typically represents an "off-time" event in the lives of those affected.

This is also usually the case for HIV caregivers. For parents, the loss of a child (even an adult child) is generally considered the most acute of all kinds of grief—primarily because it is an off-time event that disrupts the natural flow and rhythm of the generations. Janice is taking care of her 28-year-old daughter, Kim, who is dying from AIDS. Janice had always envisioned that at this time in her life she would be a grandmother helping take care of Kim's babies, rather than seeing Kim die before she even became a mother.

The extent to which caregiving is a "normative" experience also appears to influence the level of stress associated with this role. Because so many HIV caregivers are young and male, this is clearly not a normative experience for most. Young caregivers also suffer from what Turner et al. (1994) refer to as the "opportunity costs" of caregiving—interference with establishing a career, developing deep and stable relationships, and entering the social and political life of the community. These costs represent disruptions in important developmental tasks—costs that would not be so important for older caregivers.

Because so many HIV disease caregivers are young and have experienced multiple losses, they may have to face spiritual and existential questions that their contemporaries may not face for decades (Brown & Powell-Cope, 1993). Finally, unlike many caregivers for other diseases, most HIV caregivers are working full-time (due to their age and, in some cases, their gender). In Folkman et al.'s (1994) study of gay caregivers, 70% of the caregiving group were working full-time, whereas 70% of their partners with AIDS no longer worked. It is likely that these working caregivers are providing the primary source of financial support, as few young people with AIDS have adequate pensions and savings, given their length of time in the work force; many lack adequate health insurance.

ASPECTS OF CAREGIVING MORE SPECIFIC
TO THE GAY COMMUNITY

The majority of partners who are caring for persons with AIDS are gay men (e.g., Brown & Powell-Cope, 1993; Folkman et al., 1994). This means that many of these men are addressing changes in their primary relationship that most heterosexual couples do not have to face until they have been together many years. Some of these changes in the relationship are due to shifting responsibilities, which may begin with the caregiver taking more responsibility for household responsibilities and eventually taking responsibility for major decisions regarding medical treatment. According to Folkman et al. (1994), this shift is upsetting and stressful to the caregiver as it signals a decline in the partner's health, increasingly necessitates that the caregiver take responsibility for highly personal decisions affecting the dying partner, and may require that the caregiver perform tasks that may exceed his perceived or actual competence.

Gay caregivers may fear that they will have to go through the dying process again with a new lover or with themselves (Brown & Powell-Cope, 1993). This is especially salient for HIV-positive caregivers who may wonder what will happen to them and who will take care of them when they get sicker. Gay men suffer a major loss when their partner dies, but society often discounts the significance of their relationship and offers none of the supports and rituals afforded those who are widowed. For example, Larry's family acknowledged that Phil was Larry's "roommate" but actively avoided ever admitting that Larry was gay or that he and Phil were partners. When Phil was dying from AIDS, Larry's family often suggested that it would make sense for Phil to go home to his family so that they could take care of him. When Phil eventually died, Larry's family barely acknowledged this event and told other relatives that one of Larry's housemates had died from cancer. By not acknowledging the bond between Larry and Phil, Larry's family discounted the significance of their relationship, both while Phil was alive and after he died.

A final issue for many gay men who are caregivers is that they may have already experienced multiple bereavements, resulting in a shrinking of their support network. Additionally, the experience of losing significant numbers of one's peers can be viewed as an off-time event.

INTERVENTIONS TO ASSIST INFORMAL CAREGIVERS

Based on their study of partner caregivers for gay men, Folkman et al. (1994) make several recommendations about how professionals can help this group:

1. Work with caregivers to define what is personally meaningful about helping their partner. What values are activated by caretaking? This approach is similar to cognitive reframing in that it shifts the focus of the caregiving experience from negative or frustrating aspects (e.g., having to change the bedsheets four times a night) to a positive value (e.g., helping my partner maintain a sense of dignity).
2. Facilitate intimacy between caregivers and partners by encour-

aging open conversations that allow exploration of hopes and fears as well as expressions of appreciation. There are many shifts that occur in intimate relationships as HIV progresses, such as changes in the sexual aspects or not being able to go out as often. Intimate conversations can be maintained in many cases throughout the course of the disease and can provide something crucial for both members—an opportunity to express love and to receive love.

3. Help caregivers learn strategies that they can use with their significant other, such as praying together, practicing deep relaxation together, or meditating together, to create deeper intimacy, reduce pain and anxiety, and open the way for talking about important issues. In his book *Who Dies?*, Levine (1982) provides some examples of meditations that can be used.

4. Help caregivers develop a capacity to be aware of brief, human moments. These moments often go unnoticed when people are busy and focused on other details of their lives. Yet an awareness of sights, smells, and touch can be important and essential in reminding PWHIVs and their significant others that they are still connected to this world in a meaningful way.

Focusing on the concept of transformed time, Brown and Powell-Cope (1993) suggest several strategies with parallels to those described by Folkman et al. (1994). For example, many of the caregivers they interviewed reported feeling "suspended in time" as their perceptions of what was important in life narrowed and the usual markers of time were not attended to. To manage transformed time, Brown and Powell-Cope suggest three strategies: (1) taking one day at a time to allow caregivers to focus on only the most immediate challenge as a way of managing stress, (2) living fully in the moment, and (3) actualizing future dreams (e.g., taking a special trip, making amends with family, spending quality time with significant others, completing an important project).

Support Groups

Others have written about the value of support groups for informal caregivers. A support group for partners of persons with AIDS was described by Land and Harangody (1990). The goal of this group was to lower stress and improve psychological functioning in caregivers. What differentiated this group from other types of support groups was the reason for termination—the death of one's partner. This experience provided a preview of what was in the future for other group members, and in many ways paralleled the process many members experience in groups for PWHIVs.

Murphy and Perry (1988) described a support group for bereaved caregivers where information on the grieving process was provided along with support. They noted that these groups address two issues that are strikingly different from other bereavement groups: the stigmatization associated with HIV disease and the youth of the majority of those affected. Because of these issues, group members often failed to get support from places where it would normally be available, such as work, friends, and family. Often group members expressed fears that they too would get HIV. Losing one's partner at a young age also created other dilemmas, such as guilt over meeting someone new, questioning religious and spiritual beliefs, and dealing with one's mortality at a young age. Because these were common themes expressed in these groups, other group members were able to address these issues in a way that might not be possible with other interventions.

Managing Family Stress

Some family-of-origin members serve as caregivers for PWHIVs. Lippmann et al. (1993) described an intervention aimed at maintaining the integrity and supportiveness of this social unit as the disease progressed. They focused on teaching about transmission to alleviate concerns about contagion, helped family members manage the unique social aspects of HIV bereavement, such as fear, stigmatization, shame, and anger, and attempted to instill a sense of hope and control in family members. One of the most important aspects of their approach was helping family members learn about and utilize community resources.

Costs for Informal Caregivers

Financial costs of caring for one person with HIV disease throughout the disease progression are often extremely high. These costs vary in part, depending on how long the PWHIV spends in the hospital. Clearly, successful informal caregivers can greatly reduce the financial costs of this disease, and there is evidence that this is occurring as AIDS deaths increasingly shift from hospitals to homes (Kelly, Chu, et al., 1993). However, benefits to the medical and economic sector are probably accompanied by considerable costs to these caregivers (Turner et al., 1994). Thus, it is important to support these informal caregivers through helpful and buffering psychological interventions.

IMPACT OF HIV DISEASE ON FORMAL CAREGIVERS

There is a striking lack of empirical literature on formal caregivers to PWHIVs, especially in describing the impact of caregiving on psychologists and psychiatrists (Silverman, 1993). One of the few studies to look at this group (as well as nurses, social workers, physicians, and dentists) surveyed stressors of working with HIV care versus other life-threatening diseases (Nashman, Hoare, & Heddesheimer, 1990). Notably, 81% of the sample felt that HIV disease was more stressful because of the stigmatization, suffering, and incurable nature of the disease. No respondents stated that they experienced less stress when caring for PWHIVs as compared with other patients with equally serious diseases. These professionals also noted that caregiving to PWHIVs provided considerable satisfaction in terms of providing comfort, support, education, and helping significant others.

In one of the few controlled studies examining the psychological impact of offering care for PWHIVs, Treiber, Shaw, and Malcolm (1987) compared nurses and physicians who were simultaneously treating a patient with AIDS and a matched patient with another life-threatening disease. Both patients were closely matched on age, race, sexual orientation, length of hospitalization, medical treatments, and psychiatric diagnosis. Work with the AIDS patient created more anxiety, more interference with nonwork activities, and more frequent negative ruminations, such as worrying about contagion.

Other researchers have examined the ways in which formal HIV caregivers cope. In a study of physicians working with patients with AIDS, Horstman and McKusick (1986) found that their respondents frequently used forms of coping that could be viewed as negative, such as getting depressed (34%), crying (21%), and drinking alcohol (13%), as well as more positive forms of coping, such as seeking support and teaching others about AIDS. They also concluded that caregiver burnout was more a function of the proportion of the professional's work devoted to patients with HIV disease than the number of years working with this population.

Ross and Seeger (1988) also looked at levels of stress, rewards, and coping mechanisms in a sample of various health care providers (primarily nurses) caring for patients with AIDS. High stress was reported by 34% of the sample and overwork by 55% of the sample. The greatest stressors in caring for PWHIVs were the youth of the patients, neurological aspects of the disease, and dying patients. Burnout was correlated with stress, the need for more information about a patient's emotional needs, need for a support program, concerns about patients' ongoing injecting drug use, depression, and anxiety. Respondents reported that peer support and support from significant others were most helpful in job-related coping. Ross and Seeger (1988) concluded that the stress and burnout associated with HIV care was primarily situational (e.g., due to the unique aspects of HIV disease rather than serious illness per se) rather than personality based. However, a study by Egan (1993) of hospital social workers found that potency, a resilience factor that includes mastery, accounted for a limited amount of the variance in burnout measures. This suggests that some characteristics of the caregiver may also influence stress.

Other researchers have also looked at burnout in professional caregivers caring for PWHIVs. Based on his review of the literature, Miller (1991) acknowledged that although burnout is difficult to conceptualize, there is evidence that working with PWHIVs causes it. His review showed that respondents described many symptoms of burnout, such as physical exhaustion, lingering somatic complaints, proneness to frustration and anger, increased alcohol use, marital and relationship problems, emotional numbness, and depression.

These concerns were attributed in part to fears about HIV transmission, treating the terminally ill, overidentification with patients their own age, identification with patients with similar life-styles, and concerns about being ostracized for working with this population. Some respondents experienced great pressure from themselves and others to become active in health policy and political advocacy for PWHIVs. For example, Ray, a psychologist, completed a brief rotation working with patients with HIV disease when he completed his predoctoral internship in a VA hospital. When he began his first job at a community hospital that did not have an established HIV program, he quickly became known as "the AIDS shrink." Every HIV case was assigned to him because he had "expertise"; he was assigned to every hospital committee that had any connection to HIV disease; and he was directed to represent the hospital to the community as an expert on HIV disease. Although Ray had wanted to address issues related to chronic mental illness, he had been forced into the role of being a mental health advocate for HIV disease.

A final issue that Miller (1991) found in his review of the literature on formal caregivers was that many patients with HIV disease and the patients' significant others were highly informed and motivated regarding their treatment, which created a high level of scrutiny of the care they offered. It is likely that many PWHIVs and their significant others cope with anxiety and uncertainty through educating themselves and seeking the best possible treatment. Thus, scrutiny may make caregivers feel challenged, although it often reflects anxiety rather than a lack of confidence in the professional caregiver.

Most of the other writings on the psychological stresses formal caregivers experience working with PWHIVs are descriptive and based on personal experiences, clinical observations, and survey questionnaires. In his review of this literature, Silverman (1993) was struck by how often caregivers reveal their aversion to this disease, the patients, and their life-styles. For example, health care workers may overestimate the risk of HIV transmission through accidental needle sticks or may say that they would ask for a transfer if assigned to a heavy load of patients with HIV disease.

Perhaps what these studies suggest is a pervasive anxiety, rather than an aversion, around the issues that are stimulated by this disease. Relatively early in this epidemic, Dunkel and Hatfield (1986) noted that professional caregivers experience fear of the unknown, fear of contagion, fear of facing their own mortality and, oftentimes, overidentification with PWHIVs. In addition, this level of emotional engagement with the disease will stimulate many issues, such as feeling helpless to halt disease progression or losing a patient to whom one is attached. Murphy and Perry (1988) poignantly describe health care providers as hidden grievers "who have lived and died a little with each dying patient for whom them have cared" (p. 454).

Unresolved issues in the caregiver's life may also be stimulated by the intensity of this work, such as grief over previous losses. Drawing a parallel to the termination process in psychotherapy, counselor loss history (e.g., whether significant losses have occurred and whether these losses have been resolved) has been shown to be a significant predictor of counselor anxiety and depression during the end phase of counseling—when the client and counselor are saying good-bye (Boyer & Hoffman, 1993). Terminations also created more anxiety for counselors when they perceived that the client was sensitive to loss and was experiencing other losses. These results support the view that the termination process is affected by both counselor and client loss variables. It is likely that these same types of caregiver and patient loss variables also affect the terminal work with PWHIVs. Many formal caregivers have experienced multiple AIDS-related deaths among their clients or patients. For example, Sarah, a social worker, found herself weeping as she presented a paper at a professional conference. As she discussed themes of loss that occur in work with PWHIVs, the extent of her own losses and the wrenching impact of saying "good-bye" to 39 clients became palpable to her, and she realized that she had not allowed herself to grieve these losses. Rather, she had focused all of her energy on the losses the PWHIV and his or her significant others were experiencing.

Themes in Formal Caregiving Literature

These studies suggest that caregiving to PWHIVs is challenging and rewarding, as well as threatening and anxiety provoking. Several significant themes run through this literature: (1) feelings of helplessness and ineffectiveness in the face of disease progression; (2) emotions associated with stigmatizatio by others for doing this type of work as well as one's own internalized homophobia and attitudes toward PWHIVs; (3) fear of contagion; (4) coping with inadequate medical and social resources to assist PWHIVs; (5) profound feelings of grief and loss; and (6) emotional reactions to repeated exposure to death and dying.

INTERVENTIONS TO ASSIST FORMAL CAREGIVERS

Several studies have suggested that peer support groups may be the most important strategy to assist professional caregivers in managing stress and burnout in their work with PWHIVs (e.g., Ross & Seeger, 1988). Although the effectiveness of this type of support group has not been empirically established, descriptions of these groups suggest that several components are helpful: (1) encouraging group members to discuss emotional reactions to HIV disease, rather than simply facts (Frost et al., 1991); (2) asking group members to keep diaries or logs describing reactions to their work as well as to the group (Frost et al., 1991; Lego, 1994); (3) identifying and discussing sources of stress in their work with PWHIVs (Lego, 1994); and (4) discussing ways of coping (both positive and negative) with the stresses associated with HIV care.

It is important to note that there is little in the literature to guide the clinician in providing interventions to assist professional caregivers. Based on his review of the literature on professional caregiver stress and burnout, Miller (1991) concluded that there was no significant data on the effectiveness of various suggested prevention strategies. Most reflected a reaction to the crisis of caring for those with HIV disease rather than a proactive strategy for assisting HIV professional caregivers. Based on suggestions from non-HIV settings for the prevention of burnout, Miller (1991) suggested the following: (1) enhanced staff selection and orientation, (2) ongoing staff support, management and professional development, and (3) assistance with nonwork (e.g., family life, exercise) adaptation. Compellingly, he suggested that burnout prevention strategies help professionals incorporate more realistic expectations about their own capabilities and their response to "failures" of treatment. This fits with the notion of emphasizing "caring" rather than "curing." In other words, supporting emotional wellness by offering compassionate and comforting care should be as valued as efforts to make the PWHIV feel physically well. It is also helpful to view interventions from an organizational persective, especially in the loss-saturated work places where HIV care often occurs (Macks & Abrams, 1992).

SUMMARY

Little attention has been directed to the experience of being an informal or formal caregiver to PWHIVs. The enormity of what HIV means in the life of the PWHIV is so compelling that often the caregiver's struggles, losses, and grief are overlooked. Yet caregivers often experience many of the same issues as the PWHIV: stigmatization by others, worry about transmission of the virus, a sense of helplessness and loss, feeling overwhelmed, and feeling isolated. Despite this, the needs of caregivers have typically not been examined through research or addressed through counseling interventions. This chapter explored some of these issues and some of the ways that counseling can address these needs. The next chapter, which explores HIV-related graduate-level and professional training for mental health providers, shows how some of the needs of formal caregivers can be addressed through training.

CHAPTER 18

Training Mental Health Professionals to Work with Clients with HIV-Related Concerns

Most important, therapists are obligated to educate themselves about AIDS, whether or not they anticipate ever working with an individual directly affected by the epidemic. One truth is that we are all affected by the epidemic.

—COCHRAN AND MAYS (1989, p. 530)

In the not-too-distant past, none of us was prepared to work with clients affected by HIV disease. Now it is difficult to imagine a therapist who would expect to go through his or her career untouched by this epidemic. Yet are mental health professionals prepared to counsel clients living with HIV disease? To be effective, counselors need to know specific information about modes of transmission and aspects of disease progression, be knowledgeable about assessing clients, and be skilled in helping clients manage the psychosocial aspects of this disease. Sensitivity in recognizing and addressing multicultural aspects of HIV disease, as well as effectively responding to ethical and case management issues that may arise when working with clients with HIV disease, are also important. Finally, counselors need to be aware of how their own reactions to HIV disease, such as internalized homophobia, willingness to explore sexual and drug practices, and anxiety about the dying process, affect the counseling relationship so that they can truly connect with their clients and provide them optimal psychological care.

TRAINING IN GRADUATE PROGRAMS

How often does HIV-specific training occur in undergraduate and graduate programs for mental health professionals? There is a paucity of literature on this important training issue, and many of the studies that exist examine training in only a few fields (e.g., psychologists, nurses, physicians, dentists). Training in medical fields typically focuses on the health and disease transmission and progression aspects of HIV, with considerably less attention paid to psychosocial variables.

Surveys of graduate-level psychology training typically focus simply on whether or not HIV-related content is taught in graduate programs. For example, a survey of APA-approved graduate programs in counseling and clinical psychology, as well as predoctoral internship programs, found that 75% of these programs did not cover HIV disease in any way in their curricula (Campos, Brasfield, & Kelly, 1989). Regarding internships, two-thirds reported offering no training experiences in clinical services for PWHIVs. However, nearly half of their sample did not respond to their questionnaire, so it is possible that far fewer than 25% of APA-approved programs in these areas offer any level of training specific to HIV disease.

More recent surveys of doctoral psychology programs have found similar results. For instance, Pingitore and Morrison (1993) found that only five (4.5%) programs offering doctoral-level training in psychology offered a formal course on HIV. In a survey of clinical psychology programs, Sayette and Mayne (1990) reported that only eight programs listed AIDS/HIV as a research area in that field. This lack of HIV-specific training in graduate programs may reflect in large part the lack of expertise of the faculty. For example, Sayette and Mayne (1990) found in their survey of 115 APA-accredited clinical psychology programs that only eight had faculty members who were conducting research on HIV disease, and only two programs provided HIV-related practicum training. It is important to note that most faculty would not have received training in HIV-related issues during their graduate work because of the relative recency of this epidemic.

Do graduate students view themselves as being competent to provide services to HIV-positive clients? This question was addressed in a study examining clinical psychology students' perceived competence in providing clinical services to PWHIVs. A modest correlation was found between perceived competence and the amount of HIV training students had received (Kindermann, Matteo, & Morales, 1993). Surprisingly, there was no significant relationship between the multicultural emphasis respondents had received in their training and their perceived competence to treat special populations affected by HIV disease. In other words, students who had received little or no multicultural training perceived themselves to be as competent to treat PWHIVs as did those students with higher levels of multicultural training. This suggests that graduate students may underestimate the complexity of multicultural issues in HIV populations and may believe that this knowledge is imparted quickly and applied relatively easily. Because students from only one program in professional psychology were surveyed and the return rate was low (24%), results of this study must be interpreted cautiously.

Other studies have also examined graduate level training in multicultural issues. Although this body of research does not specifically address the issue of HIV training, one component of HIV training would be an emphasis on multicultural issues. In a survey of American Psychological Association members who had received their doctorates from counseling and clinical psychology programs between 1985 and 1987, only a limited number of respondents reported high levels of competence in providing services to persons in most of the ethnic and diverse groups examined (Allison, Crawford, Echemendia, Robinson, & Knepp, 1994). Respondents described their graduate level training in terms of training exposure and perceived level of competence in working with diverse clients. More than 50% of respondents felt very or extremely competent in providing services to whites, women, and economically disadvantaged individuals. However, for many other client groups there were major discrepancies between the percentage of respondents serving a particular group and their felt level of competence (e.g., 93% had seen African American clients but only 38% felt very or extremely competent. These discrepancies were most notable when rating experience versus felt competence with the following groups: African Americans, Asian Americans, Latinos, Native Americans, and gay clients. This study suggests that many psychologists serve specific client groups despite viewing themselves as limited in their competence to serve these groups. Although this study did not specifically address the issue of HIV disease, it is useful because competence in working with diverse client populations is necessary in this field.

Other research using a sample of psychology doctoral interns has shown that multicultural competencies correlated with certain educational variables (Pope-Davis, Reynolds, Dings, & Ottavi, 1994). Specifically, attending multicultural seminars or workshops, taking a multicultural course, or receiving supervision in a multicultural setting were significantly related to multicultural competence. Although this study did not specifically address HIV disease, the finding that multicultural training was needed to become multiculturally competent has implications for working with PWHIVs.

These few studies on graduate-level training specific to HIV disease suggest that this type of training is rare. Yet, many of the issues that define the HIV epidemic—sexual and drug practices, multicultural, social, and political factors, spirituality, and mortality—are relevant to other problems that mental health professionals address. It is possible that these issues are discussed in graduate training programs in contexts such as multicultural counseling. It is not clear if inattention to this topic is due to lack of faculty interest, or to difficulties determining whether and how HIV should be placed within the broader context of training (Werth & Carney, 1994). I believe that there may be several other reasons why HIV-specific graduate-level training is rare. For example, I think that many faculty did not expect HIV disease to be a longstanding problem. There was initially great optimism that this disease would be successfully addressed through medical interventions such as vaccines. I think that there is also confusion about whether HIV disease should be addressed primarily from a health perspective or a psychosocial perspective. In other words, where should training occur? Finally, HIV disease has unevenly affected different parts of the country so that it is a much more salient issue in some areas where graduate-level training for mental health professionals occurs than in others.

TRAINING NEEDS OF MENTAL HEALTH PROFESSIONALS WORKING WITH HIV DISEASE

To understand what types of HIV-relevant training should occur in graduate training as well as in ongoing professional training, it is helpful to see what employed mental health professionals report. Based on a random survey of clinical and counseling psychologists from Division 29 (Psychotherapy) of the American Psychological Association, Trezza (1994) concluded that many respondents lacked accurate information on some aspects of HIV transmission and prevention. About 25% of his respondents had worked with at least one client with HIV disease. Although these psychologists were relatively nonhomophobic, homophobia was correlated significantly with AIDS stigma. This study suggests that psychologists need training that includes information about transmission and prevention of HIV disease, as well as a focus on homophobia and stigmatization.

Gillman (1991) surveyed social work practitioners in the Philadelphia area to assess their experiences and attitudes toward working with clients with HIV disease. About 50% of her respondents had worked with HIV-positive clients, either directly through their clinical work or as a supervisor. Fewer than 10% of respondents had worked with 10 or more clients with HIV. Approximately 33% of respondents expressed some degree of resistance to working with HIV-positive clients, and 20% indicated that they would prefer not to work with any clients with HIV. The primary reasons for not wanting to work with this group of clients were as follows: (1) did not want to work with terminally ill clients, (2) did not want to work with injecting drug users, and (3) did not know enough about HIV disease.

Few respondents had received HIV-relevant training (in graduate school or on the job) on clinical issues, case management, attitudes about HIV, or death and dying issues. It is interesting to note that high HIV knowledge scores were associated with having received HIV training, a willingness to work with HIV-positive clients, and the belief that HIV has a high impact on one's present work. The findings of this survey suggest that lack of adequate knowledge about issues relevant to HIV disease may be one reason why some mental health professionals are uncomfortable working with HIV-positive clients.

It is also helpful to examine the training needs of mental health professionals who are extensively involved in working with PWHIVs. In a survey of 2000 professionals (representing many mental health disciplines) who were experienced in working with HIV-positive clients (*HIV Frontline*, July/August 1993e), the vast majority expressed an interest in receiving additional training in the following areas (in order of frequency): (1) psychosocial issues of specific groups (especially women, teens, and heterosexual men); (2) presentation of models of successful treatment and counseling programs; (3) information on how to influence psychological aspects of HIV; (4) information regarding how to decrease client depression and anxiety; (5) the treatment team approach; (6) discussion of "difficult" cases; (7) decreasing fear in clients; (8) decreasing prejudice in individuals or groups; (9) increasing hope in clients; and (10) information on how working with people of other ethnicities affects practitioners. These experienced professionals expressed little interest in receiving additional training in medical updates on new treatments and on infection control.

Results of this study suggest that even mental health professionals who are experienced in working with HIV-positive clients continue to have significant unmet training needs. Many of their needs are similar to those of graduate students and less experienced professionals (e.g., multicultural training, stigmatization). It seems that much of the training for counseling clients with HIV-related concerns occurs "on the spot"—with actual PWHIVs. In other words, training to meet the psychosocial needs of PWHIVs is often reactive, or in response to a need, rather than based on a proactive training plan. This may be one of the reasons why mental health professionals in this area often feel that they are constantly responding to crises, which can result in a high degree of job stress.

TRAINING RECOMMENDATIONS
FOR GRADUATE STUDENTS AND PROFESSIONALS

Several important themes emerge from the experiences of professionals working with HIV disease and from the research on graduate training programs. Others have also discussed the importance of many of these themes in counselor training (Hoffman, 1991b; Werth, 1993). Werth's (1993) review of the literature on training needs of counselors is particularly helpful.

Themes to be included in both graduate-level and professional training include the following:

1. Knowledge of HIV transmission, including an understanding of sexual and drug practices, disease progression including neurocognitive effects, and medical interventions.
2. Knowledge of psychosocial issues that accompany or predispose one to acquiring HIV disease (e.g., substance abuse, cultural norms regarding sexual practices).
3. Skill in designing and delivering psychotherapeutic interventions to assist those with HIV and their significant others.
4. Awareness of and sensitivity to the social, cultural, economic, and political forces that affect responses to HIV, from the perspectives of the client, the client's social network and community, and the country at large.
5. Skill in designing and implementing prevention interventions for HIV-positive clients as well as uninfected clients.
6. Awareness of ethical, professional, and case management issues related to HIV disease.
7. Self-awareness of one's attitudes toward diverse client groups (e.g., gay men, injecting drug users, people in racial and ethnic groups other than one's own) and behaviors relevant to HIV transmission (e.g., sexual and drug practices).

8. Comfort with exploring issues related to death and dying, including end-of-life discussions, such as rational suicide.

Training can occur in the context of a course specific to HIV disease, or within the context of courses addressing related issues such as sexuality, multiculturalism, or health promotion (Hoffman, 1991b). Werth and Carney (1994) also suggest that HIV-related issues might be discussed in four different types of courses: (1) ethical, legal, and professional issues, (2) counseling diverse populations, (3) assessment and diagnosis, and (4) research design.

Training may also occur as a part of practica, internships, or clinical rotations. Professional development and ongoing supervision provide other avenues for obtaining HIV-relevant training. For example, the American Psychological Association has sponsored training in this area utilizing a "train the trainer" model (American Psychological Association Ad Hoc Committee on Psychology and AIDS, 1993).

WORKING WITH A CASE CONSULTATION TEAM

For counselors who are inexperienced in working with HIV-related concerns, it is helpful to seek consultation or supervision with an experienced professional for help in refining risk-assessment skills. For mental health professionals who are working with clients with HIV disease, it is essential to collaborate with other professionals who are involved in the client's care.

Winiarski (1991) provides a comprehensive description of the HIV case consultation team and suggests that the following professionals should typically be involved:

- Physician
- Neurologist, when the central nervous system is impaired
- Ophthalmologist, to check eyes every 6 months, so damage due to cytomegalovirus can be detected and treated
- Pulmonologist, when respiratory disorders occur
- Infectious disease specialist
- Hospital system personnel, if hospitalized
- Nonhospital social services agencies
- Pharmacist
- Dentist, willing to treat and knowledgeable about HIV
- Spiritual advisor or clergyperson
- Occupational and physical therapist
- Nutritionist

- Home care agency
- Psychologist (or mental health professional)
- Family (of origin or of choice)

Winiarski (1991) presents a comprehensive list that I view as a "wish list" for those with HIV disease. It is likely that motivation, time, and resources, as well as perceived and actual access to professionals and services, severely limits the size and level of involvement of the case management team for many individuals with HIV.

However, the concept of a case management team is extremely important in providing services to those with HIV. The array of services and types of expertise and support that are needed at various points in the disease progression suggest that one provider cannot serve all of the needs of the HIV-positive individual. Indeed, not even the best team of "experts" can provide for all of the needs of the PWHIV. Rather, ensuring "safe passage" involves not only medical and psychological care, but the care of significant others and the community.

SUMMARY: TRAINING PROFESSIONALS
FOR THE HIV EPIDEMIC

HIV-specific training is rare in mental health provider training programs. Few programs even require training in issues that are central to the AIDS epidemic, such as multiculturalism, sexuality, and substance abuse. HIV disease will continue to be a significant psychosocial issues in the foreseeable future, so it is important that training programs find ways to address this concern. Although some counselors may not expect to encounter clients with HIV-related concerns in their clinical practice or in their supervision of other professionals, it is unlikely that this issue will never touch their professional lives. In addition, prevention of HIV disease is an important focus of clinical work with nearly all clients. Therefore, training is important to prepare counselors to address HIV-related concerns.

PART IV

PREVENTION: RISK FACTORS, MODELS OF INTERVENTION, AND COMMUNITY-BASED INTERVENTIONS

Prevention is presently the only way to curb the AIDS epidemic. An obvious goal of prevention efforts is to keep uninfected people from becoming infected. Another important goal is to help PWHIVs prevent the spread of the virus to others. To do this, it is important to begin by exploring how your client became HIV-positive. This exploration goes beyond obvious explanations (e.g., having unprotected sex) to truly immersing yourself in your client's subjective experience. Questions to be explored might include the following: "What kinds of experiences provide a sense of intimacy, connection, and pleasure?" "What other functions, such as soothing, does sex serve?" "In what ways has the client's family, culture, and self-identity influenced his or her behavior and attitudes?" It is essential to understand the client's motivations and needs and to be able to explore alternative ways of fulfilling these needs, other than through risky behaviors. For example, many clients find that sex is a way to feel soothed. Some may take risks because they have not found other ways to create this experience of being soothed. Still others may find risk taking stimulating.

Exploring these motivational themes provides valuable insight into aspects of the client's life that may be distressing or self-defeating and therefore important to address in counseling. Moreover, these themes often need to be understood before PWHIVs can successfully prevent the spread of the virus to others.

Finally, prevention should become an integral part of counseling with all clients. Primary prevention focuses on helping clients maintain an HIV-negative status and therefore differs from prevention directed toward those who are already HIV-positive. With HIV-negative clients it is important to explore motivational themes to understand risk taking that might lead to HIV disease (Odets, 1992), as well as to support behaviors and attitudes that promote safety.

With these counseling goals in mind, prevention is explored from three different perspectives, all of which are important in addressing this issue in the most effective way. Chapter 19 looks at specific attitudinal and behavioral variables that are relevant to the risk of acquiring HIV disease. In contrast, Chapter 20 presents models of risk reduction that consider multiple attitudinal and behavioral variables. These models represent comprehensive approaches. Chapter 21 addresses prevention efforts on a community, rather than an individual, basis. Focusing on community-based prevention efforts is important because it is very difficult for individuals to make and maintain HIV-related behavior changes without support from the system or community with which they identify. Moreover, it is neither cost-efficient nor likely that large numbers of people will have the opportunity to receive individual or group prevention interventions. Community-based efforts have the potential to reach many people, and the prevention approach can be tailored to target a specific population or group.

These three chapters on prevention are based more on empirical research than were the previous chapters, for several reasons. First, HIV prevention approaches have drawn heavily from fields such as health education and social psychology, which do not rely on psychotherapeutic interventions. Next, only recently have approaches specific to HIV disease been explored. Consequently, relatively few prevention interventions or approaches have been systematically applied to clinical settings. Finally, most prevention approaches have met with mixed success. Nevertheless, these studies and approaches are very useful to counselors because they provide an important foundation for understanding what needs to be explored and appreciating why it is so difficult for clients to change their risk behaviors and maintain these changes over time.

CHAPTER 19

Counseling for Prevention: Understanding Risk Factors

Prevention of HIV disease needs to become an
integral part of our clinical work with all clients.
This has become increasingly clear as the concept
of "risk groups" has been replaced by the concept
of "risk behaviors."

—HOFFMAN (1991a, p. 534)

Although HIV disease is typically caused by behaviors under voluntary
control, these behaviors are often difficult to change because they can be
gratifying. This makes successful prevention interventions difficult.
Gratification includes sexual pleasure, escape, intimacy, and getting a
drug "fix." Other times risky behaviors reflect cultural or sex-role expectations. Because of the strong link between HIV risk behaviors and
psychosocial variables that are important to explore in counseling, it is
helpful to consider prevention and risk factors with clients who are
HIV-positive as well as those who are not. The more obvious focus of
prevention is keeping uninfected people from becoming infected. But it
is also important to understand how seropositive clients acquired HIV
disease. This provides valuable information about issues such as risk
taking, patterns of intimacy, substance use and abuse, and sexual self-
efficacy. Exploring these areas is important for the PWHIV's psychosocial growth and is critical in assisting him or her in preventing the spread
of HIV to others.

It is helpful to think of prevention in a complex way by considering multiple behavioral and attitudinal factors. These factors will be grouped into five broad clusters: knowledge about transmission and prevention, attitudes about transmission, behaviors related to transmission, health cofactors that make transmission more efficient, and contextual variables that help define situations in which risk taking is more likely to occur. Although earlier research often looked only at the link between knowledge and behavior, many recent studies have looked at several of the above clusters in predicting risk behaviors.

TRANSMISSION AND PREVENTION KNOWLEDGE

Does knowledge translate into health-protective behaviors? Research examining this link has focused both on knowledge about transmission and on prevention (e.g., how to prevent HIV while remaining sexually active or while injecting drugs). Studies have shown a high level of knowledge paired with risky behaviors, such as inconsistent or no condom use, in some populations, such as college students.

In a series of studies involving college students, Edgar, Freimuth, and Hammond (1988) found that the majority of students were reasonably knowledgeable about the transmission of HIV. However, only a minority translated their knowledge into behavioral changes such as condom use. Likewise, Baldwin and Baldwin (1988) concluded that the majority of undergraduates they surveyed had accurate knowledge about HIV, but that most were not engaging in safer sexual practices. Similarly, Sunenblick (1988) found a high level of understanding about the transmission of HIV in a sample of undergraduates, but no significant relationship between knowledge and actual sexual behaviors. Finally, similar results were found in a study of young adults from large, urban areas, where knowledge levels (regarding transmission) were high, but knowledge was not linked to changes in risk behavior (Stiffman, Earls, Dore, & Cunningham, 1992).

While one could argue that the majority of participants in these studies were heterosexuals who may not have perceived themselves to be at risk, similar findings have been found among gay men (Siegel, Bauman, Christ, & Krown, 1988). Apparently, many gay men in some AIDS epicenters modified their behavior as a result of intensive educational campaigns (see review by Stall et al., 1988), but recent reports suggest that gay men (especially young men) are returning to higher levels of risky behaviors (Kelly & Murphy, 1992).

Other populations have shown relatively low levels of knowledge about HIV transmission. Discussing the results of a series of studies of working-class gay men, Dowsett (1994) reported that these men were less accurate in their HIV-related knowledge than more affluent gay men. Many relied on informal sources, such as their own experience, rather than on formal information sources, such as pamphlets and safer sex workshops. Dowsett concluded that socioeconomic status was as important a defining variable in these men's lives as was being gay.

In another study looking at socioeconomic level, race, and HIV knowledge, socioeconomic status predicted lower levels of knowledge about transmission than did race (Peruga & Rivo, 1992). In general, knowledge about proven transmission methods was high and did not vary much; however, socioeconomic status was predictive of low levels of knowledge about preventive measures. Socioeconomic status also corresponded to low levels of AIDS knowledge in a sample of pregnant, inner-city women (Hobfoll, Jackson, Lavin, Britton, & Shepherd, 1993). Transmission knowledge as well as prevention knowledge was poor for both African American and white women.

This overview suggests that knowledge does not always (or often) translate into behavior change or into safer behaviors. Therefore, it appears that the mere acquisition of knowledge about HIV is not sufficient to bring about desired and necessary behavior changes.

A study of the sexual behavior of adults in the United States offers some insight into why education alone does not necessarily translate into behavior change (Leigh, Temple, & Trocki, 1993). In this study, many respondents engaged in unprotected sex with multiple partners over the course of a year, yet perceived their risk of contracting HIV disease to be small. The researchers suggest that some of these respondents may not have believed they were taking a risk—for example, if a partner told them he or she was HIV-negative. Some may have actually been practicing serial monogamy and thus may not have viewed themselves as fitting the risk category of "having multiple partners." Leigh et al. (1993) concluded that there may be a distinction between behavioral risk indices (as AIDS educators view them) and individuals' perceptions of their own risk. In other words, many people may base their perceptions of risk on the emotional aspects of their relationships rather than on the sexual aspects.

This conclusion is supported by Hobfoll et al.'s (1993) study of inner-city pregnant women, who based their lack of personal risk perception on their having a single sexual partner, whose current or past behavior was not seen as putting them at risk. This suggests that emotional factors (e.g., feeling committed to one's partner) are important and that knowledge alone may not help people to accurately assess their own risk or make them feel personally susceptible to HIV disease. If knowledge of risk does not predict health-protective behaviors, what other factors need to be considered?

ATTITUDES AND BELIEFS
RELATED TO HIV TRANSMISSION

People need to feel susceptible or perceive that they are at risk in order to be motivated to protect their health, especially if it means making changes that are logistically, psychologically, or interpersonally difficult. What other attitudinal variables are relevant in bringing about or maintaining health-protective behaviors? Three other clusters of attitudes or beliefs will be discussed. Barriers refer to perceptions of logistical (e.g., cost, lack of availability) or psychological (e.g., feeling that condoms are unnatural or not pleasurable) impediments to making and maintaining HIV health-protective behaviors. Self-efficacy is a person's level of believing that he or she can exert control over his or her motives and behaviors and social environment. Finally, peer or cultural norms are important in understanding the context that shapes a person's attitudes about HIV transmission.

Risk Perception and Susceptibility

Why do some people perceive themselves to be at risk for being exposed to and acquiring HIV disease whereas others do not? Is risk perception based on an accurate assessment of one's risk? People may underestimate their risk because of their developmental stage: For example, adolescents often feel immortal and therefore invulnerable (Elliott, 1993). Other individuals may underestimate their risk through the process of denial (Sandfort & van Zessen, 1992). Still others may believe they are not at risk because they have only one partner or practice serial monogamy (Hobfoll et al., 1993; Leigh et al., 1993). Underestimating one's risk is sometimes referred to as unrealistic optimism (Weinstein, 1989). Of course, other people overestimate their risk and expend great worry and expense agonizing over their HIV status and getting tested multiple times. However, this latter response is much less common.

A closer look at research that has examined risk perceptions provides some insight into how people make assessments of their own susceptibility to or risk of acquiring HIV disease. Studies have consistently found that in most populations (gay men being one exception) people underestimate their risk, even in cases where they are infected but unaware. For example, in an urban African American cohort, Brunswick et al. (1993) found that the vast majority of men and women who were found to be HIV-positive were unaware and unsuspecting of their status. This is especially striking because this study sampled persons living in the New York City area, an epicenter of the AIDS epidemic. Yet engaging in unprotected sex and other risky sexual behaviors did not lead to perceptions of personal risk for most of these respondents.

Research on college students suggests that they, too, show unrealistic optimism in their perceptions of personal risk and susceptibility. In a study of heterosexually active college students, Wulfert and Wan (1993) concluded that neither being well informed about HIV transmission nor engaging in risky sexual behaviors corresponded to feeling at risk.

Other researchers have examined risk perception in samples of people who are at obvious risk of exposure to HIV. In a study of women receiving substance abuse treatment in methadone clinics (the majority were injecting drug users), 84% perceived that it was unlikely that they would acquire AIDS, yet 66% never used condoms, and only 22% used them "more often than not" (Kline & Strickler, 1993). In addition to their own injecting drug use, 46% said that their current sexual partner was a former or current injecting drug user. This group was more realistic in their self-perceptions of their risk from injecting drug use, but underestimated their risk from sexual behavior. Kline and Strickler concluded that the women seemed to define their sexual risk more in terms of who they had sex with (in other words, the quality and duration of the relationship) than in terms of the actual risk associated with the sexual behaviors. Thus, emotional aspects of relationships may often define perceptions of risk or may make concerns about risk less salient.

Does the relative accuracy of risk assessment differ for samples varying in actual risk? This question was addressed in a study of heterosexual men and women with private partners, heterosexual men and women with prostitution partners, and gay men (van der Velde, van der Pligt, & Hooykaas, 1994). Although all three groups of men showed an optimistic bias, perceptions of risk were related to actual risk behaviors only in the two high-risk groups. In other words, gay men and both men and women with prostitution partners had a fairly accurate assessment of their risk based on their sexual behaviors. However, very little of the variance was explained, suggesting the importance of looking at other variables. Heterosexual men and women with multiple private partners estimated their susceptibility or risk to be quite low.

This brief review of the literature on risk perception suggests that perceived susceptibility varies across populations and is in part shaped by sociocultural factors. If there is a common thread running through these studies on risk perception, it is that engaging in certain behaviors related to HIV transmission often leads to fairly accurate perceptions of risk: for example, men having sex with men (probably unprotected anal intercourse), injecting drug use (probably sharing needles with others), and being involved in prostitution as either a prostitute or a customer (probably unprotected intercourse). Where underestimates seem to occur is in heterosexual relationships and in relationships that are viewed as monogamous, even if it is serial monogamy. The reasons for underestimates are not known but likely involve basing risk estimates on the emotional quality of the relationship rather than its sexual aspects, and not wishing to challenge or threaten a primary relationship.

Barriers to Risk Reduction

People often perceive physical, psychological, and interpersonal barriers to risk reduction. Physical barriers include discomfort buying condoms (e.g., women, teens), not having money to buy condoms, and not having access to clean or sterile needles. Many physical barriers can be readily addressed by HIV prevention programs. Psychological and interpersonal barriers are more complex and more difficult to impact. For example, emotional and material dependency have been cited as reasons why low-income, ethnic minority women may underestimate or deny the risk their sexual partners may present (Worth, 1990). Moreover, risky sexual behavior involves two people, so that one's sexual partner is often a barrier to making behavior changes. This is especially true if there are differences in power and dependency in the relationship.

There are often psychological costs to changing behaviors. How sexual enjoyment or gratification is perceived may be a contextual barrier to adopting and maintaining safer sex practices. The research on condom use (or disuse) that will be discussed shortly suggests that many people are not embracing condoms as an acceptable alternative to unsafe sex. For example, some people believe that sex should be spontaneous and unplanned or that condoms make sex less pleasurable. Disinhibition or sensation seeking has also been linked to unsafe sexual practices (Hoffman, 1994). Further, dangerousness or risk is a central component of sexual expression for some people (Marks, 1993). Clearly, perceiving that safer sex does not offer sufficient sexual enjoyment or excitement is a major barrier to changing sexual practices.

Sexual Self-Efficacy

Self-efficacy, the belief that one can exert control over his or her motives and behaviors and social environment, is included in several models of HIV risk reduction. Self-efficacy refers to beliefs about capabilities that affect effort, choices, perseverance, thought patterns, depression, and stress (Bandura, 1990). Although self-efficacy has been examined in the context of a wide range of other health behaviors, relatively few studies have looked at this variable in HIV risk reduction (Wulfert & Wan, 1993). Yet low self-efficacy has been viewed as an important barrier to sexual risk reduction for women who may not believe that they have sufficient power or control to induce their male partner to use a condom (Worth, 1990).

In one of the few empirical studies investigating the relationship of self-efficacy to safer sex practices, Kelly et al. (1994) studied women at high risk for HIV disease. They found that increases in sexual communication and negotiation skills led to a significant decline in unprotected intercourse and an increase in condom use. In another study, self-efficacy was found to relate to condom use outcome expectancies (Wulfert & Wan, 1993). Surveying heterosexually active college men and women, Wulfert and Wan found that diminished self-efficacy was correlated with the belief that using condoms had negative consequences, such as diminished pleasure. Condom use associated with positive consequences such as disease and pregnancy prevention was related to greater self-efficacy (and increased condom use). Furthermore, respondents who viewed themselves as using condoms at least as often as their peers also reported greater self-efficacy. This last finding, about the importance of peers and social networks, leads to the final attitudinal variable that will be considered.

Social and Cultural Norms

Social influence is one of the most powerful and pervasive forces shaping behavior—especially behaviors involving interactions between people. According to Fisher (1988), people conform to the attitudinal and behavioral norms of their reference group and have a fear of nonconformity. Basically, this is because people are motivated to be liked and accepted by significant others, and an important process of acceptance is to avoid being dissimilar in meaningful ways. Several studies looking at the role that social or cultural norm groups play in influencing and shaping behavior relevant to HIV transmission illustrate this concept.

Dowsett (1994) is one of the few researchers to carefully examine how cultural norms, other than being gay, influence gay men's behaviors. In a study of working-class gay men in Australia, he found that this group of men differed from middle-class gay men in several significant ways. For example, they responded more positively to HIV prevention materials that focused on "intimate" touch rather than "hot" or explicit sexual scenarios. Another difference was that most of them lived in local working-class communities, often near their families of origin, rather than in urban gay-centered communities. Although Dowsett concluded that these men were influenced by their gay subculture, he emphasized the strong role that their local working-class community played in shaping their behaviors.

Studying urban, inner-city African American adolescents (referred to as the "hip hop" generation, after a popular style of music), McLaurin and Juzang (1993) viewed this group as alienated from Eurocentric values and, to a large extent, from African American values. Instead, these young people had evolved a culture where peers have the greatest power to influence or persuade—where success is measured in terms of peer influence, and where power is the ability to shape the tastes and values of the group. McLaurin and Juzang (1993) labeled this culture as "macho" because risk taking, including sex with many partners, was central.

In subcultures such as hip hop, risk taking may not be viewed as risk taking per se, but rather as a means of bonding with the values and beliefs of the group. This may be similar to the bonding and camaraderie that some injecting drug users share when they share their "works" or needles. It may be akin to the 1960's ritual of passing around a marijuana pipe.

Furthermore, what may be viewed as risk taking by counselors and heath professionals may also be viewed as a way of showing trust, confidence, and intimacy with one's primary sexual partner. In my work with adolescents, many said that they used condoms (at least at times) with casual partners, but would never do that with their main partner because it would show disrespect and a lack of trust. My observations have been supported by research on other populations. For example, Osmond et al. (1994) found that serodiscordant gay couples were as likely as seroconcordant couples to practice unprotected anal intercourse. They attributed this behavior to issues such as intimacy, trust, and sharing risk, which may work against risk reduction in close relationships.

Beliefs, values, or social norms may also help explain a theme running through most cultures that undermines women's power to negotiate sexual behaviors. Marks (1993), in describing the 1993 International AIDS Conference, mentioned several studies detailing the lack of power women across cultures have in sexual matters. For example, East Indian women do not discuss sex with their husbands and typically cover their eyes during sex. These behaviors are unlikely to lead to sexual negotiation around condom use. Studies on women who are financially, emotionally, or socially dependent on their partners also suggest that women in these situations view negotiation of safer sex as directly conflicting with normative expectations (Gentry, 1993; Middlestadt, 1992).

The influence of peers or one's normative group has also been shown in studies of injecting drug users. One study reported that the best predictor of HIV-related behavior change was whether or not the injecting drug user perceived that his or her user friends had changed their behavior in response to AIDS (Friedman et al., 1987). This is because transmission of HIV in injecting drug users often occurs within the context of a social relationship (Friedman et al., 1990). This relationship may be with a partner or with others who utilize the same shooting gallery.

Studies detailing the impact of celebrities announcing that they are HIV-positive also suggest that people are most responsive to role models representing their culture or peer group. For example, when Magic Johnson publicly announced that he had HIV disease, requests for antibody testing rose dramatically in many cities (Kalichman & Hunter, 1992; Taylor, 1993). This was especially true for requests from African American men. However, white men did not appear to respond to this announcement. It will be interesting to see if Pedro Zamora, a young gay man who recently died from HIV disease and who appeared (playing himself) on the MTV show *The Real World*, will have a similar impact on requests from teens and young adults to get tested for HIV.

Unfortunately, the effects of Magic Johnson's announcement, and that of Arthur Ashe, quickly peaked and rapidly subsided. The initial impact, most pronounced among black men, supports the importance of peer groups but also highlights the transient effects of interventions if mechanisms are not found to actually alter peer or social norms.

CONTEXTUAL VARIABLES

Understanding and altering the contexts in which unsafe sexual and drug practices occur is a promising area for counseling interventions. Contextual variables include social norms, expectations of others, self-efficacy in specific situations, and expectations of pleasure associated with certain behaviors and certain situations. In other words, this perspective considers the interpersonal and situational dimensions of unsafe behaviors as well as the individual dimensions. For example, an individual may associate drinking heavily with feeling comfortable in social situations. Heavy drinking may also lower inhibitions about sexual activity and reduce the individual's ability and motivation to practice safer sex. To be successful, a prevention intervention would also need to address the "drinking to socialize" context in which the unsafe sexual behaviors occurred. Other contextual variables were previously described in the section discussing barriers to change.

BEHAVIORS THAT POSE RISK
OF TRANSMISSION OF HIV

Ultimately, the goal of HIV prevention interventions is to help people achieve and maintain health-protective and other-protective behaviors. Most transmission of HIV occurs through unprotected vaginal and anal intercourse and sharing needles for injecting drug use. It is also possible that many injecting drug users become infected through sexual means rather than through sharing needles. Quite simply, if people correctly and consistently used condoms and did not share needles, transmission of HIV would drop precipitously. This course of action sounds so easy, yet the following literature review will show that it is not.

Sexual Behavior of Adults in the United States

What are the sexual behaviors of adults in the United States? Knowing this helps the counselor understand some of the barriers to risk reduction. Yet, it is very difficult to get accurate and complete information about sexual behaviors, including use of condoms, because of the intimate and private nature of sexual behavior. This lack of current data is one reason why the information on sexual behavior collected by Kinsey and his colleagues over 40 years ago is still often used by public health officials in understanding various aspects of HIV (Leigh et al., 1993).

Although a number of surveys have been conducted since Kinsey, they have limited usefulness in drawing conclusions regarding HIV transmission factors. For example, they may not study representative samples or may include only limited measures of sexual behavior (Leigh et al., 1993). To address these concerns, Leigh et al. conducted a survey of what they described as a nationally representative sample of adults in the United States that included detailed measures of different aspects of sexuality, including sexual practices associated with HIV transmission. This study is very helpful in putting sexual practices in a useful context when considering HIV risk factors.

A total of 2058 individuals were interviewed in their homes (unless other arrangements were made to ensure privacy) during 1990 (a response rate of 70.3%). Detailed information was collected on sexual behavior, alcohol use, and drug use. Two percent of the sample reported being gay or lesbian (which is similar to Kinsey's 1970 data). However, sexual orientation is an example of an area where it is probably difficult to get an accurate estimate, both because of possible sampling bias (e.g., nearly 30% of the sample did not respond to the survey) and because some respondents may be unwilling to reveal this information. Of the respondents, 90% had been sexually active in the past 5 years. Most reported having only one partner in the past year, with 18% of the sexually active reporting more than one sexual partner. Of married respondents, approximately 4% reported having more than one sexual partner in the past year. Only 23% of respondents with multiple partners used a condom every time with their nonprimary partners.

This higher-risk group was comprised primarily of males, those younger than 30 years, and people who had never been married or who were divorced. Of those with one primary partner, 77% inconsistently or never used condoms. Finally, only 25% used a condom the first time they had sex with a new partner. For the most part, respondents' levels of concern about AIDS, behavior change in response to AIDS, and perceptions of risk for AIDS were low. However, those with more than one partner reported more worry and saw themselves as more susceptible. Even those who did not use condoms consistently reported that AIDS had made an impact on their behavior.

Leigh et al. (1993), as have other researchers, point out the difficulty of conceptualizing and measuring sexual risk. Although they were able to assess the reported number of sexual partners, they were not able to assess the relevant characteristics of these partners and their previous partners (this was likely unknown to the respondents in most cases) or what exactly the person did with each partner. Further, respondents may not have always provided accurate information because of memory distortion and unreliability in estimating frequencies of various behaviors.

What is helpful about this study is the snapshot it provides into the sexual practices of a sample of American adults. Several important conclusions can be drawn that are useful for therapists helping clients with risk reduction: The vast majority of people do not use condoms with primary partners; nearly as many do not use condoms with nonprimary partners; relatively few people use a condom the first time they have sex with a new partner (only 25% in this sample); most people do not consider themselves at risk for HIV (although it is important to note that those with multiple partners do perceive some risk, but it does not appear to directly translate into condom use for many); and most people consider themselves to be monogamous (or possibly serially monogamous). It appears that perceiving oneself as monogamous, even if this means having more than one partner in a year but one at a time, has a major impact on condom use and on perceptions of risk. These conclusions seem supported by previously discussed studies examining perceived risk or susceptibility to HIV (e.g., Kline & Strickler, 1993).

I have chosen to focus on the Leigh et al. (1993) national survey on adult sexual behaviors because of its emphasis on understanding behaviors and attitudes relevant to HIV transmission. However, a more recent survey of adult sexual behaviors supports many of the findings of Leigh et al. in terms of numbers of sexual partners, rates of monogamy, and percentages of respondents who report being gay or lesbian (Michael, Gagnon, Laumann, & Kolata, 1994). In contrast to Leigh et al., this survey minimized the risk of HIV spread beyond gay and drug-using communities. This is puzzling given some of the findings. For example, 8% of 18 to 24- year-olds admitted having five or more partners within the last year. It is likely that many of these encounters involved unsafe sex because of the low rate of reported condom use. This suggests that a significant minority of respondents in a national sample engage in behaviors associated with HIV transmission.

Condom Use/Nonuse

The Leigh et al. (1993) study shows that in a largely heterosexual sample, relatively few people consistently use condoms. Similarly, results of another study showed that only 10% of heterosexuals with four or more sexual partners in the previous year always used condoms with nonprimary partners (Dolcini, Coates, Catania, Kegeles, & Hauck, 1995). In a study of married heterosexuals, only 8% of those having extramarital affairs reported consistent condom use (Choi, Catania, & Dolcini, 1994). Yet condoms have been shown to be an effective barrier against HIV disease. Other than abstinence, engaging only in noninsertive sexual activities, or sex between two uninfected, monogamous partners, condoms remain the only protection against sexual HIV transmission.

While the Leigh et al. (1993) study reported on a national sample of primarily heterosexual adults, what is known about condom use in other populations? Given that HIV disease has been a salient issue in the gay community for some time as well as the relative risk of unprotected anal intercourse, gay men are an important group to study in understanding condom use. Studies of gay men in HIV epicenters (e.g., San Francisco) have typically shown that about 10% of men engage in unprotected receptive anal intercourse (Ekstrand & Coates, 1990; McKusick, Coates, Morin, Pollack, & Hoff, 1990). Men who were more likely to engage in this practice were younger, reported having more sex partners, reported that their friends were more likely to engage in high-risk sexual activity, were low in perceived efficacy to change sexual behaviors, and reported that unprotected anal intercourse was their favorite sexual activity (Ekstrand, 1992; Ekstrand & Coates, 1990; McKusick et al., 1990). These findings suggest that many factors influence condom use in gay men, including pleasure, peer norms, sexual efficacy, and age.

Injecting drug users represent another population with a high rate of HIV disease. Studies have typically shown that this group reports a relatively low rate of condom use. For example, only 19% of injecting drug users being treated at a methadone clinic reported using condoms all of the time (Kleinman, Millman, & Robinson, 1992).

Other populations also report relatively low rates of condom use. For example, approximately 13–20% of sexually active college students report using condoms (Baldwin & Baldwin, 1988; Butcher, Manning, & O'Neal, 1991). Campbell, Peplau, and DeBro (1992) examined attitudes about condoms in an attempt to understand why many college students do not use condoms. Overall, their respondents believed that condoms provided effective protection but detracted from sexual sensation. Women were more favorable toward condoms than were men.

Similar rates of condom use were also found in a sample of Latino adolescents, in which 26% of respondents estimated that they used condoms every time they had intercourse in the previous 6 months and nearly half never used condoms during this period (Smith, McGraw, Crawford, Costa, & McKinlay, 1993). Interestingly, the greater the respondents' frequency of sexual intercourse, the less frequently they used condoms. To assess the validity of condom usage estimates, respondents were asked whether they had a condom in their possession at the time of the interview.

The Smith et al. (1993) study on Latino adolescents is important in that the researchers tried more than one method of establishing how frequently respondents used condoms. Most of the research on sexual practices simply asks respondents whether or how frequently they use condoms, which may lead to inaccurate estimates for a variety of reasons. For example, when undergraduates were asked if they had ever used a condom during intercourse, 83% reported that they had. However, when asked whether they had used a condom the last time they had intercourse, only 31% reported having done so. Similarly, only about half of adults having intercourse with someone they had just met at a bar used a condom (Herold & Mewhinney, 1993). Leigh et al.'s (1993) respondents reported an even lower rate of condom use the first time with a new partner—25%.

Condom Failure Rates

Because condoms represent the only protection from HIV during intercourse when one partner is HIV-positive or the serostatus of either partner is unknown, it is important to examine condom failure rate. This topic was previously discussed in chapter 9, so research will only be briefly summarized here. Frequency of condom use and estimated condom failure rates were studied in a sample of gay men in New York City, with respondents reporting on four sexual acts over a 12-month time period (Thompson et al., 1993). Condom failure rate (e.g., breaking or falling off) was relatively high (15%) in receptive anal intercourse for men who used a condom only once in the year before the interview. In contrast, failure rates decreased to 1.5% for men who had used a condom four or five times and to below 1% for men who had used a condom more than 10 times. Condoms failed less frequently in oral sex, with a 6% failure rate for men who had used them once for this sexual behavior and 0.2% for those using condoms more than 15 times. Clearly, increased practice and experience significantly increases the effectiveness of condoms.

Other studies have found reported breakage rates of 2% or less for vaginal or anal intercourse (Cates & Stone, 1992). Although no clinical studies have established the rate of protection from HIV provided by the female condom, the estimated 12-month failure rate for pregnancy prevention was 26% (Centers for Disease Control, 1993b). This implies that the female condom is either difficult to use correctly or has a high failure rate even when used correctly.

Studies on condom failures suggest that experience and knowledge about proper use is linked to a low failure rate. Given the severity of the possible consequences of condom failure, interventions that provide explicit instructions on how to correctly use condoms are essential.

Negotiated Sex

Some people negotiate with sexual partners who share their HIV antibody status to forgo practicing safer sex. For example, an HIV-negative man might agree to have a monogamous relationship with another seronegative man and agree not to use condoms. This approach will usually minimize, but may not eliminate, risk. The success of this approach depends on accurate knowledge of one's current antibody status and the fidelity of both partners.

Conclusions about Condom Use

Several conclusions can be drawn from literature on condom use. Most people do not report regularly using condoms in relationships with their primary partners. In most samples, the majority of respondents do not regularly use condoms even with casual partners. The exception may be gay men, who report a much higher rate of condom use. What is important is that most risk-reduction interventions are "condom centered," yet relatively few people find condoms either acceptable and/or necessary. The reasons for this vary from population to population but often include interference with pleasure, partner preferences, and low perceptions of susceptibility. Successful interventions need to move beyond only providing factual information and to begin to address emotional, social, cultural, and contextual issues that affect condom acceptability and consistent use.

Sharing Needles

Sharing injecting drug needles is risky and is one of the primary modes in which HIV is transmitted, yet this behavior remains prevalent among many injecting drug users. A study comprised primarily of minority inner-city drug users found that 80% of injecting heroin users and 69% of injecting heroin and cocaine users had shared needles during the previous year (Kramer, Ottomanelli, & Bihari, 1992). However, sharing needles used to inject drugs intramuscularly (such as in injecting steroids) is also risky.

Why do people share needles? There are several primary reasons: lack of access to individual sterile needles, lack of information or supplies to sterilize needles, lack of motivation in the context of an addiction, and lack of awareness of risk. But there are also psychological and cultural reasons. For example, the sharing of needles or "works" may be viewed as a form of bonding or trust, or as a rite of initiation within the injecting drug culture (Des Jarlais & Friedman, 1988).

Pairing Alcohol and/or Drugs with Sexual Activity

Research has consistently found a strong link between sexual behavior and the use of alcohol. In one study of adolescents, 64% of those who were sexually active had sex after or while drinking, and 49% reported that they were more likely to have sex if they and their partner had been drinking (Strunin & Hingson, 1992). Similarly, by the time college students were over 21, only 19% reported never having had sex when intoxicated (Butcher et al., 1991). However, the relationship between substance use and high-risk sexual behavior is less clear (Leigh & Stall, 1993).

Many studies have examined this issue using samples of gay men. For example, substance use in conjunction with sexual activity has been strongly linked to unsafe sexual practices (Stall et al., 1988). However, Ostrow (1994) found that only the use of "poppers" (volative nitrites) showed a consistent and strong cross-sectional association with high-risk receptive anal intercourse. Additionally, poppers used in conjunction with cocaine and marijuana showed the highest level of unsafe sexual behaviors. Other substances (e.g., alcohol, marijuana) showed some association with high-risk behaviors, but not consistently so. Most striking, Ostrow (1994) concluded that over 90% of the substance use reported by his respondents occurred within the specific context of sexual encounters. This research suggests that for gay men, substance use typically occurs within the context of sexual situations, but that use is not consistently linked to unsafe sexual practices.

Much less is known about the link between substance use and sexual practices in substance-using (noninjecting drug users) hetero-sexuals. In a study looking at both homosexual and heterosexual adults (ages 18 to 50) in the San Francisco city area, drinking habits, drug use, sexual behavior, and attitudinal data were collected (Leigh, 1990). Re-sults showed that for heterosexuals, the more often a person used alcohol or other drugs with sex, the more risky his or her behavior overall. Similar results were found in a sample of adolescents, where failure to use a condom at last intercourse was associated with use of alcohol or drugs during that encounter (Collins, Holtzman, Kann, & Kolbe, 1993).

These studies suggest that alcohol and other drugs have a disin-hibiting effect and often are associated with sexual contexts, such as feeling more assertive or less anxious in interpersonal situations. For example, Brown (1985) concluded that alcohol expectancies, specifically the expectation of social and physical pleasure, significantly contributed to the prediction of alcohol use among college students.Similarly, other researchers have concluded that the expectation of pleasure is a strong predictor of alcohol use (e.g., Mooney, Fromme, Kivlahan, & Marlatt, 1987). Alcohol and drugs may also be seen as creating a romantic mood, and drugs such as cocaine and nitrites are viewed as being aphrodisiacs (Leigh, 1990). Pleasure, enhancement of sexual response, and disinhibi-tion are important reasons why substances are so often used in sexual contexts.

Being Unaware of HIV-Positive Status

Another theme found in the literature on prevention is the large percent-age of people who are HIV-positive but are both unaware and unsus-pecting of their status (e.g., Brunswick et al., 1993; Reardon et al., 1993). There are likely multiple reasons why this is so: misperceptions about who is at risk for HIV (e.g., only gay men); misperceptions about what types of sexual practices lead to HIV; believing that monogamy (even serial) prevents HIV; denial; trust in one's partner; and not knowing how to assess one's own or one's partner(s)' risk history. It is unlikely that people who are unsuspecting, and therefore not perceiving themselves as at risk, will readily embrace prevention behaviors. Therefore, people who are unaware of their positive antibody status may put their partners at risk of infection.

Clusters of High-Risk Behavior

Research has also shown that some high-risk behaviors cluster together. In heterosexual adolescents, infrequent use of condoms, sex with multiple partners, sex with persons one does not know well, sex with non-monogamous partners, and a positive sexually transmitted disease history were highly intercorrelated in all samples (Metzler, Noell, Biglan, & Oregon Research Institute, 1992). Many of the studies discussed in this chapter also support this pattern. For example, several studies showed that respondents who had the most sex partners were also more likely to engage in risky sexual practices.

The reasons why some people engage in multiple high-risk behaviors are likely varied, and few studies have specifically addressed this issue. For example, persons with drug addictions may trade sex for drugs or be so disinhibited because of their addiction that they are not thinking about consequences. A study of gay and bisexual adolescents found that youths with an involvement in commercial sexual activity (prostitution) were significantly less likely than those not involved in prostitution to reduce the number of unprotected same-sex anal and oral acts (Rotheran-Borus, Reid, & Rosario, 1994). These youths may have been financially dependent on the wishes of their customers and were likely to have been prostituting themselves to support a drug habit.

Some people may take risks because their culture does not accept their sexual orientation. For example, Spanish-speaking Latino men were more likely than those who were English-speaking to withhold their HIV-positive serostatus and their gay or bisexual orientation from significant others (Mason, Marks, Simoni, Ruiz, & Richardson, 1995). One could speculate that these "culturally sanctioned secrets" might lead these men to have taken HIV-related risks that led to becoming seropositive. In addition, they may continue to put others at risk for this same reason.

Other people may find dangerous sex or risk taking stimulating. Still others may not know how to relate to others and how to find intimacy in other ways than through sex. This pattern of multiple risk factors puts many people at high risk for HIV transmission and is an important issue to address in both counseling and research.

TRANSLATING HIV RISK REDUCTION
INTO COUNSELING WITH ALL CLIENTS

When should therapists focus on risk assessment and risk prevention with HIV-negative clients? It is important to assess all clients (beginning around early adolescence) with regard to their HIV-risk attitudes and behaviors. This might begin with an informal assessment. For example, a counselor might conclude that further risk assessment and interventions are not necessary if the client is a non-drug using man in a monogamous, long-term relationship of 20 years' duration.

In contrast, the specific risk behaviors of a man or woman having frequent, high-risk sexual encounters warrants a more comprehensive assessment of risk. Such assessment may include the following: What types of sexual behaviors is the client engaging in (e.g., does he or she always use a latex condom for insertive sex)? What sexual activities are preferred (e.g., receptive anal intercourse without a condom)? What is his or her level of self-efficacy in managing sexual situations? Is sexual activity paired with alcohol or drugs so that there is less likelihood of practicing safer sex? What function does sexual activity play in his or her life (e.g, intimacy in the absence of ongoing relationships, self-soothing/medicating, escape, release, alternative to boredom)? Is coercion of any kind involved? Is the client concerned about a pattern of engaging in casual sex, and if so, why? Does he or she want to change this pattern? Is he or she worried about becoming HIV-infected? These same questions can be explored with clients who are HIV-positive. This exploration can help the client make desired changes in sexual practices, increase sexual self-efficacy, and enhance interpersonal functioning.

Many men and women are also uncomfortable with their sexuality—be it heterosexual, homosexual, or bisexual—and this discomfort may be expressed through high-risk sexual behaviors. For example, many people drink to feel comfortable and assertive in social situations that they know might lead to sex. Often, when drinking and sexual activity are paired, safer sex is not practiced. Others may express unresolved conflicts, low self-esteem, or low self-efficacy through high-risk behaviors and self-destructive behaviors. Because of the interface of risky behaviors with other psychosocial concerns, I have found it to be most helpful to view HIV prevention within the broader context of health-protective behaviors, attitudes, and values. Addressing these areas typically precedes helping clients practice safer sex and drug behaviors.

CHAPTER 20

Models of Intervention

> The exhortations to intervene and
> recommendations for interventions far
> outnumber credible interventions that
> have been subject to statistical evaluation.
>
> —FISHER AND FISHER (1992, p. 456)

Specific behaviors and attitudes related to HIV disease acquisition, and therefore disease prevention, were discussed in the previous chapter. Because behaviors and attitudes often cluster together, prevention interventions are most effective when they consider multiple risk variables. This chapter will explore some of the most promising models or theories of health-protective behaviors. However, to varying degrees, these models fail to capture some of the variables that are important in understanding risk reduction, a topic that will be discussed at the end of the chapter. It is also important to note that these models have not been extensively examined in relationship to HIV prevention. Most of them originated in response to other health problems or decision making in general. Moreover, many of the studies that have examined HIV prevention have done so by looking at aspects of a particular model rather than the model in its entirety. Nevertheless, they are useful to illustrate the importance of considering multiple variables, such as motivation, perceptions, attitudes, and behaviors when implementing risk-reduction interventions.

THE HEALTH BELIEF MODEL

One theory that has been used to explain why some people have not changed their sexual behavior is the health belief model (HBM), which has been used for many years to explain why people knowingly jeopardize their health through practices like smoking (Hayes, 1991; Janz & Becker, 1984; Maiman & Becker, 1974). According to Leventhal, Zimmerman, and Gutmann (1984), the health belief model has been described as the cognitive model most frequently used in studies of health behavior and compliance. This model has also been used in developing health-behavior interventions.

Four predictors of health-risk behavior comprise the basic model: (1) perceived (personal) susceptibility to a negative health consequence such as a disease, (2) perceptions of the severity of this condition, (3) perceived benefits (effectiveness) of making certain health changes, and (4) perceived barriers to making these changes. More recently, some researchers have added a fifth component, perceived self-efficacy, to the model (Kirscht & Joseph, 1989; Strecher, DeVillis, Becker, & Rosenstock, 1986). This component can also be conceptualized as a type of barrier to change. These beliefs are hypothesized to produce some degree of psychological readiness to act (Kirscht & Joseph, 1989). Nevertheless, researchers like Rosenstock (1974) suggest that a cue may be required to initiate a health-related action; in other words, the beliefs must become salient by being called into awareness or action. Finally, most research has treated these components as being additive (Weinstein, 1993).

Although the health belief model originated prior to the AIDS epidemic to explain a variety of health behaviors, the model's components are relevant to HIV disease. This can be seen from the following descriptions of the components from the perspective of HIV disease.

1. *Perceived susceptibility.* This dimension refers to the individual's feelings of personal vulnerability to becoming (or being) infected with HIV. According to Janz and Becker (1984), it refers to the subjective perception of risk of contracting an illness, disease, or condition. Researchers have speculated that because the odds of becoming HIV-infected are relatively small when engaging in any single instance of at-risk behavior, individuals tend to minimize their perceived susceptibility (Bauman & Siegel, 1987; Edgar et al., 1988). Similarly, Weinstein (1989) described "unrealistic optimism" as the false belief that one is invulnerable (or less vulnerable than others) to health risks. For example, a number of adolescents I have counseled believe that they "have

an immunity" to HIV disease because they have had unprotected sex a number of times and have not become infected. This inflated sense of invulnerability is especially prevalent in adolescents (DiClemente, Zorn, & Temoshok, 1986) and young adults, as well as in heterosexuals who have perceived this disease as one primarily affecting gay men and injecting drug users.

2. *Perceived severity (of the consequences of a threat).* This dimension refers to how serious a threat (in this case, HIV disease) is perceived to be in terms of health consequences (e.g., death, pain, disability) and/or in terms of social consequences (e.g., discrimination, stigmatization, effect on relationships) (Janz & Becker, 1984). Although perceived severity of the consequences of HIV disease appears to be a strong predictor of behavior change among gay males, it does not appear to be so for injecting drug users (Friedman & Des Jarlais, 1991). Nor does perceived severity appear to alter the behavior of many heterosexuals.

3. *Perceived benefits.* This dimension refers to the beliefs individuals hold about the effectiveness of various actions available to protect themselves from a particular disease as well as the feasibility of these actions (Janz & Becker, 1984). An individual's belief about the effectiveness of safer sex guidelines is an example of this dimension.

4. *Perceived barriers.* This dimension refers to the perceived costs or barriers to engaging in health-promoting behaviors. The effectiveness of actions is weighed against the individual's perceptions that these actions may be unpleasant, difficult, expensive, or inconvenient (Janz & Becker, 1984). More recently, attention has focused on normative behavior as an important example of a perceived barrier to change. For example, many high-risk behaviors related to HIV transmission involve normative, interpersonal dimensions, such as rituals around needle sharing, and are often "overlearned" behaviors (Friedman & Des Jarlais, 1991). Additionally, sexual activity is often paired with alcohol and/or drug use, which might present a barrier to safer sex practices.

5. *Perceived self-efficacy.* This dimension is somewhat similar to that of barriers, but relates more specifically to individuals' beliefs that they can alter their behaviors, that their efforts will result in positive consequences, and that they have the personal power to not only control their own actions, but to influence the actions of significant others (Bandura, 1990). Several studies have supported this link between self-efficacy and HIV-related behavior

change (e.g., McKusick, Coates, Morin, Pollack, & Hoff, 1990; Namir et al., 1987).

Relatively few studies have tested the efficacy of the health belief model in terms of HIV transmission by examining all four components (with or without also looking at self-efficacy). Rather, many studies have looked at two or three components. Often a component has been examined using only one item, and there is little consistency between studies in terms of how the components (as they relate to AIDS/HIV) are conceptualized.

To address this issue, Hoffman (1994) developed a measure called The Health Belief Model–HIV Questionnaire. Based on a sample of college students, health-protective attitudes on the dimensions of self-efficacy, barriers, and susceptibility were significant predictors of condom use. In contrast, low self-efficacy and perceiving more barriers were predictive of pairing alcohol or drugs with sexual activity. Respondents with higher disinhibition scores attributed more barriers and fewer benefits to health-protective behaviors. The results of this study suggest that for this sample of college students, health beliefs may be a useful way to understand why some students do not make health-protective behavior changes.

PROTECTION-MOTIVATION THEORY

Protection-motivation theory (Maddux & Rogers, 1983; Prentice-Dunn & Rogers, 1986; Rogers, 1983), like the health belief model, was developed specifically to explain health-protective behavior. This theory is closely related to the health belief model, but has developed more explicit hypotheses regarding reactions to threat (Kirscht & Joseph, 1989).

Like all of the risk prevention models, protection-motivation theory begins with the individual perceiving or anticipating a threat of a negative health outcome and making an assessment of the noxiousness or severity of the threat. An assessment or appraisal of the likelihood of the threat occurring is made (conditional probability), which parallels "susceptibility" in the health belief model. This perception of the severity of the health threat and one's susceptibility (if one's behavior does not change) determines the level of motivation to take action. Motivation is also affected by the belief that the action can reduce or eliminate the severity of the risk, or, in other words, that the action is effective (similar to "benefits" in the health belief model). Up to this point, protection-motivation theory closely parallels the health belief model.

Unlike the health belief model, however, protection-motivation theory separates perceived costs (or barriers to making the change) from self-efficacy. In other words, self-efficacy is explicitly referred to by this theory, whereas it is only implied in the barriers dimension of the health beief model. However, the barriers to action dimension of the latter is highly similar to self-efficacy (Weinstein, 1993), and several recent studies have included self-efficacy as a separate component of the health belief model.

In addition to explicitly referring to self-efficacy, protection-motivation theory includes variables that might intervene between the perceived attractiveness of a health precaution and actually adopting that health precaution. These are the loss of current internal rewards (IR) and external rewards (ER) that will result from a specific behavioral change (Weinstein, 1993). In other words, a man who enjoys the feeling of sexual intercourse without a condom (IR) will now balance that reward with his perception of the severity of HIV and his own susceptibility to HIV disease.

THEORY OF REASONED ACTION

The theory of reasoned action (Ajzen & Fishbein, 1980; Fishbein & Ajzen, 1975) is based on the assumption that humans are reasonable and that they systematically process and utilize information that is made available to them (Fishbein & Middlestadt, 1989). Changes in behavior are the result of changing the cognitive structure underlying the behavior. Thus, the theory of reasoned action is essentially a cognitive theory, as are both the health belief model and the protection-motivation theory.

Similar to the theories that have been discussed, the theory of reasoned action hypothesizes that an individual's anticipation of a negative outcome that might result from a specific behavior leads to intentions to change that behavior. This theory then diverges by positing that the individual's subjective norms also lead to intentions to change behaviors. Subjective norms are the person's belief that specific individuals or groups with whom he or she wants to identify or conform think he or she should or should not perform the behavior. To illustrate, an adolescent male's peer group may find condom use acceptable with nonprimary partners, but may view them as showing a lack of trust and caring when used with a primary partner.

Overall, the theory of reasoned action views an individual's attitudes and subjective norms as being the sole determinants of intentions to change a behavior (Weinstein, 1993). This theory differs from the health belief model and the protection-motivation theory in that it considers a much wider range of consequences (beyond health consequences), if the specific behavior were to continue or be altered. For example, the other two theories consider explicit costs of changing one's behavior and the benefits of decreasing health risks. In contrast, the theory of reasoned action might also consider interpersonal costs or benefits (such as maintaining one's status in a group or in a relationship, living to raise one's children, and not infecting one's partner). This theory posits that the individual identifies the main consequences of action or inaction (Weinstein, 1993) and balances the likelihood that these consequences will occur with the expected value of making a behavior change.

The theory of reasoned action is also unlike the health belief model and the protection-motivation theory in that it looks at social influences (which are an aspect of subjective norms). However, social influences may implicitly be an aspect of the barriers dimension of the health belief model. Finally, the theory of reasoned action views intentions as sufficient to predict behavior. Weinstein (1993) suggests that this aspect of the theory does not necessarily account for intervening issues. However, Ajzen and Fishbein (1980) do state that intentions only predict behavior when that behavior is under the volitional control of the individual. For example, a woman who is economically dependent on her husband and physically afraid of him may not believe that she has a choice in whether or not to practice safer sex. Thus, there is acknowledgment of at least one important type of intervening variable.

BANDURA'S THEORY OF SELF-EFFICACY

Bandura posits that translating health knowledge into effective self-protection against HIV disease requires people to exercise influence over their own motivation and behavior, to have adequate social skills to make the necessary behavioral and interpersonal changes, and to have a sense of personal power to exercise control over the situation (Bandura, 1990). People need to be given not only reasons (e.g., knowledge or education) to alter risky behaviors but also the means and resources to do so. People's self-efficacy beliefs about their capabilities affect not only what they choose to do, but how much effort they expend, how long they persevere when encountering difficulties, whether they engage in positive or negative thought patterns, and the amount of stress they experience in difficult and challenging situations.

Bandura (1990) described four components that are necessary for effective self-directed change.

1. *Information.* People need to have an awareness and knowledge of the severity of the threat of HIV disease. This includes

information about modes of transmission, what constitutes risky sexual and drug practices, and specific information on avoiding infection. The informational component of the model includes two main factors: The informational content must be presented in an understandable, credible, and persuasive manner, and, it must be effectively disseminated to reach its audience.

2. *Development of self-protective skills and controlling self-efficacy.* Once people are convinced that they need to change risky behaviors, they also need to translate their concerns into efficacious behaviors. In other words, knowledge alone typically does not translate into behavior change. How do people learn self-protective skills and increase their self-efficacy? Social modeling can teach both self-regulatory and risk-reduction strategies for managing a variety of situations. Further, the impact of various methods of influence on health behavior is partly mediated through effects on perceived self-efficacy (Bandura, 1989). In other words, modeling strategies should not only convey rules and approaches for dealing effectively with situations, but should also be designed to increase self-assurance. Bandura (1986) has shown that models are more effective if they match the target audience in salient ways, such as age, gender, or sexual orientation.

3. *Enhancement of social proficiency and resiliency of self-efficacy.* People need extensive practice (with opportunities for feedback and skills refinement) to effectively manage interpersonal aspects of sexuality and drug use. Initially, this may occur in simulated or role-play situations. Feedback is received and corrective changes can be made. This process continues until skills performance is proficient and spontaneous. Benefits from this practice are due to skill enhancement as well as increases in self-efficacy.

4. *Social support for personal change.* Change occurs within a network of social influences that can assist or undermine efforts at change. Interpersonal, sociocultural, economic, and religious factors can put constraints on self-protective behaviors. According to Bandura, these constraints often fall on women, who may find it difficult to adopt self-protective behaviors in the face of emotional and economic dependence, having less power than men, facing coercive threats, and cultural prescriptions about appropriate compliant roles. Another example would be a man or woman whose religion puts constraints on using condoms.

Bandura's theory includes cognition (awareness of severity of threat), skill building in terms of both behaviors and attitudes, and a recognition of social context. He does not address to the same extent as do the protection-motivation theory and the theory of reasoned action how an appraisal of threat (leading to motivation to change health behaviors) is made. However, he is more explicit than the other theories about how people acquire and refine new skills (eg, social modeling). Additionally, most theories or models of health-protective behavior change now acknowledge the importance of self-efficacy as a component of successful behavior change.

AIDS RISK-REDUCTION MODEL

Designed specifically to address HIV disease, the AIDS risk-reduction model provides a conceptual framework for organizing the factors that appear to influence people's ability to change high-risk sexual behaviors (Catania, Kegeles, & Coates, 1990). This model builds on several models of change, including the health belief model, self-efficacy theory, and the theory of reasoned action. The AIDS risk-reduction model organizes general predictors of health behavior (e.g., perceived susceptibility) and specific predictors of sexual behavior (e.g., sexual enjoyment), then considers some of the unique influences of the HIV epidemic (e.g., knowing someone with HIV).

This model is described by Catania et al. (1990) as broader in scope than models that emphasize cognitive determinants of health behaviors. Although cognitive factors are viewed as important, Catania et al. believe that it is unknown whether beliefs that affect the onset of behavior change will also affect the maintenance of these new behaviors over time. This distinction is important because lapses and relapse are so common in behavior change. Additionally, they suggest that the social context in which sexual behaviors occur are not understandable solely in terms of beliefs or attitudes. In this regard, the AIDS risk-reduction model is somewhat similar to Bandura's self-efficacy theory.

The AIDS risk-reduction model hypothesizes the following stages of change:

1. Recognizing and labeling one's sexual behavior as high risk for contracting HIV (this is similar to perceived susceptibility of one's behavior and perceived severity of HIV).
2. Making a commitment to reduce high-risk sexual contacts and increase low-risk activities (this process might be influenced by perceptions of enjoyment, self-efficacy, or attitudes toward condoms).
3. Seeking and enacting strategies to obtain these goals (this might include communication with partner, informal networking, or formal help-seeking).

These stages are not viewed as unidirectional or invariant (Catania et al., 1990). One valuable aspect of their model is the emphasis on both cognition and emotions. For example, this model addresses the important role that sensation seeking or sexual enjoyment may play in maintaining high-risk behaviors, such as unprotected anal intercourse. This emphasis is important because a number of studies have shown that HIV-positive gay men whose preferred sexual activity was unprotected receptive anal intercourse prior to learning of their seropositive status were significantly more likely than other groups of seropositive gay men to continue this practice after learning of their HIV-positive status. This model is also one of the few attempts to develop a risk-prevention model specific to HIV disease.

A recent study using the AIDS risk-reduction model to reduce HIV risk in a group of unmarried heterosexual adults with an HIV risk factor illustrates how this model can be used in prevention programs (Catania, Coates, & Kegeles, 1994). For example, high levels of condom use, with both primary and secondary partners, were associated with greater condom commitment, greater enjoyment, and health-protective sexual communication. Each of these correlates of condom use could easily be addressed in a prevention program.

SUMMARY: DISCUSSION OF RISK-REDUCTION MODELS

It is not possible at this time to determine which theory of risk reduction is best, both because of the limited amount of research on each of these models that specifically addresses HIV disease (Fisher & Fisher, 1992) and because only rarely is one theory pitted against another (Weinstein, 1993). As Fisher and Fisher (1992) compellingly show in their review of the AIDS risk-reduction literature, exhortations to intervene outnumber credible interventions. Their review of this body of literature also shows that the vast majority of this research is based on informal conceptualizations (as opposed to theories or models) of risk reduction and behavior change. Because tests of these models have primarily utilized convenience samples of gay and bisexual men, it is less clear how they might reduce risk in other populations.

Based on their review of this literature, Fisher and Fisher (1992) did conclude that risk-reduction studies that were conceptually based and group specific, and that provided information, motivation, and behavioral skills had the greatest impact on reducing risky behaviors. This finding suggests that risk-reduction models should, at a minimum, include these components to be effective in bringing about important behavior changes.

Another criticism of the risk-reduction models and theories that have been discussed is that most do not explicitly discuss an important aspect of the change process—relapse. According to Marlatt and Gordon (1985), lapses (e.g., unprotected anal intercourse with a partner whose serostatus is unknown) are expected components of the change process, and are important in understanding the corrections or refinements that need to be made to strengthen and maintain positive health-behavior changes. What is critical is the individual's reaction to a lapse, or the "abstinence violation effect." Is it viewed as a response to a specific situation (e.g., feeling momentarily overwhelmed), or is it viewed as a personal failure or weakness? In the latter case, the risk of relapse (and a return to baseline) is much greater. For example, Kirk, an HIV-negative, gay health professional, had consistently practiced safer sex for over 8 years. One night, in Kirk's own words, "I got swept away." Kirk was able to look at 8 years of safer sex and view this one time as an atypical response to a specific situation and focus on understanding what it was about that situation that put him at risk. However, unlike with most behaviors, lapses in HIV-related behaviors can have disastrous consequences.

The cognitive-behavioral literature on other types of health changes, such as maintaining weight loss, exercise programs, and dietary restrictions, is replete with examples of achieving target behaviors relatively easily in comparison with the difficulties most people have in maintaining these behaviors over time. This supports the importance of building the concept of relapse into interventions, having brief, follow-up interventions to help maintain behavior change and to manage lapses, and intervening on a community level so that changes are supported by the individual's social environment.

Finally, it is important to note that these models do not capture all of the variables that are important in risk reduction. Perhaps one reason is that it is difficult to create or re-create the actual contexts in which sexuality and drug use play out. For example, behavioral skills might be taught and role-played in the safety of a workshop where there is a group expectation that safer practices are desirable and beneficial. In contrast, an individual's actual experience may be quite different when encountering pressures in his or her environment. These models also rely heavily on rational approaches to risk reduction (the AIDS risk-reduction model does this to a lesser extent). In other words, they assume that people will logically and rationally evaluate the costs and benefits of behavior change. Yet most HIV risk behaviors occur in interpersonal contexts that are not defined by logic and reason. Prevention models that consider the importance of these interpersonal factors, and the contexts in which these relationships occur, are needed to reduce HIV risk behaviors.

CHAPTER 21

Community-Based Interventions

Finally, it is important to consider the processes
that underlie changes at the community level.
The relevance of this issue is obvious when we
consider that only a fraction of all people
practicing high-risk behavior will ever directly
contact our intervention programs.

—CATANIA ET AL. (1989, p. 248)

If the HIV epidemic is to be contained in the near future, the best hope
is through interventions that alter the behaviors of both individuals and
of communities. Traditionally, the focus of health interventions has been
on the individual (Chesney, 1993). Because of the interpersonal nature
of HIV disease, which is influenced by individuals, peers, and community norms, interventions need to encompass all of these contexts to be
optimally effective. Counselors can play important roles in helping
design and implement community services as well as prevention interventions by drawing from their work with individual and group clients.
Communities may be represented by neighborhoods, by affiliations
such as being gay or being an injecting drug user, by schools, by ethnicity,
or by a combination of identifying factors.

Community-based interventions that alter social norms to encourage risk avoidance and to discourage risk-taking behaviors that can
spread HIV disease represent one promising community approach
(Kelly, Murphy, Sikkema, & Kalichman, 1993b). Kelly et al. (1994) rec-

ommend multifaceted community approaches that combine community activation, social marketing, and mass media. Similarly, Fisher and Fisher (1992) noted in their review of the HIV risk-reduction literature that those interventions that are conceptually based and group specific and that provide information, motivation, and behavioral skills have the greatest impact on changing risky behaviors. Yet as will be seen from the following literature review, this is not the case in the majority of interventions relevant to service delivery.

OVERVIEW OF EMPIRICAL LITERATURE
ON INTERVENTIONS AND SERVICES

What is presently known about the effectiveness of HIV interventions for specific populations? More is known about HIV risk-reduction intervention, and consequently service delivery, for the gay population than any other population (Fisher & Fisher, 1992). Although many of the interventions described in the literature were successful in reducing risky behaviors, some common methodological limitations reduce the definitiveness of this research. According to Fisher and Fisher (1992), these limitations include using as participants men who were so highly motivated that they willingly attended 7 to 13 intervention sessions, lack of control groups, and the exclusive use of self-report measures.

Research on adolescents and on injecting drug users and their partners is next in frequency in the literature. However, most of these interventions were not based on formal approaches (such as one of the models or theories discussed in the previous chapter on risk reduction), relied on self-report, and, in the case of adolescents, were primarily informational in nature. Interventions for injecting drug users have often confounded psychosocial interventions with medical interventions (e.g., testing). However, for both of these populations, the few studies that contained multiple components (e.g., informational, motivational, and/or behavioral) did show some success.

Perhaps more so than for any other population, the majority of interventions targeted at university students have been based on nontheoretical formulations and have focused on delivering information rather than on increasing motivation or learning relevant health-protective skills. Despite these limitations, information appears to have a greater impact on the behaviors of college students than it does in some other populations.

Finally, there have been few empirical examinations of interventions directed at other groups, such as people seeking services for STDs, prostitutes, and the general public. Most risk-reduction interventions directed at the general public have been based on informal (e.g., ads, posters) approaches and have been informational only.

It is clear from this overview of the empirical literature on HIV risk-reduction interventions that exhortations and recommendations to intervene in relevant and meaningful ways for specific, targeted populations have not resulted in a definitive body of research to guide service delivery. Fisher and Fisher (1992) drew several themes from their review of this risk-reduction literature. (1) There is a need for conceptually based interventions, as most have been informal. (2) Formal research to identify group- appropriate interventions is rare, although many researchers stress the importance of tailoring interventions to meet the needs of specific target groups. (3) Many writers allude to the importance of interventions including informational, motivational, and behavioral skills components, yet such a broad and inclusive focus is uncommon. (4) Many researchers stress the importance of systematic evaluation research to monitor the effectiveness of interventions, yet there were almost always problems with aspects of the research, such as the absence of control groups, reliance on reactive, self-report measures, high rates of participant self-selection, high attrition rates, and confounded interventions. These methodological limitations make it difficult to know if the intervention even caused the effects, or which specific component of the intervention caused an effect. On a positive note, those interventions that were conceptually based and group specific and that provided information, motivation, and behavioral skills had the greatest impact.

The previous chapter on models of risk reduction described a number of conceptual models or theories that could provide an adequate conceptual base for community-based interventions and that include informational, motivational, and behavioral skills components. But how does one design interventions that are "group specific"? Before effective interventions can be designed, group-specific gaps in knowledge about transmission and prevention must first be identified. In other words, what information and misinformation do various groups have about HIV transmission and prevention? Once this information is obtained, it can then be used to design group-specific interventions.

Group-specific information about HIV should be obtained in a manner that provides few cues as to the correct responses, so as to get a complex and accurate view of gaps in knowledge and barriers to change (Fisher & Fisher, 1992). This might be done through open-ended questions and through the use of focus groups. Focus groups allow a small number of people to informally discuss specific topics. For example, focus groups for poor women who are financially and emotionally dependent on men might reveal that the women know that condoms prevent HIV and know how to use them, but fear asking their partners to use them. Using this example, interventions that focus solely on information about condoms and HIV transmission and on how to use condoms will not be as effective as discovering and eliminating the barriers to condom use for this group of women. These barriers might include feeling powerless, feeling constrained by sex roles, or lacking self-efficacy. Understanding the needs of the target group has become increasingly important as the demographics shift from primarily gay men, whose interventions were often researched and designed by other gay men, to economically impoverished people of color whose needs and perspectives may not be as well understood by those who offer them services.

The importance of interventions being "group specific" has been one of the weakest links in the empirical literature on service delivery. Often the researchers decide what the informational, motivational, and behavioral skill needs of a specific group are rather than going through a process (e.g., focus groups, needs assessments) to determine this. Therefore, in drawing conclusions and making recommendations about community-based interventions to reduce HIV disease, it is also helpful to review the theoretical and the applied literature.

ATTENDING TO SOCIAL AND COMMUNITY VARIABLES OF THE TARGET GROUP

Bandura (1990) includes "social supports for personal change" as the final component of his self-efficacy model of behavior change. He discusses the role of interpersonal, sociocultural, religious, political, and economic factors that create constraints on the individual's ability (and motivation) to learn and maintain self-protective behaviors. In other words, subcommunity or community norms can support or hinder attempts to make health-protective changes. Ignoring or minimizing these factors can lead to intervention failures.

Similarly, Fisher (1988) discussed the importance of reference group based social influence. In other words, the reference group of the individual (e.g., other gang members) can increase the likelihood of an intervention being effective if it is in line with reference group norms, or it can cause the intervention to be ineffective if it is not. In order for HIV-preventive behavior changes to occur, reference group norms need to be relatively consistent with the desired behavior.

Moderator variables are also viewed as important in determining the success of an intervention. For example, the centrality of a value or behavior to the core of a group's assumptive world will affect the success or failure of a particular intervention. Designing an intervention around "always using condoms when having intercourse" will almost certainly fail if the target population is a group of married Latina women who are devout Catholics. Other moderators include level of trust toward the group or institution proposing the change, and the target group's previous experience and success with making changes. How can HIV-protective behaviors be made "value consistent"? Fisher offers some interesting and useful ideas, such as reframing the intervention so it appears consistent with group norms. For example, this might involve finding ways for condom use to seem "macho" in a macho subculture.

Croteau, Nero, and Prosser (1993) also acknowledged the importance of social and cultural sensitivity when designing group-specific HIV prevention programming. They suggested that failing to work from a socially and culturally sensitive base can continue a pattern of oppression already experienced by many groups. Focusing on four target groups (African Americans, Latinos, women, and gay men), they proposed that three key ideas should be considered in designing socially and culturally sensitive interventions.

1. Negative misinformation about the sexuality of certain groups are barriers to effective prevention efforts. For example, African Americans and Latinos are often viewed as "hypersexual," gay men as "promiscuous," and women as "objects" for the sexual enjoyment of men.

2. Individuals in these groups may hold a variety of group-specific misconceptions about HIV that create barriers to change. For example, many individuals may believe that HIV is a genocide attempt by the dominant white heterosexual culture (some African Americans believe that AIDS is planned biological warfare against blacks, and some gays view institutional indifference as a form of genocide against gays). Some groups may also view HIV as a "white gay male thing," or be misinformed about virus transmission.

3. Individuals who hold membership in two or more of these groups may face added difficulties in adopting preventive behaviors because of multiple stigmatization or discrimination.

These three perspectives offer compelling reasons why the social and cultural context of a targeted group must be considered, understood, and valued in order to design, implement, and optimize the chances of bringing about positive health-protective behavior changes. It is something akin to empathic attunement in our clinical work—the importance of coming to an in-depth understanding of the inner world of another person, or, in this case, a group of people.

CHARACTERISTICS OF EFFECTIVE
COMMUNITY INTERVENTIONS

A number of researchers have described their observations of characteristics of effective community interventions. There are striking parallels between these perspectives, even though they often originate from work with vastly different populations.

Coates and Greenblatt (1988) propose several basic principles for community-based interventions: (1) pragmatic—use all avenues and all types of helpers indigenous to the community; (2) *simpatico*—selected interventions and methods of delivery need to be consistent with the dominant values of the community; (3) persistent—to be effective, interventions need to occur and recur frequently over time so that the diffusion process is maximized and so as to shape new community norms; and (4) grass roots—it is essential to include community leaders and help sources in planning and implementing interventions.

Bandura (1990) also emphasizes the importance of using indigenous (e.g., community) sources, as they can help mobilize formal and informal networks of influence and help create a motivational base for change. Indigenous leaders also serve as models of new skills and help establish health-protective behaviors as the normative standard of conduct. Similarly, Croteau et al. (1993) also suggest including target group members as full partners in interventions. For example, peer leaders can serve as advocates for prevention and often serve as opinion leaders who diffuse interventions to others in the network.

Deriving their recommendations from culturally sensitive interventions found in the literature, Croteau et al. (1993) discuss the importance of including culturally relevant content, media, and settings when designing and delivering interventions. For example, interventions for women might include some discussion of the role of sexism in the socialization of women and how that affects health-protective behaviors. Media includes aspects such as reading level, appropriate language, appropriate models, and the depiction of meaningful real-life situations. Settings for interventions should be natural gathering places where people feel safe and at home. This might be in a bar, a church, or a community center.

Both Kelly, Murphy, et al. (1993) and De La Cancela (1989) offer many of the same or similar suggestions already described, based on their reviews of the literature. However, De La Cancela (1989) attended more explicitly to social-class factors and to communities that may be dealing with multiple sources of discrimination, such as economically impoverished communities of color. His recommendations for minority prevention interventions include (1) use of natural support systems, information networks, and educational centers such as churches, barbershops, and small restaurants; (2) use of professional human services centers such as schools, and health and youth centers; (3) use of self-help and community-based organizations such as tenant and political groups; (4) use of credible, professional speakers and community leaders who can appropriately relate to the target group; (5) use of nonjudgmental print materials and public service announcements; (6) placement of HIV information in a context that locates its risk in relation to other risks in the community; and (7) the active education of staff who live in the community, so that they become informal community educators.

SUMMARY OF RECOMMENDATIONS FOR COMMUNITY INTERVENTIONS

Several common components emerge from these sets of recommendations. First, it is essential to utilize indigenous resources, including peer or opinion leaders as well as existing agencies and institutions. Community leaders serve the critical functions of being credible conveyors of information, models of new skills, and diffusers of new norms. Next, interventions need to be congruent with the values, beliefs, and resources of the community. Then, delivery of interventions should occur in culturally relevant and comfortable settings. Finally, grass roots efforts, firmly grounded in the community, are essential to maintain the targeted behavior changes. In addition, Kelly, Murphy, et al. (1993) emphasize the importance of utilizing print, broadcast, and other mass media in getting a message out to the target population.

EXAMPLES OF EFFECTIVE COMMUNITY-BASED HIV-RELATED INTERVENTIONS

It is helpful to describe actual community-based interventions that are culturally relevant and apparently effective in addressing important community or group needs. The first four were identified by Croteau et al. (1993) and are described as exemplar programs that include a sensitivity to social and cultural contexts. Additionally, two other community-based interventions will be described, which address critical prevention and service needs in other populations. Both Fisher and Fisher (1992) and Kelly, Murphy, et al. (1993), have also published excellent reviews of successful community-based HIV prevention interventions.

Opinion Leaders in Gay Clubs

Peer-identified opinion leaders in gay clubs in three cities were taught HIV information and trained to initiate conversations with other club patrons in which they presented health-promoting messages (Kelly et al., 1991). This resulted in a significant reduction in risk behavior when compared with a control group, an effect attributed to the effectiveness of opinion leaders to produce or accelerate change.

Theater Productions by Latino Youth

Theater presentations involving Latino teens as actors and discussants were described by Matiella (1988). These presentations offered bilingual skits depicting a variety of unresolved problems, including some related to HIV transmission, followed by discussions with the audience. The audience's role was to generate creative means of responding to the problems.

Rap Music Contests

In another intervention aimed at teens, Martin and Stroud (1988) described a rap music contest titled "Rap'n down AIDS" held in the San Francisco area. Entrants wrote songs related to HIV topics such as routes of transmission, and cash prizes were given. The winning raps were then developed into radio and television public service announcements.

Student Leaders on College Campuses

An intervention designed by Croteau, Morgan, Henderson, and Nero (1992) targeted student leaders of the African American, Latino, feminist, and lesbian and gay college campus organizations. During a weekend retreat, leaders participated in activities including awareness of the experience of oppression, films and lectures about HIV, and culture-specific performances in music and theater. The purpose of the intervention was to empower the leaders to serve as advocates in their communities for HIV-prevention activities and attitudes. Both positive attitudes toward HIV disease and leadership behaviors involving HIV prevention increased.

Street Youth

Springer described her intervention with street youths, many of whom are prostitutes, as reaching the unreachable (*HIV Frontline*, July/August

1994d). In this intervention taking place on the streets of New York City, street youths educated their peers in HIV risk-reduction using an approach based on the harm-reduction model. This approach does not require abstinence from sex or drugs but reduces the harmful consequences. For example, one might continue to inject drugs but only use sterile needles that are not shared, or he or she may continue to prostitute but always use condoms. Called the Clinton Peer AIDS Education Coalition, the goal is to help street youth change what they do rather than who they are.

Rural HIV Services

The final intervention differs from the others that have been described as its primary goal is to provide services to those with HIV and their significant others. However, this intervention is noteworthy because it is a model of how to bring services to a rural, sparsely populated area that would likely have few, if any, services otherwise. The HIV/AIDS Wellness—Grand Traverse Area, Inc., is a network of volunteers covering a 14-county area in Michigan, organized to help those with AIDS and their significant others cope with isolation, discrimination, and stigmatization (*HIV Frontline*, July/August 1994c). An impressive variety of services are offered, including a monthly education group, a buddy program, housecleaning and other support services, bedside support, transportation services, and financial support.

Although this program addresses the needs of those who already have HIV, it is likely that it has a broader impact on the community at large because of its modeling of a compassionate, caring response to the problem of HIV disease. Raising awareness and lessening of stigmatization are critical as increasing numbers of PWHIVs return to rural areas to be with their families or communities of origin as they become ill.

SUMMARY: SERVICE DELIVERY
AND COMMUNITY-BASED PREVENTION

This review of the literature on community-based HIV-prevention interventions suggests that barriers to effective prevention strategies exist for many people. Many interventions have been modeled on the needs of gay white men, who represented the first wave of the epidemic. The needs of these men differ in many ways from the needs of other persons needing prevention interventions today. There is consensus that service delivery can be enhanced by understanding cultural values and behavioral patterns for subgroups of clients that are relevant both to HIV transmission as well as to coping with HIV disease.

Finally, service delivery is very limited in some parts of the country where demand is great and resources limited, or where there are few cases of HIV disease. This is particularly true in smaller towns and in rural areas. Persons seeking services in these areas also risk greater stigmatization, as anonymity may be compromised when they seek services. While, on the other hand, major cities with a high incidence of HIV-infected persons may offer an array of medical and psychosocial services, these may not be perceived as addressing the specific sociocultural needs of many subgroups in these larger urban areas. Moreover, because many service networks are already straining to meet the ever-increasing demand, access to services, particularly for people with limited resources such as income, health insurance, and transportation, may be quite difficult.

Major changes in service delivery will need to occur to accommodate those in need of prevention strategies as well as those who are already living with HIV disease. Interventions that are group specific and that meet minimum criteria for effectiveness need to be developed, implemented, and refined. According to Bandura (1990), the greatest impediment to prevention efforts is viewing behavior change as a stopgap measure until a vaccine is developed.

Epilogue: What We Can Learn from HIV Disease

HIV disease, like many other health epidemics, reflects an array of biological, social, political, and psychological factors in terms of who becomes ill, the resources of the infected to manage their disease, and societal and political responses to the disease. In addition, HIV is the most intensively studied virus ever (Greene, 1993). This is in part because of the fatality of the virus and the resultant devastation of many lives, as well as the profound impact this virus has had worldwide. Therefore, HIV disease provides an opportunity to understand how health crises might unfold in the future.

Chesney (1993), describing the HIV pandemic as a harbinger of things to come, posits that HIV has introduced researchers to five trends and issues that have broad implications for worldwide health in the future: (1) early identification (and intervention) of people who are at risk for disease; (2) rising expectations for successful behavior change programs; (3) growing populations of those who are coping with chronic disease; (4) increasing shift to include community and public health perspectives; and (5) emerging need to address health problems on a global scale. Although Chesney is specifically viewing these trends from the perspective of the health community, these trends also have important implications for mental health professionals.

For example, attitudinal and behavioral changes are at present the best ways to reduce the transmission of HIV disease. These efforts will be most successful when targeted at communities, rather than at individuals. For those who have already acquired HIV disease, it is likely that earlier identification and increased longevity will mean that many people will be living for years with a chronic disease. This has important implications for helping people and their significant others cope with the effects of chronic illness. HIV has also shown us that many health issues now have the potential to become global concerns. For example, prior to jet travel and urbanization, HIV disease might have stayed contained within small, isolated communities.

In addition to the trends described by Chesney (1993), I would add several other trends or issues that I believe are especially salient for mental health professionals:

1. HIV disease should be viewed within the context of the individual's life. HIV represents only one aspect of the person's life rather than his or her entire life. Other problems (e.g., poverty, addictions) may be more pressing or urgent. Therefore, attention should focus on other life events in order to effectively address HIV disease.

2. Counseling interventions should focus on both the individual and the individual's system or community so that behavioral and attitudinal changes are supported and maintained. Interventions will also be more effective if they consider contextual variables such as subculture and community norms and behaviors.

3. Communities need to become actively involved in HIV risk-reduction interventions as well as interventions for those who have already acquired HIV disease. Interventions are more effective when mental health professionals and others work in partnership with community leaders.

4. Much of what we know about HIV disease in the United States is based on gay men. Additionally, much of what we know is based on quantitative research, rather than qualitative research, which may not be the best or only way to learn about some aspects of HIV and about some populations.

5. It is likely that in the near future, HIV will be viewed as a chronic, but not necessarily life-threatening, disease. However, the possibility of a fatal outcome is but one aspect of a chronic disease. For example, PWHIVs will likely continue to be infectious, which will have implications for interpersonal relationships and life goals such as becoming a parent. Chronic diseases also require many other adaptations, such as accepting the disease as part of one's identity and experiencing fears or restrictions as a result of the disease.

6. Finally, therapeutic work can be enhanced by reframing what we can offer to clients with HIV that is valuable. I believe that

healing can occur through the therapeutic relationship and alliance. This type of healing is based not on curing, but rather on the power of caring.

Many do not expect HIV disease to be the last pandemic. The conditions that created this pandemic have the potential to perpetuate others. Because of this, we can use HIV disease to help us prepare for future epidemics. Our response to HIV disease can serve as a template for responding to other health crises. Will HIV prepare us to respond effectively to other health challenges? Will we have learned effective strategies that prevent the spread of disease? Will we have learned psychosocial interventions that alleviate the distress of those who are infected and their significant others? Most important, will we have learned to view those affected by diseases such as HIV in a more compassionate way that reflects that we are all in this together, that what happens to others also affects us?

Appendix: Resources for Mental Health Professionals Working with Clients with HIV Disease

ORGANIZATIONS

American Foundation for AIDS Research (AMFAR)
733 Third Avenue, 12th Floor
New York, NY 10017
Phone: (212) 682-7440

Funds research and publishes information about resources and treatment and provides many other services.

Gay Men's Health Crisis (GMHC)
129 W. 20th Street
New York, NY 10011-0022
Phone: (212) 807-6655

One of the first organizations to provide comprehensive HIV services. Offers a hotline, counseling, and other social services as well as publications about HIV disease.

Names Project
2362 Market Street
San Francisco, CA 94114
Phone: (800) USA-NAME

This organization has created the quilt that remembers those who have died of AIDS.

National Association of People With AIDS
2025 I Street, NW, Suite 415
Washington, DC 20006
Phone: (202) 429-2856

National Gay and Lesbian Task Force
1517 U Street, NW
Washington, DC 20009
Phone: (202) 332-6483

Pediatric AIDS Foundation
1311 Colorado Avenue
Santa Monica, CA 90404
Phone: (800) 488-5000

San Francisco AIDS Foundation
333 Valencia Street
San Francisco, CA 94101-6182
Phone: (415) 861-3397

University of California—San Francisco AIDS Health Project
Box 0884
San Francisco, CA 94143-0884
Phone: (415) 476-6430

Whitman–Walker Clinic
1407 S. Street, NW
Washington, DC 20009
Phone: (202) 797-3590

One of the first clinics to provide comprehensive HIV services including a hotline, counseling, social services, and outreach.

RESEARCH AND INFORMATIONAL NEWSLETTERS

Focus: A Guide to AIDS Research and Counseling
UCSF AIDS Health Project
Box 0884
San Francisco, CA 94143-0884
Phone: (415) 476-6430

CDC AIDS Weekly Subscription Office
P.O. Box 830409
Birmingham, AL 35283-0409
Phone: (800) 633-4931

HIV Frontline
NCM Publishers, Inc.
200 Varick Street
New York, NY 10014

This newsletter is supported by an educational grant from Burroughts Wellcome Co. Copies of the newsletter are available to counselors by calling (800) 722-9292, ext. 54511, and specifying program BW-YO5663.

Psychology and AIDS Exchange
American Psychological Association
Office on AIDS
750 First Street, NE
Washington, DC 20002-4242
Phone: (202) 336-6042

This newsletter is published quarterly and includes articles, resources, and information on conferences and workshops.

Reality
c/o Antigone Hodgins
Project AHEAD
375 Woodside Avenue, Building W-1
San Francisco, CA 94127
Phone: (415) 753-7875

This is a quarterly newsletter by and for young people with HIV disease.

INFORMATIONAL AND TRAINING SERVICES

AIDS Information Network
32 North 3rd Street
Philadelphia, PA 19106
Phone: (215) 922-5120.

This network maintains a library of HIV information and will conduct a literature search.

Centers for Disease Control and Prevention
National AIDS Clearinghouse
P.O. Box 6003
Rockville, MD 20849-6003
Phone: (800) 458-5231

The clearinghouse collects, classifies, and distributes up-to-date information and provides expert assistance to HIV-prevention professionals including information about more than 17,000 organizations that provide HIV-related services, assistance with networking, and comprehensive on-line services.

HOPE Program
American Psychological Association
Office of AIDS
750 First Street, NE
Washington, DC 20002-4242
Phone: (202) 336-6057

This is a training program that prepares mental health professionals to work with PWHIVs and to train other mental health professionals.

Learning AIDS: An Informational Resources Directory
R.R. Bowker
245 West 17th Street
New York, NY 10011
Phone: (800) 521-8110

SPECIAL INTERESTS INFORMATION

Affording Care
429 E. 52nd Street, #4G
New York, NY 10022-6431
Phone: (212) 371-4740

Provides information on financial aspects of living with HIV (run by David Peterson).

Gay Men's Health Crisis (GMHC)
129 W. 20th Street
New York, NY 10011-0022
Phone: (212) 807-6655

Kairos Support for Caregivers
114 Douglas Street
San Francisco, CA 94114
Phone: (415) 861-0877

Kairos offers various services to help caregivers manage stress including a caregiver's booklet and guidelines for developing local support groups.

Minority Task Force on AIDS
123 W. 115th Street
New York, NY 10026
Phone: (212) 663-7772

Women AIDS Network
San Francisco AIDS Foundation
333 Valencia Street
San Francisco, CA 94101
Phone: (415) 864-4376

Women and AIDS Resource Network
P.O. Box 020525
Brooklyn, NY 11202
Phone: (718) 596-6007

National Library of Medicine
National Institutes of Health
Bethesda, MD 20894
Phone: (301) 496-6308

The library provides several online computer services including AIDSLINE (in Medline) and a bibliography of research on HIV disease.

Project Inform
Phone: (800) 822-7422

Provides information about the Concorde and other studies on antiretroviral treatments.

TELEPHONE INFORMATION AND HOTLINES

Center for Substance Abuse Prevention (CSAP) National Clearinghouse for Alcohol and Drug Information: (800) 729-6686.

Centers for Disease Control and Prevention National STD (Sexually Transmitted Diseases) Hotline: (800) 227-8922.

Clinical Trials Information Hotline, National Institutes of Health: (800) TRIALS-A.

National AIDS Hot Line: (800)-342-AIDS; Spanish: (800) 344-SIDA; Hearing Impaired AIDS Hotline: (800) 243-7889.

National Drug Information and Referral Line, National Institute of Drug Abuse: (800) 662-HELP.

National Native American AIDS Prevention Center, Indian AIDS Hotline: (800) 283-AIDS.

Pediatric AIDS Information Line: (800) 488-5000.

Project Inform Information Hotline National: (800) 822-7422; California (except San Francisco): (800) 334-7422, San Francisco: (415) 558-9051.

References

Adler, G., & Beckett, A. (1989). Psychotherapy of the patient with an HIV infection: Some ethical and therapeutic dilemmas. *Psychosomatics, 30,* 203–208.

Ajzen, I., & Fishbein, M. (1980). *Understanding attitudes and predicting behavior.* Englewood Cliffs, NJ: Prentice-Hall.

Allers, C. T., & Katrin, S. E. (1988). AIDS counseling: Psychosocial model. *Journal of Mental Health Counseling, 10,* 235–244.

Allison, K. W., Crawford, I., Echemendia, R., Robinson, L., & Knepp, D. (1994). Human diversity and professional competence: Training in clinical and counseling psychology revisited. *American Psychologist, 49,* 792–796.

American Association for Counseling and Development Governing Council. (1988, July 14–17). *AACD position statement on Acquired Immune Deficiency Syndrome.* Symposium conducted by the AACD Governing Council.

American Psychological Association. (1991). *American Psychological Association AIDS-related policy statements.* Washington, DC: American Psychological Association.

American Psychological Association Ad Hoc Committee on Psychology and AIDS. (1993). APA HOPE program moves west! *Psychology and AIDS Exchange, 12,* 14.

Americans with Disabilities Act of 1990, Pub. L. No. 101–336, §2,104 Stat. 328 (1991).

Anderson, R. M., & May, R. M. (1992). Understanding the AIDS pandemic. *Scientific American, 266,* 58–61, 64–66.

Antoni, M. H., Baggett, L., Ironson, G., LaPerriere, A., August, S., Klimas, N., Schneiderman, N., & Fletcher, M. A. (1991). Cognitive-behavioral stress management intervention buffers distress responses and immunologic changes following notification of HIV-1 seropositivity. *Journal of Consulting and Clinical Psychology, 59,* 906–915.

Antoni, M. H., Schneiderman, N., Fletcher, M. A., Goldstein, D. A., Ironson, G.,

& Laperriere, A. (1990). Psychoneuroimmunology and HIV-1. *Journal of Counseling and Clinical Psychology, 58*, 38–49.

APA [American Psychiatric Association] Ad Hoc Committee on AIDS Policy. (1988). AIDS policy: Confidentiality and disclosure. *American Journal of Psychiatry, 145*, 541–542.

Aronson, E., Fried, C., & Stone, J. (1991). Overcoming denial and increasing the intention to use condoms through the induction of hypocrisy. *American Journal of Public Health, 81*, 1636–1638.

Atkinson, J. H., & Grant, I. (1994). Natural history of neuropsychiatric manifestations of HIV disease. *Psychiatric Clinics of North America, 17*, 17–31

Attig, T. (1983). Respecting the dying and bereaved believers. *Newsletter of Forum for Death Education and Counseling, 6*, 16.

Baiss, A. (1989). A peer counseling program for persons testing H.I.V. antibody positive. *Canadian Journal of Counseling, 23*, 127–132.

Baker, J. (1993). Treatment of mood disorders. *FOCUS: A Guide to AIDS Research and Counseling, 8*(8), 1–4.

Baker, R. (1994). Prospects for a new strategy for HIV treatment. *FOCUS: A Guide to AIDS Research and Counseling, 9*, 1–4.

Baldwin, D., & Baldwin, I. (1988). AIDS information and sexual behavior on a university campus. *Journal of Sex Education and Therapy, 14*, 24–28.

Baltimore, D. (1995). Lessons from people with nonprogressive HIV infection. *New England Journal of Medicine, 332*, 259–260.

Baum, M., Cassetti, L., Bonvehi, P., Shor-Posner, G., Lu, Y., & Suberlich, H. (1994). Inadequate dietary intake and altered nutrition status in early HIV-1 infection. *Nutrition, 10*, 16–20.

Baum, M., Shor-Posner, G., Bonvehi, P., Cassetti, L., Lu, Y., Mantero-Atienza, E., Beach, R. S., & Sauberlich, H. E. (1992). Influence of HIV infection on vitamin status and requirements. *Annals of the New York Academy of Sciences, 669*, 165–173.

Bennett, T. A., & Hendrickson, M. (1993). Pastoral counseling. *FOCUS: A Guide to AIDS Research and Counseling, 8*(7), 5–6.

Bandura, A. (1986). *Social foundations of thought and action: A social cognitive theory.* Englewood Cliffs, NJ: Prentice- Hall.

Bandura, A. (1989). Self-efficacy mechanism in physiological activation and health-promoting behavior. In J. Madden, IV, S. Matthysee, & J. Barchas (Eds.), *Adaptation, learning, and affect.* New York: Raven Press.

Bandura, A. (1990). Perceived self-efficacy in the exercise of control over AIDS infection. *Evaluation and Program Planning, 13*, 9–17.

Barret, R. L. (1989). Counseling gay men with AIDS: Human dimensions. *Journal of Counseling and Development, 67*, 573–575.

Bartnof, H. S. (1988). Health care professional education and AIDS. In AIDS: Principles, practices, and politics [Special issue]. *Death Studies, 12*, 547–562.

Bauman, L. J., & Siegel, K. (1987). Misperceptions among gay men of the risk for AIDS associated with their sexual behavior. *Journal of Applied Social Psychology, 17*, 329–350.

Beckett, A., & Rutan, J. S. (1990). Treating persons with ARC and AIDS in group psychotherapy. *International Group Psychotherapy, 40*, 19–29.

Beckett, A., & Shenson, D. (1993). Suicide risk in patients with human immunodeficiency virus infection and acquired immunodeficiency syndrome. *Harvard Review of Psychiatry, 1,* 27–35.

Beckham, D. (1988). Group work with people who have AIDS. *Journal of Psychosocial Oncology, 6,* 213–218.

Behnke, J., & Bok, S. (1975). *The dilemmas of euthanasia.* Garden City, NY: Doubleday.

Belcher, A. E., Dettmore, D., & Holzemer, S. P. (1989). Spirituality and sense of well-being in persons with AIDS. *Holistic Nurse Practitioner, 3,* 16–25.

Bell, N. K. (1989). AIDS and women: Remaining ethical issues. *AIDS Education and Prevention, 1,* 22–30.

Bellemare, D. (1988). AIDS: The challenge to pastoral care. *Journal of Palliative Care, 4,* 58–60.

Bialer, P. A., Wallacke, J. J., & Snyder, S. L. (1991). Psychiatric diagnosis in HIV-spectrum disorders. *Psychiatric Medicine, 9,* 361–375.

Bloom, J. R. (1982). Social support, accommodation to stress, and adjustment to breast cancer. *Social Science Medicine, 16,* 1329–1338.

Bloom, P., & Carliner, G. (1988). The economic impact of AIDS in the United States. *Science, 239,* 604–609.

Bor, R., & Miller, R. (1988). Addressing "dreaded issues": A description of a unique counseling intervention with patients with AIDS/HIV. *Counseling Psychology Quarterly, 4,* 397–406.

Bor, R., Miller, R., & Goldman, E. (1993). *Theory and practice of HIV Counseling: A systemic approach.* New York: Brunner/Mazel.

Bosnak, R. (1994). Dreamwork and AIDS. *FOCUS: A Guide to AIDS Research and Counseling, 9*(2), 5–6.

Boyer, S. P., & Hoffman, M. A. (1993). Therapists' affective reactions to termination: Impact of therapist loss history and client sensitivity to loss. *Journal of Counseling Psychology, 40,* 271–277.

Britton, P. J., Zarski, J. J., & Hobfoll, S. E. (1993). Psychological distress and the role of significant others in a population of gay/bisexual men in the era of HIV. *AIDS Care, 5,* 43–54.

Brodkey, H. (1994, February 7). Dying: An update. *The New Yorker,* pp. 70–84.

Brookmeyer, R. (1991). Reconstruction and future trends of the AIDS epidemic in the United States. *Science, 253,* 37–42.

Brown, M. A., & Powell-Cope, G. (1993). Themes of loss and dying in caring for a family member with AIDS. *Research in Nursing and Health, 16,* 179–191.

Brown, S. A. (1985). Expectancies versus background in the prediction of college drinking patterns. *Journal of Consulting and Clinical Psychology, 53,* 123–130.

Bruhn, J. G. (1989). Counseling persons with a fear of AIDS. *Journal of Counseling and Development, 67,* 445–457.

Brunswick, A. F., Aidala, A., Dobkin, J., Howard, J., Titus, S. P., & Banaszak-Holl, J. (1993). HIV-1 seroprevalence and risk behaviors in a urban African-American community cohort. *American Journal of Public Health, 83,* 1390–1394.

Bulman, R. J., & Wortman, C. B. (1977). Attributions of blame and coping in the "real world": Severe accident victims react to their lot. *Journal of Personality and Social Psychology, 35,* 351–363.

Burack, J. H., Barrett, D. C., Stall, R. D., Chesney, M. A., Ekstrand, M. L., & Coates, T. J. (1993). Depressive symptoms and CD4 lymphocyte decline among HIV-infected men. *Journal of the American Medical Association, 270,* 2568–2573.

Burns, D. N., Kramer, A., Yellin, F., Fuchs, D., Wachter, H., DiGioia, R. A., Sanchez, W. C., Grossman, R. J., Gordin, F. M, Biggar, R. J., & Goedert, J. J. (1991). Cigarette smoking: A modifier of Human Immunodeficiency Virus Type 1 infection? *Journal of Acquired Immune Deficiency Syndromes, 4,* 76–83.

Butcher, A. H., Manning, D., & O'Neal, E. C. (1991). HIV-related sexual behaviors of college students. *Journal of American College Health, 40,* 115–118.

Butters, N., Grant, I., Haxby, J., Judd, L. L., Martin, A., McClelland, J., Pequegnat, W., Schacter, D., & Stover, E. (1990). Assessment of AIDS-related cognitive changes: Recommendations of the NIMH workshop on neuropsychological assessment approaches. *Journal of Clinical and Experimental Neuropsychology, 12,* 963–978.

Cadwell, S. (1991). Twice removed: The stigma suffered by gay men with AIDS. *Smith College Studies in Social Work, 61,* 236–246.

Cadwell, S. A. (1994). Over-identification with HIV clients. *Journal of Gay and Lesbian Psychotherapy, 2,* 77–99.

Campbell, S. M., Peplau, L. A., & DeBro, S. C. (1992). Women, men, and condoms: Attitudes and experiences of heterosexual college students. *Psychology of Women Quarterly, 16,* 273–288.

Campos, P. E., Brasfield, T. L., & Kelly, J. A. (1989). Psychology training related to AIDS: Survey of doctoral graduate programs and predoctoral internship programs. *Professional Psychology Research and Practice, 20,* 214–220.

Cao, Y., Qin, L., Zhang, L., Safrit, J., & Ho, D. (1995). Virologic and immunologic characteristics of long-term survivers of human immunodeficiency virus Type 1 infection. *New England Journal of Medicine, 332,* 201–207.

Carson, V. (1993). Prayer, meditation, exercise, and special diets: Behaviors of the hardy person with HIV/AIDS. *Journal of the Association of Nurses in AIDS Care, 4,* 18–21.

Carson, V., Soeken, K. L., & Shanty, J. (1990). Hope and spiritual well-being: Essentials for living with AIDS. *Perspectives in Psychiatric Care, 26,* 28–34.

Catania, J. A., Coates, T. J., & Kegeles, S. M. (1994). A test of the AIDS Risk Reduction Model: Psychosocial correlates of condom use in the AMEN cohort survey. *Health Psychology, 13,* 548–555.

Catania, J. A., Coates, T. J., Kegeles, S. M., Ekstrand, M., Guydish, J. R., & Bye, L. L. (1989). Implications of the AIDS risk-reduction model for the gay community: The importance of perceived sexual enjoyment and help-seeking behaviors. In V. M. Mays, G. W. Albee, & S. F. Schneider (Eds.), *Primary prevention of AIDS: Psychological approaches.* Newbury Park, CA: Sage.

Catania, J. A., Gibson, D. R., Chitwood, D. D., & Coates, T. J. (1990). Methodological problems in AIDS behavioral research: Influences on measurement error and participation bias in studies of sexual behavior. *Psychological Bulletin, 108,* 339–362.

Catania, J. A., Kegeles, S., & Coates, T. J. (1990). Towards an understanding of risk behavior: An AIDS risk reduction model (AARM). *Health Education Quarterly, 17,* 53–72.

Cates, W., & Stone, K. M. (1992). Family planning, sexually transmitted diseases, and contraceptive choice: A literature update. *Family Planning Perspectives, 24,* 75–84.

CDC AIDS Weekly. (1988, October 3). p. 2

Centers for Disease Control. (1992a). 1993 revised classification system for HIV infection and expanded surveillance case definition for AIDS among adolescents and adults. *Morbidity and Mortality Weekly Report, 41,* 1–19. (RR-17)

Centers for Disease Control (1992b). Projections of the number of persons diagnosed with AIDS and the number immunosuppressed HIV-infected persons—United States, 1992–1994. *Morbidity and Mortality Weekly Report, 41,* 1–21. (RR-18)

Centers for Disease Control. (1993a). 1993 sexually transmitted diseases treatment guidelines. *Morbidity and Mortality Weekly Report, 42,* 11. (RR-14)

Centers for Disease Control. (1993b). Update: Barrier protection against HIV infection and other sexually transmitted diseases. *Morbidity and Mortality Weekly Report, 42,* 589–591.

Centers for Disease Control and Prevention. (1995). HIV/AIDS surveillance report. *HIV/AIDS Surveillance Report, 6*(2), 1–16.

Centers for Disease Control. (1994). Zidovudine for the prevention of HIV transmission from mother to infant. *Morbidity and Mortality Weekly Report, 43,* 285–287.

Chesney, M. A. (1993). Health psychology in the 21st century: Acquired immunodeficiency syndrome as a harbinger of things to come. *Health Psychology, 12,* 259–268.

Chesney, M. A., & Folkman, S. (1994). Psychological impact of HIV disease and implications for intervention. *Psychiatric Clinics of North America, 17,* 163–173.

Choi, K., Catania, J., & Dolcini, M. (1994). Extramarital sex and HIV risk behavior among US adults: Results from the national AIDS behavioral survey. *American Journal of Public Health, 84,* 2003–2007.

Christ, G., & Wiener, L. (1985). Psychosocial issues for AIDS. In V. Devita, Jr., S. Hellman, & S. Rosenberg (Eds.), *AIDS.* Philadelphia: Lippincott.

Chu, S. Y., Buehler, J. W., Lieb, L., Beckett, G., Conti, L., Costa, S., Dahan, B., Danila, R., Fordyce, E. J., Hirozawa, A., Shields, A., Singleton, J. A., & Wold, C. (1993). Causes of death among persons reported with AIDS. *American Journal of Public Health, 83,* 1429–1432.

Chuang, H. T., Devins, G. M., Hunsley, J., & Gill, M. J. (1989). Psychosocial distress and well-being among gay and bisexual men with human immunodeficiency virus infection. *American Journal of Psychiatry, 146,* 876–880.

Clarke, P. J. (1981). Exploration of countertransference toward the dying. *American Journal of Orthopsychiatry, 51,* 71–77.

Clever, L. H. (1988). AIDS: A special challenge for health care workers. In AIDS: Principles, practices, and politics [Special issue]. *Death Studies, 12,* 519–529.

Coates, T. J., & Greenblatt, R. (1990). Behavioral changes using interventions at the community level. In K. K. Holmes, P. Mardh, P. F. Sparling, & P .J. Wiesner (Eds.), *Sexually transmitted diseases*. New York: McGraw-Hill.

Coates, T. J., Stall, R., & Hoff, C. (1988). *Changes in sexual behavior of gay and bisexual men since the beginning of the AIDS epidemic*. Report prepared for Office of Technology Assessment, U.S. Congress.

Coates, T. J., Stall, R. D., Mandel, J. S., Boccallari, A., Sorenson, J. L., Morales, E. F., Morin, S. F., Wiley, J. A., & McKusick, L. (1987). AIDS: A psychosocial research agenda. *Annals of Behavioral Medicine, 9*, 21–28.

Coates, T. J., Temoshok, L., & Mandel, J. (1984). Psychosocial research is essential to understanding and treating AIDS. *American Psychologist, 39*, 1309–1314.

Cochran, S. D., & Mays, V. M. (1989). Women and AIDS related concerns: Roles for psychologists in helping the worried well. *American Psychologist, 44*, 529–535.

Cohen, E. D. (1990). Confidentiality, counseling, and clients who have AIDS: Ethical foundations of a model rule. *Journal of Counseling and Development, 68*, 282–286.

Cohen, J. (1994). The Duesberg phenomenon. *Science, 266*, 1642–1644.

Cohen, J. B., Hauer, L. B., & Wofsy, C. B. (1989). Women and IV drugs: Parenteral and heterosexual transmission of Human Immunodeficiency Virus. *Journal of Drug Issues, 19*, 39–56.

Cohen, M. A. (1990). Biopsychosocial approach to the human immunodeficiency virus epidemic: A clinician's primer. *General Hospital Psychiatry, 12*, 98–123.

Coleman, V. E., & Harris, G. N. (1989). A support group for individuals recently testing HIV positive: A psycho-educational group model. *Journal of Sex Research, 26*, 539–548.

Colleen, C., Hoff, B. A., & McKusick, L. (1992). The impact of HIV antibody status on gay men's partner preferences: A community perspective. *AIDS Education and Prevention, 4*, 197–204.

Collins, J., Holtzman, D., Kann, L., & Kolbe, L. (1993). Predictors of condom use among U.S. high school students, 1991. *International Conference on AIDS, 9*, 94.

Concorde Coordinating Committee. (1994). Concorde: MRC/ANRS randomised double-blind controlled trial of immediate and deferred zidovudine in symptom-free HIV infection. *Lancet, 34*, 871–880.

Constitutional rights of AIDS carriers. (1986). *Harvard Law Review, 99*, 1274–1292.

Consumer Reports. (1995, May). How reliable are condoms? pp. 320–325.

Council on Ethical and Judicial Affairs. (1988). Ethical issues included in the growing AIDS crisis. *Journal of the American Medical Association, 259*, 1360–1361.

Cote, T. R., Biggar, R. J., & Dannenberg, A. L. (1992). Risk of suicide among persons with AIDS: A national assessment. *Journal of the American Medical Association, 268*, 2066–2068.

Council on Ethical and Judicial Affairs. (1988). Ethical issues included in the growing AIDS crisis. *Journal of the American Medical Association, 259*, 1360–1361.

Croteau, J. M., Morgan, S., Henderson, B., & Nero, C. I. (1992). Race, gender and sexual orientation in the HIV/AIDS epidemic: Evaluating an intervention for leaders of diverse communities. *Journal of Multicultural Counseling and Development, 20,* 168–180.

Croteau, J. M., Nero, C. I., Prosser, D. J. (1993). Social and cultural sensitivity in group-specific HIV and AIDS programming. *Journal of Counseling and Development, 71,* 290–296.

Curtis, J. R., Patrick, D. L. (1993). Race and survival time with AIDS: A synthesis of the literature. *American Journal of Public Health, 83,* 1425–1428.

Dalton, H. L. (1989). AIDS in blackface. *Daedalus, 118,* 205–227.

Daniolos, P. (1993). How professional associations view confidentiality. *FOCUS: A Guide to AIDS Research and Counseling, 8*(5), 5–6.

Dean, L., Hall, W. E., & Martin, J. L. (1988). Chronic and intermittent AIDS: Related bereavement in a panel of homosexual men in New York City. *Journal of Palliative Care, 4,* 54–57.

De La Cancela, V. (1989). Perspectives: Minority AIDS prevention: Moving beyond cultural perspectives towards sociopolitical empowerment. *AIDS Education and Prevention, 1,* 141–153

Des Jarlais, D. C., & Friedman, S. R. (1994, February). AIDS and the use of injected drugs. *Scientific American, 270,* 82–88.

Des Jarlais, D. C., & Friedman, S. R. (1988). The psychology of preventing AIDS among intravenous drug users: A social learning conceptualization. *American Psychologist, 43,* 865–870.

Devins, G. M., Mann, J., Mandin, H., Paul, L. C., Hons, R. B., Burgess, E. D., Taub, K., Schorr, S., Letourneau, P. K., & Buckle, S. (1990). Psychosocial predictors of survival in end-stage renal disease. *Journal of Nervous and Mental Disease, 178,* 127–133.

DiClemente, Zorn, & Temoshok (1986). Adolescents and AIDS: A Survey of Knowledge, attitudes and beliefs about AIDS in San Francisco. *American Journal of Public Health, 76,* 1443–1445.

Dilley, J. W., Ochitill, H. N., Perl, M., & Volberding, P. A. (1985). Findings in psychiatric consultations with patients with acquired immune deficiency syndrome. *American Journal of Psychiatry, 142,* 82–86.

Dolcini, M. M., Coates, J., Catania, J. A., Kegeles, S. M., & Hauck, W. W. (1995). Multiple sexual partners and their psychosocial correlates: The population-based AIDS in multiethnic neighborhoods (AMEN) study. *Health Psychology, 14,* 22–31.

Donlou, J. N., Wolcott, D. L., Gottlieb, M. S., & Landsverk, J. (1985). Psychosocial aspects of AIDS and AIDS-related complex: A pilot study. *Journal of Psychosocial Oncology, 3,* 39–55.

Dowsett, G. W. (1994). Working-class gay communities and HIV prevention. *FOCUS: A Guide to AIDS Research and Counseling, 9*(3), 1–4.

Driscoll, J. M. (1992). Keeping covenants and confidence sacred: One point of view. *Journal of Counseling & Development, 70,* 704–708.

Drolet, C., Reaidi, G. B., Taggart, M. E., & Reidy, M. (1993). Nutritional status of HIV-infected patients: Anthropometric, biochemical and dietetic methods for clinical assessment. *International Conference on AIDS, 9*(1), 529.

Dunkel, J., & Hatfield, S. (1986). Countertransference issues in working with people with AIDS. *Social Work, 2,* 114–117.

Dunphy, R. (1987, May). Helping persons with AIDS find meaning and hope. *Health Progress, 68,* 58–63.

Dunshee, S. J. (1994). Compassion in dying. *FOCUS: A Guide to AIDS Research and Counseling, 9*(5), 5–6.

Edgar, T., Freimuth, V. S., & Hammond, S. L. (1988). Communicating the AIDS risk to college students: The problem of motivating change. *Health Education Research, 3,* 59–65.

Edwards, G. M. (1993). Art therapy with HIV-positive patients: Hardiness, creativity and meaning. *The Arts in Psychotherapy, 20,* 325–333.

Egan, M. (1993). Resilience at the front lines: Hospital social work with AIDS patients and burnout. *Social Work Health Care, 18,* 109–125.

Eichner, E. R., & Calabrese, L. H. (1994). Immunology and exercise. *Medical Clinics of North America, 78,* 377–388.

Eidson, T. (Ed.). (1993). *The AIDS caregiver's handbook.* New York: St. Martin's Press.

Ekstrand, M. L. (1992). Safer sex maintenance among gay men: Are we making any progress? *AIDS, 8,* 875–877.

Ekstrand, M. L., & Coates, T. J. (1990). Maintenance of safer sexual behaviors and predictors of risky sex: The San Francisco men's health study. *American Journal of Public Health, 80,* 973–977.

Elias, M. (1988, August 15). Many lie about AIDS risk. *U.S.A. Today,* p. D-1.

Elliot, A. S. (1993). Counseling for HIV-infected adolescents. *FOCUS: A Guide to AIDS Research and Counseling, 8*(9), 1–4.

Erickson, S. H. (1990). Counseling the irresponsible AIDS client: Guidelines for decision making. *Journal of Counseling and Development, 68,* 454–455.

Erikson, E. H. (1950). *Childhood and society.* New York: Norton.

Faulstich, M. E. (1987). Psychiatric aspects of AIDS. *American Journal of Psychiatry, 144,* 551–556.

Fernandez, F., & Levy, J. K. (1994). Psychopharmacology in HIV spectrum disorders. *Psychiatric Clinics of North America, 17,* 135–147.

Ferrara, A. J. (1984). My personal experience with AIDS. *American Psychologist, 39,* 1285–1287.

Fineberg, H. V. (1988, October). The social dimensions of AIDS. *Scientific American, 259,* pp. 128–134.

Fishbein, M., & Ajzen, I. (1975). *Belief, attitude, intention and behavior: An introduction to theory and research.* Reading, MA: Addison-Wesley.

Fishbein, M., & Middlestadt, S. E. (1989). Using the theory of reasoned action as a framework for understanding and changing AIDS-related behaviors. In V. M. Mays, G. W. Albee, & S. F. Schneider (Eds.), *Primary prevention of AIDS: Psychological approaches.* Newbury Park, CA: Sage.

Fisher, J. D. (1988). Possible effects of reference group-based social influence on AIDS-risk behavior and AIDS prevention. *American Psychologist, 43,* 914–920.

Fisher, J. D., & Fisher, W. A. (1992). Changing AIDS-risk behavior. *Psychological Bulletin, 111,* 455–474.

Fleishman, J. A., & Fogel, B. (1994). Coping and depressive symptoms among people with AIDS. *Health Psychology, 13,* 156–169.

Folkman, S., Chesney, M. A., & Christopher-Richards, A. (1994). Stress and coping in caregiving partners of men with AIDS. *Psychiatric Clinics of North America, 17,* 35–53.

Folkman, S., Chesney, M. A., Pollack, L., & Phillips, C. (1992). Stress, coping and high-risk sexual behavior. *Health Psychology, 11,* 218–222.

Folkman, S., Lazarus, R. S., Gruen, R., & DeLongis, A. (1986). Appraisal, coping, health status, and psychological symptoms. *Journal of Personality and Social Psychology, 50,* 571–579.

Fortunato, J. E. (1993). A framework for hope. *Focus: A Guide to AIDS Research and Counseling, 8*(7), 1–4.

Fox, R., Ostrow, D., Valdiserri, R., VanRaden, B., & Polk, B. F. (1987). *Changes in sexual activities among participants in the Multicenter AIDS Cohort Study.* Paper presented at the Third International Conference on AIDS, Washington, D.C.

Francis, D. P., & Chin, J. (1987). The prevention of acquired immunodeficiency syndrome in the United States. *Journal of American Medical Association, 257,* 1357–1366.

Frank, J. D., & Frank, J. B. (1991). *Persuasion and healing: A comparative study of psychotherapy* (3rd Ed.). Baltimore: Johns Hopkins University Press.

Frankl, V. (1973). *Man's search for meaning: An introduction to logotherapy.* New York: Pocket Books.

Freudenberg, N., Lee, J., & Silver, D. (1989). How black and Latino community organizations respond to the AIDS epidemic: A case study in one New York City neighborhood. *AIDS Education and Prevention, 1,* 12–21.

Friedman, S. R., & Des Jarlais, D. C. (1991). HIV among drug injectors: The epidemic and the response. *AIDS Care, 3,* 239–250.

Friedman, S. R., Des Jarlais, D. C., Sothern, J. L., Garber, J., Cohen, H., & Smith, D. (1987). AIDS and self-organization among intravenous drug users. *International Journal of the Addictions, 22,* 201–220.

Friedman, S. R., Des Jarlais, D. C., & Sterk, C. E. (1990). AIDS and the social relations of intravenous drug users. *Milbank Quarterly, 68,* 85–109.

Frost, J. C., Makadon, H. J., Judd, D., Lee, S., O'Neill, S. F., & Paulsen, R. (1991). Care for caregivers: A support group for staff caring for AIDS patients in a hospital-based primary care practice. *Journal of General Internal Medicine, 6,* 162–167.

Fullilove, M. T. (1989). Anxiety and stigmatizing aspects of HIV infection. *Journal of Clinical Psychology, 50*(11), 5–8.

Futterman, D., Hein, K., Reuben, N., Dell, R., & Shaffer, N. (1993). Human immunodeficiency virus-infected adolescents: The first 50 patients in a New York City program. *Pediatrics, 91,* 730–735.

Gallantino, M. L., & Pizzi, M. (1991). Occupational and physical therapy for persons with HIV disease and their caregivers. *Journal of Home Health Care Practice, 3,* 46–57.

Gallo, R. C., & Montagnier, L. (1988). AIDS in 1988. *Scientific American, 259,* 40–51.

Gambe, R., & Getzel, G. S. (1989). Group work with gay men with AIDS. *Social Casework, 70,* 172–179.

Gelso, C. J., & Carter, J. A. (1985). The relationship in counseling and psychotherapy: Components, consequences, and theoretical antecedents. *Counseling Psychologist, 15,* 155–244.

Gentry, J. H. (1993, Winter). Women and AIDS. *Psychology and AIDS Exchange, 11,* 1–9.

Georgianna, C., & Johnston, M. W. (1993). Duty to protect: The gay community response. *FOCUS: A Guide to AIDS Research and Counseling, 8*(5), 1–4.

Gillman, R. (1991). From resistances to rewards: Social workers' experiences and attitudes toward AIDS. *Journal of Contemporary Human Services, 2,* 593–601.

Ginzberg, E. (1991). Access to health care for Hispanics. *Journal of the American Medical Association, 265,* 238–241.

Ginzburg, H. M., & Gostin, L. (1986). Legal and ethical issues associated with HTLV-III diseases. *Psychiatric Annals, 16,* 180–185.

Goffman, E. C. (1963). *Stigma: Notes on the management of spoiled identity.* Englewood Cliffs, NJ: Prentice-Hall.

Goldblum, P., & Moulton, J. (1986). AIDS-related suicide: A dilemma for health care providers. *FOCUS: A Guide to AIDS Research and Counseling, 2*(1), 1–2.

Gonzalez, F. J. (1995). Why are Latino gay and bisexual men at risk? *FOCUS: A Guide to AIDS Research and Counseling, 10,* 1–4.

Gostin, L. O. (1990). The AIDS litigation project. *Journal of the American Medical Association, 263,* 2086–2093.

Grace, W. C. (1994). HIV counseling research needs suggested by psychotherapy process and outcome studies. *Professional Psychology: Research and Practice, 25,* 403–409.

Graham, N. M., & Tang, A. M. (1993). Vitamins could slow AIDS onset. *HIV Frontline, 17,* 3.

Grant, D., & Anns, M. (1988).Counseling AIDS antibody-positive clients: Reactions and treatment. *American Psychologist, 43,* 72–74.

Grant, I., & Heaton, R. K. (1990). Human immunodeficiency virus-type I (HIV-I) and the brain. *Journal of Consulting and Clinical Psychology, 58,* 22–30.

Gray, L. A., & Harding, A. K. (1988). Confidentiality limits with clients who have the AIDS virus. *Journal of Counseling and Development, 66,* 219–223.

Green, G. (1993). Social support and HIV [Editorial review]. *AIDS Care, 5,* 87–103.

Greene, W. C. (1993, September). AIDS and the immune system. *Scientific American,* pp. 99–105.

Hall, N. R. S. (1988). The virology of AIDS. *American Psychologist, 43,* 907–913.

Handelsman, M. M., & Galvin, M. D. (1988). Facilitating informed consent for outpatient psychotherapy: A suggested written format. *Professional Psychology Research and Practice, 19,* 223–225.

Haney, P. (1988). Providing empowerment to the person with AIDS. *Social Work, 33,* 251–253.

Hansell, P. S., Budin, W. C., & Russo, P. (1994). Seronegative children in HIV-affected families. *FOCUS: A Guide to AIDS Research and Counseling, 8,* 5–6.

Harding, A. K., Gray, L. A., & Neal, M. (1993). Confidentiality limits with clients who have HIV: A review of ethical and legal guidelines and professional policies. *Journal of Counseling and Development, 71*, 297–305.

Hayes, J. A. (1991). Psychosocial barriers to behavior change in preventing human immunodeficiency virus (HIV) infection. *Counseling Psychologist, 19*, 585–602.

Hayes, J. A., & Gelso, C. J. (1993). Male counselors' discomfort with gay and HIV-infected clients. *Journal of Counseling Psychology, 40*, 86–93.

Hays, R. B., McKusick, L., Pollack, L., & Hilliard, R. (1993). Disclosing HIV seropositivity to significant others. *AIDS, 7*, 425–431.

Hayslip, B., Luhr, D. D., & Beyerlein, M. M. (1991). Levels of death anxiety in terminally ill men: A pilot study. *OMEGA, 24*, 13–19.

Heaton, R. K., Velin, R. A., McCutchan, J. A., & Gulevich, S. J. (1994). Neuropsychological impairment in human immunodeficiency virus-infection: Implications for employment. *Psychosomatic Medicine, 56*, 18–19.

Heider, F. (1958). *The psychology of interpersonal relations.* New York: Wiley.

Henderson, D. K., Fahey, B. J., Willy, M., & Schmitt, J. M. (1990). Risk for occupational transmission of human immunodeficiency virus type I (HIV-I) associated with clinical exposure. *Annals of Internal Medicine, 113*, 740–746.

Herek, G. M. (1990). Illness, stigma, and AIDS. In P. T. Costa & G. R. VandenBos *Psychological aspects of serious illness.* Washington, DC: American Psychological Association.

Herek, G. M., & Capitanio, J. P. (1993). Public reactions to AIDS in the United States: A second decade of stigma. *American Journal of Public Health, 83*, 574–0577.

Herek, G. M., & Glunt, E. K. (1988). An epidemic of stigma: Public reactions to AIDS. *American Psychologist, 43*, 886–891.

Herold, E. S., & Mewhinney, D. K. (1993). Gender differences in casual sex and AIDS prevention: A survey of dating bars. *Journal of Sex Research, 30*, 36–42.

Higgins, D. L., Galavotti, C., O'Reilly, K. R., Schnell, D. J., Moore, M., Rugg, D. L., & Johnson, R. (1991). Evidence for the effects of HIV antibody counseling and testing on risk behaviors. *Journal of the American Medical Association, 266*, 2419–2429.

Hill, C. E. (1996). *Working with dreams in psychotherapy.* New York: Guilford Press.

Hill, C. E., Thompson, B. J, Cogar, M. C., & Denman, D. W. (1993). Beneath the surface of long-term therapy: Therapist and client report of their own and each other's covert processes. *Journal of Counseling Psychology, 40*, 278–287.

HIV Frontline. (1993a, July/August). Earlier intervention, *14*, 7.

HIV Frontline. (1993b, November/December). Frontliners talk about how they prevent AIDS-related burnout, *15*, 4–6.

HIV Frontline. (1993c, November/December). Group helps patients plan finances, *15*, 3.

HIV Frontline. (1993d, November/December). NASW guidelines encourage "end-of-life" discussions, *15*, 1–4.

HIV Frontline. (1993e, July/August). What do you need? *14*, 1–8.

HIV Frontline. (1994a, July/August). Dealing with patients in denial, *19*, 5.

HIV Frontline. (1994b, March/April). Finding the right balance: Counselors reveal how they set professional boundaries while still extending themselves to clients, *17*, 4–6.

HIV Frontline. (1994c, July/August).How one group brought AIDS services to rural Michigan, *19*, 1–6.

HIV Frontline. (1994d, July/August). Street youths educate peers with risk-reduction model, *19*, 1–6.

Ho, D. D., Neumann, A. U., Perelson, A. S., Chen, W., Leonard, J. M., & Markowitz, M. (1995). Rapid turnover of plasma virions and CD4 lymphocyles in HIV-1 infection. *Nature, 373,* 123–126.

Hobfoll, S. E., Jackson, A. P., Lavin, J., Britton, P. J., & Shepherd, J. B. (1993). Safer sex knowledge, behavior, and attitudes of inner-city women. *Health Psychology, 12,* 481–488.

Hoelter, J. W. (1979). Multidimensional treatment of fear of death. *Journal of Consulting and Clinical Psychology, 47,* 996–999.

Hoffman, A. (1986). Impact of AIDS. *Hospital and Community Psychiatry, 37,* 943–944.

Hoffman, M. A. (1991a). Counseling the HIV-infected client: A psychosocial model for assessment and intervention. *Counseling Psychologist, 19,* 467–542.

Hoffman, M. A. (1991b). Training mental health counselors for the AIDS crisis. *Journal of Mental Health Counseling, 13,* 264–269.

Hoffman, M. A. (1993). Multiculturalism as a force in counseling clients with HIV-related concerns. *Counseling Psychologist, 21,* 712–731.

Hoffman, M. A. (1994). *Development and validation of the Health Belief Model for HIV Questionnaire.* Unpublished manuscript, University of Maryland.

Hoffman, M. A., & Driscoll, J. M. (1993). *Psychosocial coping in persons with HIV disease.* Unpublished manuscript, University of Maryland.

Horstman, W., & McKusick, L. (1986). The impact of AIDS on the physician. In L. McKusick (Ed.), *What to do about AIDS.* Berkeley: University of California Press.

Janz, N. K., & Becker, M. H. (1984). The health belief model: A decade later. *Health Education Quarterly, 3,* 59–65.

Jewett, J. F., & Hecht, F. M. (1993). Preventive health care for adults with HIV infection. *Journal of the American Medical Association, 269,* 1144–1153.

Jones, J. R., & Dilley, J. W. (1993). Rational suicide and HIV disease. *FOCUS: A Guide to AIDS Research and Counseling, 8*(8), 5–6.

Jonsen, A. R., Stryker, J., & National Research Council. (1993). *The social impact of AIDS in the United States.* Washington, DC: National Academy Press.

Jordan, A. E., & Meara, N. M. (1990). Ethics and the professional practice of psychologists: The role of virtues and principles. *Professional Psychology: Research and Practice, 21,* 107–114.

Kahn, R. L., & Antonucci, T. C. (1980). Convoys over the life course: Attachment, roles, and social support. In P. B. Baltes & O. C. Brim (Eds.), *Life-span development and behavior.* New York: Academic Press.

Kain, C. D. (1988). To breach or not to breach: Is that the question? A response to Gray and Harding. *Journal of Counseling and Development, 66,* 224–225.

Kaisch, K., & Anton-Culver, H. (1989). Psychological and social consequences of HIV exposure: Homosexuals in Southern California. *Psychology and Health, 3*, 63–75.

Kalichman, S. C., & Hunter, T. L. (1992). The disclosure of celebrity HIV infection: Its effects on public attitudes. *American Journal of Public Health, 82*, 1374–1376.

Kaplan, H. B., Johnson, R. J., Bailey, C. A., & Simon, W. (1987). The sociological study of AIDS: A critical review of the literature and suggested research agenda. *Journal of Health and Social Behavior, 28*, 140–157.

Karan, L. D. (1989). AIDS prevention and chemical dependence treatment needs of women and their children. *Journal of Psychoactive Drugs, 21*, 395–399.

Kass, N. (1990). Perceived discrimination in health care and employment among homosexual men. *International Conference on AIDS, 6*, 329.

Kass, N., Faden, R., Fox, R., & Dudley, J. (1992). Homosexual and bisexual men's perceptions of discrimination in health services. *American Journal of Public Health, 82*, 1277–1279.

Kass, N. E., Munoz, A., Chen, B., Zucconi, S. L., & Bing, E. G. (1994). Changes in employment, insurance, and income in relation to HIV status and disease progression. *Journal of Acquired Immune Deficiency Syndrome, 7*, 86–91.

Katoff, L., & Dunne, R. (1988). Supporting people with AIDS: The Gay Men's Health Crisis model. In AIDS [Special issue]. *Journal of Palliative Care, 4*, 88–95.

Katz, I., Hass, R. G., Paris, N., Astone, J., McEuaddy, D., & Lucido, D.J. (1987). Lay people's and health care personnel's perception of cancer, AIDS, cardiac, and diabetic patients. *Psychological Report, 60*, 615–629.

Katz, M. H. (1994). Effect of HIV treatment on cognition, behavior, and emotion. *Psychiatric Clinics of North America, 17*, 229–231.

Keeling, R. P. (1993). HIV disease: Current concepts. *Journal of Counseling and Development, 71*, 261–274.

Kegeles, T., Catania, J., & Coates, T. (1988). Intentions to communicate positive HIV status to sex partners [Letter to the editor]. *Journal of the American Medical Association, 259*, 216–217.

Kelly, J. A., Murphy, D. A., Washington, C. D., Wilson, T. S., Koob, J. J., Davis, D. R., Ledezma, G., & Davantes, B. (1994). The effects of HIV/AIDS intervention groups for high-risk women in urban clinics. *American Journal of Public Health, 84*, 1918–1922.

Kelly, J. A., & Murphy, D. A. (1992). Psychological interventions with AIDS and HIV: Prevention and treatment. *Journal of Consulting and Clinical Psychology, 60*, 576–585.

Kelly, J. A., Murphy, D. A., Sikkema, K. J., & Kalichman, S. C. (1993). Psychological interventions to prevent HIV infection are urgently needed. *American Psychologist, 48*, 1023–1033.

Kelly, J. A., & St. Lawrence, J. S. (1988). AIDS prevention and treatment: Psychology's role in the health crisis. *Clinical Psychology Review, 8*, 255–284.

Kelly, J. A., St. Lawrence, J. S., Brasfield, T.L., Kalichman, S. C., Smith, J. E., & Andrew, M. E. (1991). HIV risk behavior reduction following intervention with key opinion leaders of population: An experimental analysis. *American Journal of Public Health, 8*, 168–171.

Kelly, J. J., Chu, S. Y., Buehler, J. W., & the AIDS Mortality Project Group. (1993). AIDS deaths shift from hospital to home. *American Journal of Public Health, 83*, 1433–1437.

Kelly, P. J. (1993). Women and HIV clinical trials. *FOCUS: A Guide to AIDS Research and Counseling, 8*(11), 1–4.

Kelly, R. J. (1985). Death anxiety, religious convictions about the afterlife, and the psychotherapist. *Death Studies, 9*, 155–162.

Kemeny, M. E. (1994). Psychoneuroimmunology of HIV infection. *Psychiatric Clinics of North America, 17*, 55–68.

Kermani, E. J., & Weiss, B. A. (1989). AIDS and confidentiality; legal concept and its application in psychotherapy. *American Journal of Psychotherapy, 63*, 25–31.

Kessler, R. C., Price, R. H., & Wortman, C. B. (1985). Social factors in psychopathology: Stress, social support, and coping processes. *Annual Review of Psychology, 36*, 531–572.

Kiecolt-Glaser, J. K., & Glaser, R. (1987). Psychosocial moderators of immune function. *Annals of Behavioral Medicine, 9*, 16–20.

Kiecolt-Glaser, J. K., & Glaser, R. (1988). Psychological influence on immunity: Implications for AIDS. In Psychology and AIDS [Special issue]. *American Psychologist, 43*, 892–898.

Kindermann, S. S., Matteo, T. M., & Morales, E. (1993). HIV training and perceived competence among doctoral students in psychology. *Health Psychology, 12*, 224–227.

Kirchhoff, F., Greenough, T. C., Brettler, D. B., Sullivan, J. L., & Desrosiers, R. C. (1995). Brief report: The absence of intact *nef* sequences in a long-term survivor with nonprogressive HIV-1 infection. *New England Journal of Medicine, 332*, 228–232.

Kirscht, J. P., & Joseph, J. G. (1989). The health belief model: Some implications for behavior change with reference to homosexual males. In V. M. Mays, G. W. Albee, & S. F. Schneider (Eds.), *Primary prevention of AIDS: Psychological approaches*. Newbury Park, CA: Sage.

Kizer, K. W., Green, M., & Perkins, C. I. (1988). AIDS and suicide in California [Letter]. *Journal of the American Medical Association, 260*, 1981.

Kleinman, P., Millman, R. B., & Robinson, H. (1992). Condom use in a methadone maintained population. *International Conference on AIDS, 8*, C288.

Kline, A., & Strickler, J. (1993). Perceptions of risk for AIDS among women in drug treatment. *Health Psychology, 12*, 313–323.

Kline, A., & Van Landingham, M. (1992). Determinants of condom use among HIV-infected women in New Jersey. *International Conference on AIDS, 8*, D422.

Knapp, S., & VandeCreek, L. (1990). Application of the duty to protect to HIV-positive patients. *Professional Psychology: Research and Practice, 21*, 161–166.

Kobasa, S. C. (1979). Stressful life events, personality, and health: An inquiry into hardiness. *Personality and Social Psychology, 37*, 1–11.

Kramer, T. H., Ottomanelli, G., & Bihari, B. (1992). IV versus non-IV drug use and selected patient variables related to AIDS risk behaviors. *International Journal of the Addictions, 27,* 477–485.

Krueger, L. E., Wood, R. W., Diehr, P. H., & Maxwell, C. L. (1990). Poverty and HIV seropositivity: The poor are more likely to be infected. *AIDS, 4,* 811–814.

Kübler-Ross, E. (1969). *On death and dying.* New York: Macmillan.

Kübler-Ross, E. (1987). *AIDS: The ultimate challenge.* New York: Macmillan.

Lamb, D. H., Clark, C., Drumheller, P., Frizzell, K., & Surrey, L. (1989). Applying *Tarasoff* to AIDS-related psychotherapy issues. *Professional Psychology: Research and Practice, 20,* 37–43.

Land, H., & Harangody, G. (1990). A support group for partners of persons with AIDS. *Journal of Contemporary Human Services, 71,* 471–481.

Landers, S. (1988). Practitioners and AIDS: Face-to-face with pain. *APA Monitor, 19,* 14–15.

LaPerriere, A., Ironson, G., Antoni, M. H., Schneiderman, N., Klimas, N., & Fletcher, M. A. (1994). Exercise and Psychoneuroimmunology. *Medicine and Science in Sports and Exercise, 26,* 182–190.

Laubenstein, L. J., Greene, J. B., Campbell, J. R., & Weisberg, M. S. (1989). Employment and the social challenges of AIDS. *International Conference on AIDS, 5,* 837.

Lazarus, R. S., DeLongis, A., Folkman, S., & Gruen, R. (1985). Stress and adaptational outcomes: The problem of confounded measures. *American Psychologist, 40,* 770–779.

Lazarus, R. S., & Folkman, S. (1984). *Stress appraisal and Coping.* New York: Springer.

Lego, S. (1994). AIDS-related anxiety and coping methods in a support group for caregivers. *Archives of Psychiatric Nursing, 8,* 200–207.

Leigh, B. C. (1990). The relationship of substance use during sex to high-risk sexual behavior. *Journal of Sex Research, 27,* 199–213.

Leigh, B. C., & Stall, R. (1993). Substance use and risky sexual behavior for exposure to HIV: Issues in methodology, interpretation, and prevention. *American Psychologist, 48,* 1035–1045.

Leigh, B. C., Temple, M. T., & Trocki, K. F. (1993). The sexual behavior of U.S. adults: Results from a national survey. *American Journal of Public Health, 83,* 1400–1408.

Levanthal, H., Zimmerman, R., & Gutman, M. (1984). Compliance: A self-regulation perspective. In D. W. Gentry (Ed.), *Handbook of behavioral medicine.* New York: Guilford Press.

Levine, C., & Dubler, N.N. (1990). Uncertain risks and bitter realities: The reproductive choices of HIV-infected women. *Milbank Quarterly, 68,* 321–351.

Levine, S. (1982). *Who dies?* New York: Doubleday.

Levy, S. M. (1990). Humanizing death: Psychotherapy with terminally ill patients. In P. T. Costa & G. R. VandenBos (Eds.), *Psychological aspects of serious illness: Chronic conditions, fatal diseases, and clinical care.* Washington, DC: American Psychological Association.

Lippman, W. A., James, W. A., & Frierson, R. L. (1993). AIDS and the family: Implications for counselling. *AIDS Care, 5,* 71–78.

Lomax, G. L., & Sandler, J. (1988). Psychotherapy and consultation with AIDS. *Psychiatric Annals, 18,* 253–259.

Lopez, D. J., & Getzel, G. S. (1984). Helping gay AIDS patients in crisis. *Social Casework: The Journal of Contemporary Social Work, 65,* 387–394.

Loring, K., & Kelen, G. (1990). Influence of the AIDS epidemic on medical students' career choices. *International Conference on AIDS, 6*(3), 308.

Lowery, B. J., Jacobsen, B. S., & McCauley, K. (1987). On the prevalence of causal search in illness situations. *Nursing Research, 36,* 88–93.

Lykestos, C. G., Hoover, D. R., Guccione, M., Senterfitt, W., Dew, M. A., Wesch, J., Van Raden, M. A., Treisman, G., & Morgenstern, H. (1993). Depressive symptoms as predictors of medical outcomes in HIV infection. *Journal of the American Medical Association, 270,* 2563–2567.

Macks, J. (Ed.). (1988, June). Women and AIDS: Countertransference issues [Special issue]. *Social Casework: The Journal of Contemporary Social Work,* 340–347.

Macks, J. A., & Abrams, D. I. (1992). Burnout among HIV/AIDS health care providers. *AIDS Clinical Review,* 281–299.

Maddux, J. E., & Rogers, R. W. (1983). Protection motivation and self-efficacy: A revised theory of fear appeals and attitude change. *Journal of Experimental Social Psychology, 19,* 469–479.

Maiman, L. A., & Becker, M. H. (1974). The health belief model: Origins and correlates in psychological theory. *Health Education Monographs, 2,* 336–353.

Maloney, B. D. (1988). The legacy of AIDS: Challenge for the next century. *Journal of Marital and Family Therapy, 14,* 143–150.

Mandel, J. S. (1986). Psychosocial challenges of AIDS and ARC: Clinical and research observation. In L. McKusick (Ed.), *What to do about AIDS.* Berkeley: University of California Press.

Mapou, R. L., & Law, W. A. (1994). Neurobehavioral aspects of HIV disease and AIDS: An update. *Professional Psychology: Research and Practice, 25,* 132–140.

Markowitz, J. C., & Perry, S. W. (1992). Effects of human immunodeficiency virus on the central nervous system. In S. C. Yudofsky & R. E. Hales (Eds.), *Textbook of neuropsychiatry.* Washington, DC: American Psychiatric Press.

Marks, G., Bundek, N. I., Richardson, J. L., Ruiz, M. S., Maldonado, N., & Mason, H. R. (1992). Self-disclosure of HIV infection: Preliminary results from a sample of Hispanic men. *Health Psychology, 11,* 300–306.

Marks, G., Richardson, J. L., & Maldonado, N. (1991). Self-disclosure of HIV infection to sexual partners. *American Journal of Public Health, 81,* 1321–1323.

Marks, R. (1993). Sexuality and AIDS. *FOCUS: A Guide to AIDS Research and Counseling, 8*(10), 7–8.

Marlatt, G. A., & Gordon, J. R. (Eds.). (1985). *Relapse prevention.* New York: Guilford Press.

Marlow, R. M., Corrigan, S. A., & Cunningham, S. C. (1993). Psychosocial factors associated with condom use among African-American drug abusers in treatment. *AIDS Education Preview, 5,* 244–253.

Marlow, R. M., West, I. A., & Corrigan, S. A. (1994). Outcome of psychoeducation for HIV risk reduction. *AIDS Education and Prevention, 6,* 113–125.

Martin, A. (1982). Some issues in the treatment of gay and lesbian patients. *Psychotherapy: Theory, Research, and Practice, 19,* 341–348.

Martin, A. C., & Stroud, F. (1988). Delivering difficult messages: AIDS prevention and Black youth. In M. Quackenbush & M. Nelson (Eds.), *The AIDS challenge: Prevention education for young people.* Santa Cruz, CA: Network Publications.

Martin, D. (1989). Human immunodeficiency virus infection and the gay community: Counseling and clinical issues. *Journal of Counseling and Development, 68,* 67–72.

Martin, J. (1988). Psychological consequences of AIDS-related bereavement among gay men. *Journal of Consulting and Clinical Psychology, 56,* 856–862.

Martin, J. L., & Dean, L. (1993). Effects of AIDS-related bereavement and HIV-related illness of psychological distress among gay men: A 7-year longitudinal study, 1985–1991. *Journal of Consulting and Clinical Psychology, 61,* 94–103.

Martin, J. L., & Vance, C. S. (1984). Behavioral and psychosocial factors in AIDS: Methodological and substantive issues. *American Psychologist, 39,* 1303–1307.

Marzuk, P. M., Tierney, H., Tardiff, K., Gross, E. M., Morgan, E. B., Hsu, M. A., & Mann, J. (1988). Increased risk of suicide in persons with AIDS. *Journal of the American Medical Association, 259,* 1333–1337.

Mason, H. R. C., Marks, G., Simoni, J. M., Ruiz, M. S., & Richardson, J. L. (1995). Culturally sanctioned secrets? Latino men's nondisclosure of HIV infection to family, friends, and lovers. *Health Psychology, 14,* 6–12.

Massagli, M. P., Weissman, J. S., Seage, G. R., & Epstein, A. M. (1994). Correlates of employment after AIDS diagnosis in the Boston health study. *American Journal of Public Health, 84,* 1976–1981.

Matiella, A. C. (1988). Developing innovative AIDS prevention programs for Latino youth. In M. Quackenbush & M. Nelson (Eds.), *The AIDS challenge: Prevention education for young people.* Santa Cruz, CA: Network Publications.

Manuel, C., Enel, P., Charrel, J., Reviron, D., Larher, M. P., Thirion, X., & Sanmarco, J. L. (1990). The ethical approach to AIDS: A bibliographical review. *Journal of Medical Ethics, 16,* 14–27.

Mays, V. M., & Cochran, S. D. (1988). Issues in the perception of AIDS risk and risk reduction activities by Black and Hispanic/Latino women. *American Psychologist, 43,* 949–957

McCain, N. L., & Gramling, L. F. (1992). Living with dying: Coping with HIV disease. *Issues in Mental Health Nursing, 13,* 271–284.

McCusker, J., Stoddard, A., Zapka, J., Zorn, M., & Mayer, K. (1989). Predictors of AIDS preventive behavior among homosexually active men: A longitudinal analysis. *AIDS, 3,* 443–448.

McKusick, L. (1988). The impact of AIDS on practitioner and client. *American Psychologist, 43,* 935–940.

McKusick, L., Coates, T. J., Morin, S. F., Pollack, L., & Hoff, C. (1990). Longitudinal predictors of reductions in unprotected anal intercourse among gay men in San Francisco: The AIDS behavioral research project. *American Journal of Public Health, 80,* 978–983.

McLaurin, P., & Juzang, I. (1993). Reaching the hip-hop generation. *FOCUS: A Guide to AIDS Research and Counseling, 8*(3), 1–4.

Meisenhelder, J. B., & La Charite, C. L. (1989). Fear of contagion: A stress response to acquired immunodeficiency syndrome. *Advances in Nursing Science, 11,* 29–38.

Melton, G. B. (1988). Ethical and legal issues in AIDS-related practice. *American Psychologist, 43,* 941–947.

Mendelson, S. T. (1995, March 19). The dying of the light. *The Washington Post,* pp. F1-F7.

Metz, S., Fox, R., Odaka, N., & McArthur, J. C. (1990). Employment status of men diagnosed with AIDS in the Baltimore MACS. *International Conference on AIDS, 6,* 293.

Metzler, C. W., Noell, J., Biglan, A., & Oregon Research Institute. (1992). The validation of a construct of high-risk sexual behavior in heterosexual adolescents. *Journal of Adolescent Research, 7,* 233–249.

Michael, R. T., Gagnon, J. H., Laumann, E. O., & Kolata, G. (1994). *Sex in America: A definitive survey.* New York: Little, Brown.

Middlestadt, S. E. (1992). The challenge of changing sexual behavior. *FOCUS: A Guide to AIDS Research and Counseling, 7*(11), 1–4.

Miller, D. (1988). HIV and social psychiatry. *British Medical Bulletin, 44,* 130–148.

Miller, D. (1991). Occupational morbidity and burnout: Lessons and warning for HIV/AIDS carers. *International Review of Psychiatry, 3,* 439–449.

Molgaard, C. A., Nakamura, C., Hovell, M. F., & Elder, J. P. (1988). Assessing alcoholism as a risk factor for Acquired Immunodeficiency. *Social Science and Medicine, 27,* 1147–1152.

Monat, A., & Lazarus, R. S. (1985). Stress and coping—Some current issues and controversies. In A. Monat & R. S. Lazarus (Eds.), *Stress and coping: An anthology.* New York: Columbia University Press.

Mooney, D. K., Fromme, K., Kivlahan, R., & Marlatt, G. A. (1987). Correlates of alcohol consumption: Sex, age, and expectancies relate differentially to quantity and frequency. *Addictive Behaviors, 12,* 235–240.

Moos, R., & Tsu, V. (1977). The crisis of physical illness: An overview. In R. Moos & V. Tsu (Eds.), *Coping with physical illness.* New York: Plenum.

Morales, E. S. (1990). HIV infection and Hispanic gay and bisexual men. *Hispanic Journal of Behavioral Sciences, 12,* 212–222.

Morrison, C. F. (1989). AIDS: Ethical implications for psychological intervention. *Professional Psychology: Research and Practice, 20,* 166–171.

Motto, J. A. (1994). Rational suicide: Then and now, when and how. *FOCUS: A Guide to AIDS Research and Counseling, 9*(5), 1–4.

Moulton, J. M., Sweet, D. M., Temoshok, L., & Mandel, J. S. (1987). Attributions of blame and responsibility in relation to distress and health behavior change in people with AIDS and AIDS-related complex. *Journal of Applied Social Psychology, 17,* 493–506.

Murphy, P., & Perry, K. (1988). Hidden grievers. *Death Studies, 12,* 451–462.

Murray, C. (1988). The coming of custodial democracy. *Commentary, 86,* 19–24.

Namir, S. (1986). Treatment issues concerning persons with AIDS. In L. McKusick (Ed.), *What to do about AIDS.* Berkeley: University of California Press.

Namir, S., Alumbaugh, M. J., Fawzy, F. I., & Wolcott, D. L.(1989). The relationship of social support to physical and psychological aspects of AIDS. *Psychology and Health, 3,* 77–86.

Namir, S., & Sherman, S. (1989). Coping with countertransference. In C. Kain (Ed.), *No longer immune: A counselor's guide to AIDS.* Alexandria, VA: American Association for Counseling and Development.

Namir, S., Wolcott, D. L., Fawzy, F. I., & Alumbaugh, M. J. (1987). Coping with AIDS: Psychological and health implications. In Acquired Immune Deficiency Syndrome [Special issue]. *Journal of Applied Social Psychology, 17,* 309–328.

Nashman, H. W., Hoare, C. H., & Heddesheimer, J. C. (1990). Stress and satisfaction among professionals who care for AIDS patients: An exploratory study. *Hospital Topics, 68,* 22–28.

National Association of Social Workers Delegate Assembly. (1990). *Acquired Immune Deficiency Syndrome/Human Immunodeficiency Virus: A social work response* [Policy statement]. Silver Spring, MD: Author.

Neugarten, B. L. (1979). Time, age, and the life cycle. *American Journal of Psychiatry, 136,* 887–894.

Neugebauer, R., Rabkin, J. G., Williams, J. B., Remien, R. H., Goetz, R., & Gorman, J. M. (1992). Bereavement reactions among homosexual men experiencing multiple losses in the AIDS epidemic. *American Journal of Psychiatry, 149,* 1374–1379.

Newmeyer, J. A. (1989). The epidemiology of HIV among intravenous drug users. In J. W. Dilley, C. Pies, & M. Helquist (Eds.), *Face to face: A guide to AIDS counseling.* Berkeley, CA: Celestial Arts.

New York Times. (June 14, 1990). Giving death a hand: Rending issue. p. A6.

Nichols, S. E. (1983). Psychiatric aspects of AIDS. *Psychosomatics, 24,* 1083–1089.

Nichols, S. E. (1986). Psychotherapy and AIDS. In T. S. Stein & C. J. Cohen (Eds.), *Contemporary perspective on psychotherapy with lesbians and gay men.* New York: Plenum.

Norsworthy, K. L., & Horne, A. M. (1994). Issues in group work with HIV-infected gay and bisexual men. *Journal for Specialists in Group Work, 19,* 112–119.

Nussbaum, N. J. (1991). HIV antibody status and employment discrimination: 1991 update. *Journal of Acquired Immune Deficiency Syndromes, 4,* 927–929.

Odets, W. W. (1992). Unconscious motivations for the practice of unsafe sex among gay men in the United States. *International Conference on AIDS, 8*(2), D418.

O'Donnell, L., O'Donnell, C. R., Pleck, J. H., Snarey, J., Snarey, R., & Richard, M. (1987). Psychological responses of hospital workers to the acquired immune deficiency syndrome (AIDS). *Journal of Applied Social Psychology, 17,* 269–285.

Osmond, D. H., Page, K., Wiley, J., Garrett, K., Sheppard, H. W., Moss, A. R.,

Schrager, L., & Winkelstein, W. (1994). HIV infection in homosexual and bisexual men 18–29 years of age: The San Francisco Young Men's Health Study. *American Journal of Public Health, 84*, 1933–1937.

Ostrow, D. G. (1994). Substance abuse and HIV infection. *Psychiatric Clinics of North America, 17*, 69–89.

Ostrow, D. G., Monjan, A., Joseph, J., VanRaden, M., Fox, R., Lawrence, K., Dudley, J., & Phair, J. (1989). HIV-related symptoms and psychological functioning in a cohort of homosexual men. *American Journal of Psychiatry, 146*, 737–742.

Pantaleo, G., Menzo, S., Vaccarezza, M., Graniosi, C., Cohen, O. J., Demarest, B. S., Montefiori, D., Orenstein, J. M., Gox, C., Schrager, L. K., Margolick, J. B., Buchbinder, S., Giorgi, J. V., & Fauci, A. S. (1995). Studies in subjects with long-term nonprogressive human immunodeficiency virus infection. *New England Journal of Medicine, 332*, 209–216.

Parkes, C. M. (1971). Psychosocial transitions: A field for study. *Social Science and Medicine, 5*, 101–115.

Pearlin, L., & Schooler, C. (1978). The structure of coping. *Journal of Health and Social Behavior, 19*, 2–21.

Pedersen, P. B. (1991). Multiculturalism as a generic approach to counseling. In Multiculturalism as a fourth force in counseling [Special issue]. *Journal of Counseling and Development, 70*, 6–12.

Penkower, L., Dew, M. A., Kingsley, L., Becker, J. T., Satz, P., Schaerf, F. W., & Sheridan, K. (1991). Behavioral, health and psychosocial factors and risk for HIV infection among sexually active homosexual men: The multicenter AIDS cohort study. *American Journal of Public Health, 81*, 194–196.

Perkins, D. O., Stern, R. A., Golden, R. N., Murphy, C., Naftolowitz, D., & Evans, D. L. (1994). Mood disorders in HIV infection: Prevalence and risk factors in a nonepicenter of the AIDS epidemic. *American Journal of Psychiatry, 151*, 233–236.

Perry, S., Fishman, B., Jacobsberg, L., Young, J., & Frances, A. (1991). Effectiveness of psychoeducational interventions in reducing emotional distress after human immunodeficiency virus antibody testing. *Archive of Geriatric Psychiatry, 48*, 143–147.

Perry, S., Jacobsberg, L. B., Fishman, B., Frances, A., Bobo, J., & Jacobsberg, B. K. (1990). Psychiatric diagnosis before serological testing for the human immunodeficiency virus. *American Journal of Psychiatry, 147*, 89–93.

Peruga, A., & Rivo, M. (1992). Racial differences in AIDS knowledge among adults. *AIDS Education and Prevention, 4*, 52–60.

Peterson, J. L., & Marin, G.(1988). Issues in the prevention of AIDS among black and Hispanic men. *American Psychologist, 43*, 871–877.

Pickrel, J. (1989). "Tell me your story": Using life review in counseling the terminally ill. *Death Studies, 13*, 127–135.

Pingitore, D. P., & Morrison, A. (1993). AIDS-related activities offered by doctoral psychology programs: Results from a national survey. *Professional Psychology: Research and Practice, 24*, 110–114.

Pope-Davis, D. B., Reynolds, A. L., Dings, J. G., & Ottavi, T. M. (1994). Multicultural competencies of doctoral interns at university counseling centers: An exploratory investigation. *Professional Psychology: Research and Practice, 25,* 466–470.

Prentice-Dunn, S., & Rogers, R. W. (1986). Protection motivation theory and preventive health: Beyond the health belief model. *Health Education Research, 1,* 153–161.

Price, R., Omizo, M.M., & Hammett, V.L. (1986). Counseling clients with AIDS. *Journal of Counseling and Development, 65,* 96–97.

Quill, T. E. (1991). Death and dignity: A case of individualized decision-making. *New England Journal of Medicine, 324,* 691–694.

Rabkin, J. G., Remien, R., Katoff, L., & Williams, J. B. (1993). Resilience in adversity among long-term survivors of AIDS. *Hospital and Community Psychiatry, 44,* 161–167.

Ramsey, P. (1970). *The patient as person.* New Haven: Yale University Press.

Rando, T. A. (1984). A comprehensive analysis of anticipatory grief: Perspectives, processes, promises, and problems. In T. A. Rando (Ed.), *Loss and anticipatory grief.* Lexington, MA: Lexington Books.

Reardon, J., Warren, N., Keilch, R., Jenssen, D., Wise, F., & Brunner, W. (1993). Are HIV-infected injection drug users taking HIV tests? *American Journal of Public Health, 83,* 1414–1417.

Redfield, R. R., & Burke, D. S. (1988). HIV infection: The clinical picture. *Scientific American, 259,* 90–98.

Reed, G. M., Kemeny, M. E., Taylor, S. E., Wang, H. J., & Visscher, B. R. (1994). Realistic acceptance as a predictor of decreased survival time in gay men with AIDS. *Health Psychology, 13,* 299–307.

Reed, P. (1987). Religiousness among terminally ill and healthy adults. *Research in Nursing and Health, 9,* 35–41.

Reiss, J. O. (1994). Recognizing denial among HIV-infected clients. *FOCUS: A Guide to AIDS Research and Counseling, 8*(9), 1–4.

Remien, R., Rabkin, J. G., & Williams, J. B., (1992). Coping strategies and health beliefs of AIDS long-term survivors. *Psychology and Health, 6,* 335–345.

Rogers, R. W. (1983). Cognitive and psychological processes in fear appeals and attitude change: A revised theory of protection motivation. In J. T. Cacioppo & R. E. Petty (Eds.), *Social psychophysiology.* New York: Guilford Press.

Room, R. (1985). AIDS and alcohol: Epidemiological and behavioral aspects. *NIAAA Consultation on AIDS and Alcohol.* Bethesda, MD: National Institutes on Alcoholism and Alcohol Abuse.

Rosenberg, C. E. (1987). *The cholera years: The United States in 1832, 1849, and 1866* (2nd ed.). Chicago: University of Chicago Press.

Rosenstock, I. (1974). Historical origins of the health belief model. *Health Education Monographs, 2,* 328–332.

Ross, M. W., & Seeger, V. (1988). Determinants of reported burnout in health professionals associated with the care of patients with AIDS. *AIDS, 2,* 395–397.

Rotheram-Borus, M. J., Reid, H., Rosario, M. (1994). Factors medicating changes in sexual HIV risk behaviors among gay and bisexual male adolescents. *American Journal of Public Health, 84,* 1938–1946.

Royce, R. A., & Winklestein, W. (1990). HIV infection, cigarette smoking and cd4+

T-lymphocyte counts: Preliminary results from the San Francisco Men's Health Study. *AIDS, 4,* 327–333.

Ryan, C. C. (1988). The social and clinical challenges of AIDS. In AIDS [Special issue]. *Smith College Studies in Social Work, 59,* 3–20.

Sandfort, T. G., & van Zessen, G. (1992). Denial as a barrier for HIV prevention within the general population. *Journal of Psychology and Human Sexuality, 5,* 69–87.

Saracco, A., Musicco, M., & Nicolosi, A. (1993). Man-to-woman sexual transmission of HIV: Longitudinal study of 343 steady partners of infected men. *Journal of Acquired Immune Deficiency Syndrome, 6,* 497–502.

Sayette, M. A., & Mayne, T. J. (1990). Survey of current clinical and research trends in clinical psychology. *American Psychologist, 45,* 1263–1266.

Saynor, J. K. (1988). Existential and spiritual concerns of people with AIDS. *Journal of Palliative Care, 4,* 61–65.

Schlesinger, H. J., Mumford, E., Glass, G. V., Patrick, C., & Sharpstein, S. (1983). Mental health treatment and medical care utilization in a fee-for-service systems: Outpatient mental treatment following the onset of a chronic disease. *American Journal of Public Health, 73,* 422–429.

Schlossberg, N. K. (1981). A model for analyzing human adaptation to transition. *Counseling Psychologist, 9,* 2–39.

Schlossberg, N. K. (1989). *Overwhelmed: Coping with life's ups and downs.* Lexington, MA: Lexington Books.

Selwyn, P. A. (1986). AIDS: What is now known. *Hospital Practice, 21,* 125–164.

Shelp, E. E., DuBose, E. R., & Sunderland, R. H. (1990). The infrastructure of religious communities: A neglected resource for care of people with AIDS. *American Journal of Public Health, 80,* 970–972.

Sheridan, K., & Sheridan, E. P. (1988). Psychological consultation to persons with AIDS. *Professional Psychology Research and Practice, 19,* 532–535.

Shilts, R. (1987). *And the band played on.* New York: St. Martin's Press.

Siegel, B. (1988). *Love, medicine and miracles.* New York: Harper & Row.

Siegel, K., Bauman, L. J., Christ, G. H., & Krown, S. (1988). Patterns of change in sexual behavior among gay men in New York City. *Archives of Sexual Behavior, 17,* 481–497.

Siegel, L. (1986). AIDS: Relationship to alcohol and other drugs. *Journal of Substance Abuse Treatment, 3,* 271–274.

Significant Losses Project. (1994). Terry Gips Art Gallery, University of Maryland, College Park, MD.

Silverman, D. C. (1993). Psychosocial impact of HIV-related caregiving on health providers: A review and recommendations for the role of psychiatry. *American Journal of Psychiatry, 150,* 705–712.

Smith, K. W., McGraw, S. A., Crawford, S. L., Costa, L. A., & McKinlay, J. B. (1993). HIV risk among Latino adolescents in two New England cities. *American Journal of Public Health, 83,* 1395–1399.

Solomon, G. F., Temoshok, L., O'Leary, A., & Zich, J. (1987). An intensive psychoimmunologic study of long-surviving persons with AIDS. *Annals of the New York Academy of Sciences, 496,* 647–655.

Sontag, S. (1989). *AIDS and its metaphors.* Toronto: Collins.

Spiegel, D., Bloom, J. R., & Yalom, I. (1981). Group support for patients with metastatic cancer. *Archives of General Psychiatry, 38,* 527–533.

St. Lawrence, J. S., Husfeldt, B. A., Kelly, J., Hood, H. V., & Smith, S., Jr. (1990). The stigma of AIDS: Fear of disease and prejudice toward gay men. *Journal of Homosexuality, 19,* 85–101.

St. Louis, M. E., Conway, G. A., Hayman, C. R., Miller, C., Petersen, L. R., & Dondero, T. J. (1991). Human immunodeficiency virus infection in disadvantaged adolescents. *Journal of the American Medical Association, 266,* 2387–2391.

Stall, R. (1988). The prevention of HIV infection associated with drug and alcohol use during sex activity. *Advances in alcohol and substance abuse, 7,* 73–88.

Stall, R. D., Coates, T. J., & Hoff, C. (1988). Behavioral risk reduction for HIV infection among gay and bisexual men: A review of results from the United States. *American Psychologist, 43,* 878–885.

Stewart, G. M., & Gregory, B. C. (in press). Themes, critical mass and termination of an ongoing AIDS support group. *Journal of Counseling and Psychology.*

Stiffman, A. R., Earls, F., Dore, P., & Cunningham, R. (1992). Changes in acquired immunodeficiency syndrome-related risk behavior after adolescence: Relationships to knowledge and experience concerning human immunodeficiency virus infection. *Pediatrics, 89,* 950–955.

Stowe, A., Ross, M. W., Wodak, A., Thomas, G. V., & Larson, S. A. (1993). Significant relationships and social supports of injecting drug users and their implications for HIV/AIDS services. *AIDS Care, 5,* 1409–1413.

Strecher, V., DeVillis, B., Becker, M., & Rosenstock, I. (1986). The role of self-efficacy in achieving health behavior change. *Health Education Quarterly, 13,* 73–92.

Strunin, L., & Hingson, R. (1992). Alcohol, drugs, and adolescent sexual behavior. *International Journal of the Addictions, 27,* 129–146.

Sunenblick, B. (1988). The AIDS epidemic: Sexual behavior of adolescents. In AIDS [Special issue]. *Smith College Studies in Social Work, 59,* 21–37.

Tarasoff v. Regents of the University of California, 17 Cal. 3d., 425, 551 P. 2d 334 (1976). (Tarasoff II).

Tardy, C. H. (1985). Social support measurement. *American Journal of Community Psychology, 13,* 187–201.

Taylor, A. D. (1993). Prevention after Magic. *FOCUS: A Guide to AIDS Research and Counseling, 8*(3), 5–6.

Taylor-Brown, S., & Wiener, L. (1993). Making videotapes of HIV-infected women for their children. *Families in Society: The Journal of Contemporary Human Services, 74,* 468–480.

Thomas, S. B., & Quinn, S. C. (1991). The Tuskegee Syphilis Study, 1932 to 1972: Implications for HIV education and AIDS risk education programs in the black community. *American Journal of Public Health, 81,* 1498–1504.

Thompson, J. L. P., Yager, T. J., & Marten, J. L. (1993). Estimated condom failure and frequency of condom use among gay men. *American Journal of Public Health, 83,* 1409–1417.

Totten, G., Lamb, D. H., & Reeder, G. D. (1990). Tarasoff and confidentiality in AIDS-related psychotherapy. *Professional Psychology, 21,* 155–160.

Treiber, F. A., Shaw, D., & Malcolm, R. (1987). Acquired immune deficiency syndrome: Psychological impact on health personnel. *Journal of Nervous and Mental Disease, 175,* 496.

Treisman, G. J., Lyketsos, C. G., Fishman, M., Hanson, A. Rosenblatt, A., & McHugh, P. R. (1993). Psychiatric care for patients with HIV infection: The varying perspectives. *Psychosomatics, 34,* 432–439.

Trezza, G. R. (1994). HIV knowledge and stigmatization of persons with AIDS: Implications for the development of HIV education for young adults. *Professional Psychology, 25,* 141–148.

Tross, S., & Hirsch, D. A. (1988). Psychological distress and neuropsychological complications of HIV infection and AIDS. In Psychology and AIDS [Special edition]. *American Psychologist, 43,* 929–934.

Tunnell, G. (1991). Complications in group psychotherapy with AIDS patients. *International Journal of Group Psychotherapy, 41,* 481–498.

Turner, H. A., Catania, J. A., & Gagnon, J. (1994). The prevalence of informal caregiving to persons with AIDS in the United States: Caregiver characteristics and their implications. *Social Science and Medicine, 38,* 1543–1552.

Turner, H. A., Hays, R. B., & Coates, T. J. (1993). Determinants of social support among gay men: The context of AIDS. *Journal of Health and Social Behavior, 34,* 37–53.

Tyler, F. (1978). Individual psychosocial competence: A personality configuration. *Educational and Psychological measurement, 38,* 309–323.

van der Velde, F. W., van der Pligt, J., & Hooykaas, C. (1994). Perceiving AIDS-related risk: Accuracy as a function of differences in actual risk. *Health Psychology, 13,* 25–33.

Wain-Hobson, S. (1995). Virological mayhem. *Nature, 373,* 102.

Walker, G. (1991). AIDS, crack, poverty, and race in the African-American community: The need for an ecosystemic approach. *Journal of Independent Social Work, 5,* 69–81.

Walkey, F. H., Taylor, A. J., & Green, D. E. (1990). Attitudes to AIDS: A comparative analysis of a new and negative stereotype. *Social Science Medicine, 30,* 549–552.

Walter, H. J., Vaughan, R. D., & Cohall, A. T. (1991). Psychosocial influences on acquired immunodeficiency syndrome-risk behaviors among high school students. *Pediatrics, 88,* 846–852.

Warner-Robbins, C. G., & Christiana, N. M. (1989). The spiritual needs of persons with AIDS. *Family and Community Health, 12,* 43–51.

Wei, X., Ghosh, S. K., Taylor, M. E., Johnson, V. A., Emini, E. A., Deutsch, P., Lifson, J. A., Bonhoeffer, S., Nowak, M. A., Hahn, B. H., Saag, M. S., & Shaw, G. M. (1995). Viral dynamics in human immunodeficiency virus type 1 infection. *Nature, 373,* 117–122.

Weinstein, N. D. (1989). Perceptions of personal susceptibility to harm. In V. M. Mays, G. W. Albee, & S. F. Schneider (Eds.), *Primary prevention of AIDS: Psychological approaches.* Newbury Park, CA: Sage.

Weinstein, N. D. (1993). Testing four competing theories of health-protective behavior. *Health Psychology, 12,* 324–333.

Weisman, A. D., & Sobel, H. J., (1979).Coping with cancer through self-instruction: A hypothesis. *Journal of Human Stress, 5,* 3–7.

Weiss, R. (1988). The experience of AIDS: Hypotheses based on pilot study interviews. In AIDS [Special issue]. *Journal of Palliative Care, 4,* 15–25.

Weiss, R. S. (1976). Transition states and other stressful situations: Their nature and programs for their management. In G. Caplan & M. Killilea (Eds.), *Support systems and mutual help.* New York: Grune & Stratton.

Weissman, J. S., Makadon, H. J., Seage, G. R., Massagli, M. P., Gatsonis, C. A., Craben, D. E., Stone, V. E., Bennett, I. A., & Epstein, A. M. (1994). Changes in insurance status and access to care for persons with AIDS in the Boston Health Study. *American Journal of Public Health, 84,* 1997–2000.

Welch, D. (1982). Anticipatory grief: Reactions in family members of adult patients. *Issues in Mental Health Nursing, 4,* 149–158.

Welman, M., & Faber, P. A. (1992). The dream in terminal illness: A Jungian formulation. *Journal of Analytical Psychology, 37,* 61–81.

Werth, J. L. (1992). Rational suicide and AIDS: Considerations for the psychotherapist. *Counseling Psychologist, 20,* 645–659.

Werth, J. L., Jr. (1993). Recommendations for the inclusion of training about persons with HIV disease in counseling psychology graduate programs. *The Counseling Psychologist, 21,* 668–686.

Werth, J. L., & Carney, J. (1994). Incorporating HIV-related issues into graduate student training. *Professional Psychology: Research and Practices, 25,* 458–465.

Werth, J. L., Duke, D. L., & Kunkel, M. A. (1994, August). *Stories about HIV disease: Different experiences and different themes.* Poster session presented at the Annual Meeting of the American Psychological Association, Los Angeles, CA.

Westbrook, M. T., & Nordholm, L. A. (1986). Reactions to patients' self- or chance-blaming attributions for illnesses having varying life-style involvement. *Journal of Applied Social Psychology, 16,* 428–446.

Whitaker, O. (1974). *Sister Death.* New York: Morehouse-Barlow.

Williams, L. S. (1986). AIDS risk reduction: A community health education intervention for minority high risk group members. *Health Education Quarterly, 13,* 407–421.

Winiarski, M. G. (1991). *AIDS-related psychotherapy.* Boston: Allyn & Bacon.

Wolcott, D. L., Namir, S., Fawzy, F. I., Gottlieb, M. S., & Mitsuyasu, R. T. (1986). Illness concerns, attitudes toward homosexuality, and social support in gay men with AIDS. *General Hospital Psychiatry, 8,* 395–403.

Woo, S. K. (1988). The psychiatric and neuropsychiatric aspects of HIV disease. *Journal of Palliative Care, 4,* 50–53.

Worth, D. (1990). Sexual decision-making and AIDS: Why condom promotion among vulnerable women is likely to fail. *Studies in family planning, 20,* 297–301.

Wulfert, E., & Wan, C. K. (1993). Condom use: A self-efficacy model. *Health Psychology, 12,* 346–353.

Wyatt, G. E. (1991). Examining ethnicity versus race in AIDS related sex research. *Social Science and Medicine, 33,* 37–45.

Yalom, I. D. (1980). *Existential psychotherapy.* New York: Basic Books.

Yalom, I. D., & Greaves, C. (1977). Group therapy with the terminally ill. *American Journal of Psychiatry, 134,* 396.

Yelin, E. H., Greenblatt, R. M., Hollander, H., & McMaster, J. R. (1991). The impact of HIV-related illness on employment. *American Journal of Public Health, 81,* 79–84.

Zich, J., & Temoshok, L. (1987). Perceptions of social support in men with AIDS and ARC: Relationships with distress and hardiness. In Acquired Immune Deficiency Syndrome [Special issue]. *Journal of Applied Social Psychology, 17,* 193–215.

Zuckerman, C., & Gordon, L. (1988). Meeting the psychosocial and legal needs of women with AIDS and their families. *New York State Journal of Medicine, 88,* 619–620.

Index

Page numbers in italics refer to tables or figures.

315